HEALING
WITH
PRESSURE POINT THERAPY

Simple, Effective Techniques for Massaging Away More Than 100 Common Ailments

JACK FOREM
AND
STEVE SHIMER, L.A.C.

PRENTICE HALL PRESS

Library of Congress Cataloging-in-Publication Data

Forem, Jack.
    Healing with pressure point therapy   /   Jack Forem and Steve Shimer.
       p.   cm.
    Includes index.
    ISBN 0-7352-0006-8 (pbk.). — ISBN 0-13-841297-9 (case).
    1. Acupressure—Popular works.   2. Acupuncture points—Popular works.
  I. Shimer, Steve. II. Title.
  RM723.A27F67   1999
  615.8'22—dc21   98-39481
                                                          CIP

Acquisitions Editor: *Doug Corcoran*
Production Editor: *Jacqueline Roulettte*
Formatting/Interior Design: *Robyn Beckerman*

© *1999 Prentice Hall*

All rights reserved. No part of this book may be reproduced in any form or by any means, without permission in writing from the publisher.

Printed in the United States of America

10 9 8 7 6

ISBN 0-7352-0006-8 (p)

This book is a reference manual based on research by the authors. All techniques and suggestions are to be used at the reader's sole discretion. The opinions expressed herein are not necessarily those of, or endorsed by, the publisher. Information is to be used as a guide to help restore balance within the body, so it can heal itself. The directions stated in this book do not constitute the practice of medicine. Nor are they intended as claims for curing a serious disease and are in no way to be considered as a substitute for consultation with a duly licensed doctor.

ATTENTION: CORPORATIONS AND SCHOOLS

Prentice Hall books are available at quantity discounts with bulk purchase for educational, business, or sales promotional use. For information, please write to: Prentice Hall Special Sales, 240 Frisch Court, Paramus, New Jersey 07652. Please supply: title of book, ISBN, quantity, how the book will be used, date needed.

PRENTICE HALL PRESS
Paramus, NJ 07652

On the World Wide Web at http://www.phdirect.com

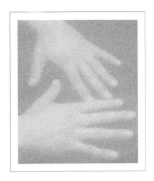

Acknowledgments

A big thank you to Roberta Forem for extensive research and preparation of a first version of Parts I and II. Her clear insights and sensitive treatment of the material brought richness and depth to the project.

We are also grateful to Doug Corcoran, Senior Editor at Prentice Hall, for superhuman patience and good humor as deadlines and extensions passed and we struggled to complete all the details of text and illustrations.

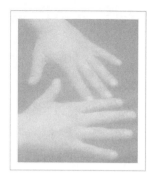

An Important Note

The remedies in this book can help you heal a wide variety of ailments. Perhaps more important, if used on a regular basis along with intelligent lifestyle choices, they can help to keep you healthy.

Although these techniques are very effective, they represent only a fraction of the knowledge in the ancient traditions they come from, systems of natural medicine, and healing that are rich and complex. To be properly trained in these healing modalities requires years of rigorous work in both theory and practice—just as in our modern Western medical schools. The techniques in this book draw from this wisdom, to help you with self-treatment for your health concerns.

One of the purposes of the book is to introduce you to these therapies. If you find these techniques helpful, you might want to pay a visit to a qualified practitioner and receive a full treatment or even a series of treatments. Or, you might want to do some further reading, or take some classes to learn more about them yourself.

The pressure point treatments and lifestyle recommendations in these pages are not meant as a substitute for medical care from a trained professional. If you have a serious or potentially serious health problem, please see a doctor. You may wish to use these suggestions in addition to the treatment prescribed by your doctor; if so, it is best to do so with his or her knowledge.

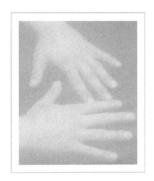

Contents

part three

PRESSURE POINT HEALING—AN "A" TO "Z" GUIDE
79

RECOMMENDED BOOKS
ON PRESSURE POINT THERAPY
380

INDEX   381

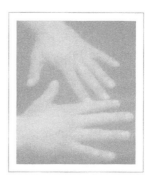

Introduction

For thousands of years, simple but very powerful finger pressure techniques have been part of the natural healing systems of China, Japan, India and other great civilizations around the globe. In this book we have gathered the hands-on healing wisdom of these ancient traditions, as well as some more recently developed Western pressure point practices, and distilled this extraordinary knowledge for you in a simple, easy-to-use format.

This book will help you claim the healing power in your own hands to bring relief from pain and eliminate a wide variety of common ailments without drugs or expensive medical procedures, and with no side effects. With the help of these pressure point therapies you will be able to safely and simply restore balance, renew energy and vitality, relieve stress and tension, and alleviate everyday aches and pains and common complaints such as headaches, menstrual cramps, neck pain, and eye strain. You will learn how to help your body heal itself.

These methods are easy to learn and enjoyable to use, whether on yourself or on someone else. The vast majority of the pressure points (with the obvious exception of some of the points on the back) can easily be reached, so self-treatment is both possible and comfortable.

In addition to their ability to quickly and safely relieve pain and alleviate many health problems, the pressure point healing systems explained in these pages help make a person stronger and less likely to become sick. They are also valuable for rebuilding the body after illness or after being treated with drugs or surgery.

These ancient treatment modalities can be used effectively in conjunction with modern Western medicine, and are being used in exactly that way in hospitals, clinics, and private practice throughout the world. Please do not consider them a substitute for Western medicine; although in some cases they may do the job, there are many other instances when drugs or surgery are the best treatment for the immediate situation.

Modern Western medicine has focused its attention almost entirely on curing disease, rather than on creating health. Its expertise lies in using surgery and medications to restore health once a person becomes ill. Many lives have been saved by this approach, sometimes almost miraculously. However, drugs often have toxic side effects which weaken the body, causing future problems which then have to be treated with more drugs.

The approach of the natural healing systems from the East is quite different. Their primary goal is not to heal disease once it occurs, but to prevent it. These systems encourage good health by paying close attention to balance in one's own life through diet, exercise, meditation, stress management, etc. If disease does occur, they aim not just to remove the symptoms, but to strengthen the body and mind and correct harmful lifestyle habits so that similar problems will not recur.

The pressure point therapies explained in these pages come from the traditional healing systems of several cultures, but all of them are based on an understanding of the human body as a dynamic, living organism, flowing with the energy of life itself. When the energy flow within a person becomes blocked or impeded or otherwise goes out of balance, the door is open for disorder and disease. When the flow of Life Energy is balanced, the body's natural defenses remain strong and health is maintained.

THE HEALING POWER OF TOUCH

The Life Energy can be enlivened by the healing power of touch. This healing power is as ancient and natural as life itself. Even animals have it. Have you ever watched a mother cat or dog licking, nudging, and cuddling her young? Generally we assume she's doing this for cleanliness. But research has revealed that this physical contact benefits all the systems of the young animal's body. The gastrointestinal, respiratory, circulatory, digestive, nervous, and endocrine systems are all stimulated and strengthened.

Research has also shown that animals that are gently touched, petted, or cuddled grow faster, have stronger immune systems, and are less fearful than animals who don't receive that physical attention. Similar results have been found with human infants, and this is no surprise. We didn't need science to teach us to caress and rock our little ones when they are upset; the natural instinct to nourish and soothe by means of touch is as old as mankind.

Indeed, touch therapy may well be the most ancient form of healing. If a place on the body hurts or feels stiff, we instinctively will touch, rub, or hold it. If another person is feeling physical or emotional pain, we spontaneously reach out to hold or touch in order to convey sympathy and support. Touch can bring reassurance, relaxation, and comfort; of course, it can have a stimulating, enlivening effect, too!

Pressure point therapies utilize the great sensitivity of our skin. A tiny section of skin, no bigger than a quarter, contains three million cells, 50 nerve endings, and three feet of blood vessels! No wonder it feels so good to be touched, and that being touched can have such a powerful effect on our health, vitality, and well-being.

THE POWER OF ATTENTION

An important and rarely considered aspect of the healing power of touch is *attention.* You may never have thought of it this way, but our awareness, the focus of our mind, is a subtle form of touch. And just as the power within the invisible energy levels of the atom is enormously greater than the power on the visible surface of things, so our subtle, invisible attention is a powerful form of healing.

Pain is the body's way of communicating an urgent need. Pain—whether in the ankle, the stomach, the throat, or the heart—says to us, "Hey! Over here! I need some attention." This is true of emotional pain as well as physical pain. And you will discover that often emotional pain and physical pain are intimately connected. Relieving one automatically has a healing effect upon the other. Just as pressure point therapy can relieve headaches, stiff necks, and allergy symptoms, it can also help to heal emotional wounds, lighten depression, and relieve anger and anxiety.

The techniques in this book will help you to use the focused energy of attention to heal. Because we offer suggestions from several different systems, you will be able to treat common health problems using a variety of methods. For any specific problem you might have, you can choose which method to use or you can try several to see which works best. With a little practice, you will develop a healing gift of touch to offer to your own body and to those dear to you.

To make the book still more complete and helpful, each chapter dealing with a specific condition also includes a section called "Additional

Suggestions." This short section offers a few simple non-pressure-point recommendations in the area of diet, exercise, herbs, etc. For example, in the chapter on Headaches we suggest drinking extra water, taking a walk, getting some fresh air, eating enough fiber to avoid constipation (a frequent cause of headaches), and so on.

You may be aware that the science of *Acupuncture* has been widely studied and accepted throughout the world in recent years. The finger pressure therapies in this book use exactly the same pressure points, and are based on the same principles as Acupuncture, except that, instead of needles, you use your fingers to stimulate the energy at these key points. Most historians actually consider Acupressure to be the older practice. Because you are using the gentle pressure of your own fingers, Acupressure may be even more effective than Acupuncture in relieving tension-related ailments and as a self-care preventive measure.

So without needles, without cost, without equipment, and in the comfort and convenience of your own home—even at your desk at work— you can take advantage of the same knowledge and methods that have been proven effective for thousands of years and are now being practiced all around the world. All you need are your own two hands and the willingness to devote a few minutes to enliven the natural selfhealing abilities of your body.

It is our desire that by using this book you will enjoy better health and greater happiness, so that you can fulfill your dreams and help others around you live a happier, healthier life.

part one

FUNDAMENTALS OF PRESSURE POINT THERAPY

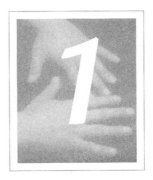

Where Do Pressure Point Therapies Come From?

Evidence of the use of pressure points for healing has been found all around the world. Acupuncture "needles" made of stone have been uncovered in Chinese tombs believed to be at least 6,000 years old. These needles were apparently used to apply pressure to specific points on the body in order to influence organs or systems related to the points.

We often associate this kind of healing therapy with the Orient, but similar needles, made of iron and perhaps equally ancient, have been found in South America and in Egypt, suggesting the use of pressure points for healing in these cultures as well. Pictographs from around 2500 B.C. in the tomb of a powerful Egyptian physician depict foot massage being performed.

In the Western medical tradition, the use of touch for healing goes back at least as far as Hippocrates, the Greek physician (5th century B.C.) generally referred to as "The father of Western medicine." He taught his students that massage would benefit tissue growth, and would be healing to the joints. The Roman emperor Julius Caesar received a daily massage to relieve the discomfort of chronic neuralgia and headaches, and Pliny, the Roman naturalist, found massage helpful to soothe his asthma.

We know that European forms of touch therapy were used in the 14th century. In the 1800s, both Europeans and Americans developed the theory and practice of zone therapy and Reflexology, which are similar to Asian methods and probably have links to ancient Chinese and Indian systems.

In the East, the traditional systems of healing have continued in an unbroken lineage for literally thousands of years. Medical texts such as *The Yellow Emperor's Classic of Internal Medicine* in China and the *Charaka Samhita* and *Sushruta Samhita* of Indian Ayurvedic medicine describe pressure point therapies and how and when to use them.

In the modern age, scientific research is re-validating the power and effectiveness of these systems of healing. In a number of Asian countries, businesses now routinely offer pressure point therapy to their employees as a preventive measure. They have found that keeping their employees healthy is cost-effective, for it reduces stress, minimizes absenteeism, and produces a more harmonious and productive work force.

Forms of pressure point therapy vary somewhat, but are fundamentally very similar. Acupressure came from China, Shiatsu from Japan, and Reflexology was developed in Europe and the United States. A system we will draw upon to a lesser degree—Yoga—was developed in India. All these methodologies are based on common underlying principles.

THE BODY AS ENERGY

Primary among these principles is that bodies are energy systems. Our modern world, influenced so strongly by the industrial age, has been dominated for 300 years by a mechanistic view of life and often looks at the body as a kind of machine. But this view is rapidly becoming obsolete as breakthroughs in science reveal a world very similar to that known and described by the ancient healers, a world of energy, relationships, and interdependence in a field of Unity.

Gradually, the nature of matter is being penetrated and revealed. We now know that cells are formed of molecules; molecules are made of atoms; atoms are composed of finer particles which, upon still deeper investigation, turn out to be energy fields. These energy fields are swirling at such tremendous speeds that they appear to be solid particles, but they are not. Remember, what we're discussing is not just matter "out there," but the deepest truth about our own body. At the atomic or "quantum" level, the body is a mass of interacting energy fields.

Leading medical thinkers (such as Deepak Chopra, Larry Dossey, Bernie Siegel, Christiane Northrup, Andrew Weill, and increasing numbers of others) are being hailed as heralds of a new medicine, revealing the interconnectedness of mind and body. Yet many of the insights that strike us as new and exciting were fundamental principles of the ancient healing systems behind pressure point therapy:

- Life is energy.
- Our bodies are complex living organisms composed of energy.
- Everything we do, eat, think, and feel affects our health and well-being.
- Therefore we can influence our health through practices (such as the finger pressure techniques in this book) which re-direct our energy and help to maintain or restore balance and vitality.

This holistic view, based on the understanding that life is energy and relationship and that everything we do affects our health, has been seen as incompatible with the modern medical view of health and disease based on the mechanistic model of the body as a machine. But things are changing.

REVIVAL OF AN ANCIENT WISDOM

When President Nixon went to China in 1972, James Reston, the *New York Times* political commentator covering the trip, had to undergo an emergency appendectomy. Following the surgery Reston reported his surprise at the pain relief he experienced from a few Acupuncture needles. His story attracted a great deal of attention in the American medical community, so much so that several doctors went to China to study the Eastern methods.

Since then, numerous film clips of treatments—including major surgery—using Acupuncture have appeared on our television screens. Research was undertaken to assess the reliability of pressure point therapy for pain relief and healing, and found it effective. Publication of this research in scientific journals has opened the door to widespread acceptance and appreciation for this knowledge.

Bill Moyers, in preparing his PBS series, *Healing and the Mind*, witnessed a brain tumor surgery in Beijing. Because of the use of Acupuncture, the patient needed only half the medication normally used for sedation. What's more, the patient remained conscious during the entire three-hour operation and actually conversed with the doctor! (Using less anesthesia means less danger for the patient as well as a faster recovery time and fewer side effects.)

Acupuncture is practiced by more than three million doctors in Asia and is used in clinics and hospitals around the world. Officially recognized by the World Health Organization as effective in treating 104 conditions including arthritis, back pain, tonsillitis, asthma, migraine headaches, and paralysis from stroke, it is being taught as a medical procedure in Russia and more than 10,000 doctors in the United States have adopted it as a tool. It has also been used extensively in treating addictions (including nicotine, alcohol, cocaine, and heroin) with great success.

Most important for you is that medical historians believe Acupuncture was derived from the simpler, finger-pressure techniques of Acupressure you will learn in these pages.

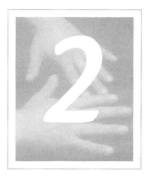

How Pressure Point Therapies Work

CH'I—THE VITAL LIFE ENERGY

The Chinese have a saying, "The tree grows because it has energy for growing." They recognized a vital energy, a Life Force that animates every living thing. In fact, just as we have learned through modern science that all matter, including inanimate objects like rocks, is made of energy, so the ancient healers perceived that Life Energy permeates all the elements of the material world, including fire, water, and rock. This energy of life is called *Ch'i* in China (sometimes spelled *Qi*), *Ki* in Japan, and *Prana* in Indian Yoga. All of these words are names for the same thing, loosely translated in the West as Life Energy or Life Force.

The Life Force is related to breath and functions similarly to electricity, yet it is more subtle than either. We can think of it as an interface, where mind and matter meet. The Chinese character for *Ch'i* is a symbol representing rice and steam, indicating that *Ch'i* is both something substantial or material, and something insubstantial at the same time.

The ancient physicians and sages perceived that this Life Energy circulates in the body along specific channels called *meridians*. These conduits are the supply lines of *Ch'i* for the body. Along each of these channels are numerous points—the Acupuncture/Acupressure points—at which the flow can be most effectively accessed and influenced.

According to this way of thinking, the flow of energy through the meridians of the body determines our health. When the flow is smooth, balanced, and unobstructed, we are healthy. Pain and disease can develop when there is a disturbance in the flow. It may, for example, become too fast or too slow, too rough or too static, too hot or too cold, too moist or too dry. By learning to apply gentle but firm pressure with your fingers to the key pressure points, you will be able to remedy these imbalances and restore health and harmony.

Pressure point therapies are based on the principle of keeping the *Ch'i* or *Prana* flowing in a balanced and harmonious way. Many of us who are basically healthy still become unbalanced at times due to overwork, injuries, or emotional stress. Lack of exercise and faulty diet can also disturb our systems, plus we have the effects of environmental pollution and chemicals in our food to contend with. Colds, allergies, headaches, backache, stomach problems, fatigue, are just a few of the ailments which commonly plague most healthy people when their flow of vital energy is weakened, disturbed, or blocked. If these minor imbalances aren't corrected, more serious health problems may develop.

CAN YOU FEEL THE ENERGY?

Many of us Westerners have some resistance to the notion of "invisible energy" running through our bodies. The idea of *Ch'i* sounds very abstract to our "see it to believe it" mentality. Yet energy is the basis for all life and is the vital factor in healing. The energy dimension of our bodies is not immediately obvious to our senses, yet it does exist, and over time and with practice you will not only develop an intuitive sense of this energy, you will begin to feel it in your hands and fingers.

You may even be able to feel it now. Try this experiment: Hold your arms out in front of you, elbows bent, hands facing each other but at a 45 degree angle (not perpendicular to the floor). Hold for a few seconds, then drop one hand part way down. Put it back. Drop it down. Put it back. Do you feel a difference? Many people can feel a subtle current of energy, a warmth or even a tingling, when the hands are facing each other, that dissipates when one hand drops down.

SCIENCE VALIDATES PRESSURE POINT THERAPY

In recent years scientists have begun to document the existence of this flow of energy as well as many of the benefits of pressure point therapy. Research has demonstrated a flow of electrical current along the pathways the ancient texts labeled as the meridians; conductivity has been found to be greater at just those key points traditionally designated as the pressure points.

In addition to research in the U.S. and other Western countries, an amazing amount of research on the practical applications of Acupuncture for various conditions is being conducted in China. Over 10,000 studies—that's not a misprint!—are published in Chinese medical journals every year. Electrocardiogram (EKG) readings have shown improvements in patients with irregular heart beats. Respiratory and digestive problems have been relieved, and substantial evidence now exists that pressure point therapy can be instrumental in regulating the nervous system and the circulatory system. Increasing circulation is always beneficial, as it both flushes toxins out of the body and brings nutrients and oxygen to all our cells.

Pressure point therapies have also been shown to trigger the brain to release endorphins, the chemical substances known to reduce pain and bring feelings of well-being.

So have confidence! Not only have millions of people directly experienced the benefits of pressure point therapy, but modern science is also documenting the power and effectiveness of these techniques.

Now let's learn a little more about *Ch'i* and its meridians and key points, so that you will have a solid foundation from which to begin using pressure point techniques. The terminology we will use is largely from the Chinese system of Acupuncture and Acupressure, but most of the principles are common to all the systems. As we explore other systems later on, any differences will be pointed out.

YIN AND YANG,
FEMININE AND MASCULINE ENERGY

Traditionally, the Life Energy (*Ch'i*) is understood to have two poles, called *yin* and *yang*. *Yin* and *yang*, which are said to be constantly fluctuating in a dynamic balance, express the interdependence and relationship of opposites. Their opposite yet complementary natures are beautifully portrayed in the ancient symbol which expresses the interactive flow of one into the other. Each participates in the other, yet maintains its distinctiveness. This symbol of *yin* and *yang* has become familiar around the world, and can be found dangling on earrings and necklaces, or incorporated into popular art.

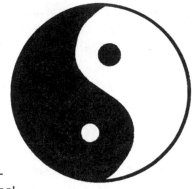

Yang and *yin* symbolize the opposites found throughout nature: light and dark, mountains and valleys, hot and cold, hard and soft, male and female, and so on. Traditional Chinese medicine sees the human body as a reflection or miniature of the natural world, so these opposites are present within us as well.

Yin (the feminine) is said to correspond to that which is dark, moist, cool, receptive, yielding, while *yang* (the masculine) is light, dry, hot, active, and penetrating. *Yin* is intuition, *yang* rationality and analysis. *Yin* is the moon, yang the sun. *Yin* is structure, *Yang* function. It is the play between these polarities, the ebb and flow of these two aspects of the one Life Energy, which creates the flowing nature of *Ch'i*. Life Energy manifests in the world through yin and yang, moving in the waves of creation.

Fig. 1—Yin/Yang

The balanced expression of these principles in the mind and body reflects a healthy condition of harmony and balance. Disease expresses imbalance and disharmony.

Some of the meridians or energy pathways are said to have a *yin* nature. These run up the front of the body. Other meridians are *yang* in nature and run down the back.

MERIDIANS—CHANNELS FOR THE FLOW OF ENERGY

Meridians are the channels or pathways through which *Ch'i* circulates. The meridian system is similar to our circulatory or nervous system. Or you might think of these channels as the wiring in the body's electrical system, carrying the vital Life Energy throughout the body.

There are twelve main meridians. Each traverses a specific path through the body, and links specific organs and physical structures. For example, the Heart meridian runs from the side of the chest (under the armpit) down the inside of the arm to the little finger. Does that sound familiar? Right—it is the path pain often follows during a heart attack.

The network of meridians is a complex and subtle system, extending throughout the body. In Western physiological terms, the meridians most likely have links with the nervous system as well as with the connective tissue and fascia. Many of the points along the meridians correspond to points used in Western physiotherapy to release tight muscles.

You don't need to have a detailed understanding of the meridian associations (heart, lungs, etc.) in order to begin using pressure points for healing. But if you have a basic understanding of the principles involved, you will feel more confident of what you are doing and why.

The 12 meridians are divided into pairs; that is, the meridians on the right and left sides of the body are identical networks which are mirror images of each other.

Six pairs run over the arms and onto the torso

Six pairs run up and down the legs and onto the trunk

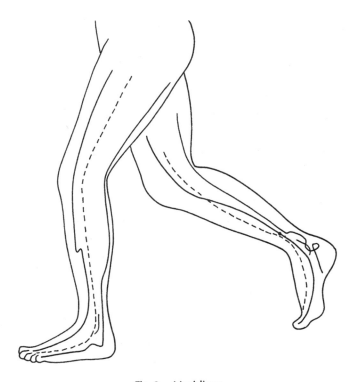

Fig. 2—Meridians

These 12 pairs of meridians influence and reflect the functioning of major organ or bodily systems.

The six leg meridians:

GB = Gall Bladder

B = Urinary Bladder

K = Kidney

Lv = Liver

S = Stomach

Sp = Spleen and pancreas

The six arm meridians:

LI = Large intestine

SI = Small intestine

H = Heart

Pc = Pericardium (protects the heart)

TW = Triple Warmer (the abdominal cavity, which maintains internal heat)

L = Lung

These 12 pairs of meridians result in 24 separate pathways.

In addition, there are two unpaired meridians which are not associated with a particular organ, but are reservoirs of *yang* and *yin* energy. They are important regulators of the entire bodily system. The Governor Vessel (GV) links the spinal column, brain, and nervous system. It runs from the tail bone straight up the back and over the top of the head to the center of the upper lip. Its main function is to govern all the yang meridians in the body. Powerful points along this meridian can help alleviate stiffness of the spine, fever, irritability, and muscle spasms of the back.

The other main unpaired meridian, the Conception Vessel (CV), is the *yin* "partner" to the Governor Vessel. The main meridian responsible for all the yin pathways, it is linked to the digestive and reproductive systems and flows up the front of the body from the perineum (a point between the anus and genitals) to the lower lip. From key points along this meridian, ailments such as cough, asthma, or urinary-genital problems can be treated.

Some *Shiatsu* practitioners place more emphasis on the meridians than on the pressure points. They feel that if you learn the location of the meridians, you will have a sense for the flow of the *Ch'i* in the body and will instinctively feel the position of the points.

Let's look at the life of just one of the meridians.

The kidneys are considered to be a storehouse of *Ch'i*. They govern sexual energy and the urinary system, as well as controlling bones and being linked with the brain. When the kidneys have an abundance of energy, the functioning of the vital organs is strong; vitality and creativity are high. On the other hand, when you feel exhausted, your store of *Ch'i* in the kidneys may be low or the Kidney meridian may be blocked.

The kidney meridian goes from the little toe to its first pressure point on the sole of the foot. It passes the heel, reaches the ankle bone on the inner side and flows up the inside of the leg past the knee and up the thigh to the coccyx. From there it goes up to the kidneys, then through the liver, diaphragm, and lungs as far as the throat and the root of the tongue. Along this meridian there are 27 main pressure points.

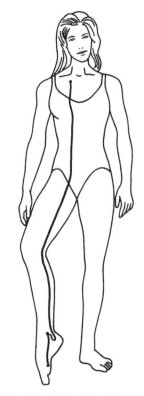

Fig. 3—The Kidney Meridian

Some symptoms one might experience due to imbalance along this meridian are asthma, breathlessness, dryness of the tongue, throat pain, edema, diarrhea, weakness of the legs, low back pain, and diminished sex drive. If points on the Kidney meridian are painful to the touch, it doesn't necessarily mean the kidney itself is weak, but that the energy in that meridian is blocked, excessive, or unbalanced. Working various points along the meridian can unblock the energy flow and help to heal various conditions.

For example, pressing on K 1 can help relieve impotence and hot flashes and is rejuvenating. Working K 2 can help relieve irregular menstruation and foot cramps. Pressure on K 6 may help relieve insomnia. And so on.

PRESSURE POINTS—THE BODY'S ENERGY TRIGGER POINTS

Along each meridian are small areas or points where the energy of the meridian is particularly close to the surface of the skin. These are the Acupressure or Shiatsu points. The ancient Chinese symbol for an Acupressure point shows a jar with a narrow neck and a cover. It is a beautiful image that looks like figure 4.

The neck of the jar represents the point on your body which leads into a reservoir of *Ch'i*. From these points you have direct access to your body's internal energy systems. They are like electrical switch points at which the power supply network can be influenced. At these points the *Ch'i* can be stimulated, pacified, or released if it is blocked.

As we mentioned above, scientific studies have shown that these points correspond to areas of particularly high electrical conductivity. Tension also tends to concentrate around these points, inhibiting circulation and causing stagnation of energy.

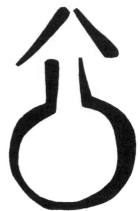

Fig. 4

These points are the places you will learn to gently but firmly press to release the tension and get your blood and Life Energy flowing freely again, to promote health and healing.

There are hundreds of pressure points. The classical Chinese texts usually list 365 "major" points. However, many are rarely used because the symptoms they can treat are highly specific and rare. Other points are used often, because they have a far-reaching influence.

The points on the feet and below the knee, and those on the hands and forearms have always been regarded as particularly helpful. This may be one of the reasons that Reflexology treatments, which focus primarily on massaging areas of the hands and feet, are so beneficial. Some of the ancient Chinese masters used to say that they could heal any sickness using just four pressure points. Others concentrated on 12 main points.

The major pressure points have poetic names which often inform us about the benefits or characteristics of that point or the systems it influences. Some of the names are "Abdominal Sorrow" (which helps relieve nausea and indigestion), "Welcoming Perfume" (which clears stuffy noses and clogged sinuses), and "Reaching Inside" (which helps resolve problems with the fetus during pregnancy). Let's look at an example, the point known as "Bubbling Springs," located at the center of the sole of the foot. You will find it at the base of the ball of your foot.

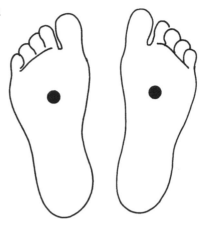

"Bubbling Springs" is the first point on the Kidney meridian. The kidneys are a storehouse for *Ch'i*; the body and all the organs need *Ch'i* to thrive, so the health and vitality of each organ depends on the energy of the kidneys. Stimulating the "Bubbling Springs" point enlivens the kidneys and is said to rejuvenate the spirit.

Also, think of the purifying work these organs are engaged in all day long. The kidneys regulate the

Fig. 5—K 1, Bubbling Springs

flow of water in the body. Each kidney has about one million tiny filtration systems called nephrons, and together the two kidneys filter about a quart of blood every minute, 15 gallons an hour, 360 gallons a day! With this background, the image of a "bubbling spring" suddenly becomes significant!

The points also have identification numbers related to their location on the meridians. For example, our "Bubbling Springs" point, as the first point on the Kidney meridian, is K 1.

But don't worry—you don't need to remember these names and numbers in order to practice the techniques in this book. Illustrations will be available pinpointing the places to press in order to care for your condition or create the effect you want to produce, such as relaxation or increased energy.

HELPER POINTS

Some beneficial points will probably be found at or near the area of your discomfort, but other helpful points may be all the way at the other end of your body. How can rubbing a spot on your foot help with a headache, or tired eyes? Because both are on the same meridian (or, in the language of

Reflexology, in the same zone) which brings energy to that particular area or organ. One example is the point called the Adjoining Valley point, located in the webbing between the thumb and index finger on the outside of your hand.

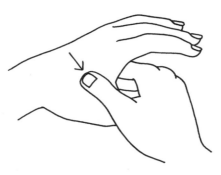

Fig. 6—Li 4, Adjoining Valley

This point, which is located on the large intestine (Li) meridian, has a multitude of effects on the body. First, it is a potent general pain reliever. Some European and American dentists have been trained to use this point in their practices to prevent pain. Stimulating this point can also have a powerful effect on the head (relieving headaches), the sinuses, and the colon. It is used to help relieve hot flashes, arthritis, allergies, and constipation, as well as to balance the entire gastrointestinal system. Its effect can be so powerful that you should not press this point during pregnancy, as it can stimulate premature contractions.

Now you know about your Life Energy, otherwise known as *Ch'i*, *Prana*, *Ki*, or *Qi*. You have learned about the meridians, the channels for this energy, and about the pressure points, which are the switch points from which the power supply network of *Ch'i* can be accessed and influenced.

Now let's briefly look at some of the benefits you can enjoy in your life from using pressure point therapy.

The Benefits: What Pressure Point Therapy Can Do for You

The simple finger pressure techniques in these pages can help you with virtually all aspects of your life. Pain relief, muscle relaxation, increased energy, emotional balance—these benefits will help you at home and at work, in relationships and in pursuit of your aspirations.

These methods will help you achieve greater balance, strength, and harmony in body and mind. When your system is strong and balanced, you will be less likely to get sick. Through practice you will gain the ability to notice the beginnings of an imbalance and correct it before it manifests as a cold or a chronic pain. You will be able to relieve pain and fatigue and promote your own health. As you become more sensitive to the state of your body, you will find yourself wanting to eat better, exercise, and get enough rest. Whatever harmful or self-destructive old habits you may have will become less attractive, and may fall away naturally.

REDUCE YOUR STRESS LEVEL

Many centuries ago, Mongolian warriors used to ritually massage themselves in order to rid themselves of fear before going into battle. Our lives generally are not quite that intense, but we certainly are challenged daily by the pollution of our air, water, and food as well as the hurry and worry of modern life. The flow of *Ch'i* can be damaged by trauma, whether emotional or physical, by infections, wrong food and drink, too much exercise, or lack of it.

Pressure point therapy can be used as an effective preventative, helping to keep your body and energy balanced so you can feel your best and do your best no matter what you have to deal with every day. It is also highly effective as a way to release tension and stress. A few minutes a day, whether in the morning to prepare your body and mind to face the challenges of the day, or in the evening to unwind and relax, can help you counteract the stress of modern living.

Major life changes are particularly stressful. Changes in jobs, in relationships, children leaving home, parents dying or becoming seriously ill— these are all times when some extra relaxation and self-nurturing are valuable.

Pressure point therapy has proven to be particularly beneficial in stress-related disorders. Estimates vary, but most experts believe at least 70% of our health disorders are related to stress and tension.

Chronic tension tends to build up around the Acupressure points and block the circulation, which sets the stage for many illnesses. It is now standard medical knowledge that many physical disorders, such as asthma, allergies, headaches, backaches, heart disease, and even high cholesterol, as well as high blood pressure and ulcers, are either caused or complicated by stress. Pressure point therapy is an effective and entirely natural way to reduce stress and therefore to prevent many illnesses from arising.

IMPROVE CIRCULATION AND ELIMINATE TOXINS

Pressure point therapy encourages the body to relax. As a result, numerous bodily functions are positively affected. Stress and tension constrict muscles and restrict blood flow in the cardiovascular system. When your muscles relax, your blood can circulate more freely and carry oxygen and nutrients to all your cells, while at the same time eliminating accumulated toxins.

INCREASE IMMUNITY

Stress and tension lower our resistance and make us more susceptible to disease. By contrast, a relaxed body is resistant to illness and more easily mobilizes its innate healing mechanisms. Research has shown that touch improves the functioning of the immune system. Pressure point therapy seems to act as a signal to the body, alerting it to activate its internal processes of healing and its preparedness to deal with oncoming challenges.

ELIMINATE UNWANTED HABITS

Because of its deep stress-releasing and energizing effects, pressure point therapy can be very helpful for people working on letting go of self-destructive habits such as smoking, over-eating, and alcohol and drug addictions. Besides the generally calming effect, there are specific points you can use to clear your mind, regulate your appetite, or balance your digestion. The increased feeling of well-being created by deep relaxation can help you overcome food cravings and add strength to your resolve to quit smoking or drop other negative habits.

RELIEVE PAIN AND HEAL CHRONIC ILLNESS

The World Health Organization has recognized that traditional systems of medicine offer valuable contributions to the health and quality of human life. It has officially recommended the use of Acupuncture for treating the pain of many conditions, such as arthritis, bursitis, tendinitis, backache, sciatica, neck and shoulder pain, and migraine and tension headaches. Remember that when you use Acupressure you are using exactly the same points used in Acupuncture.

Finger pressure therapy has also been remarkably successful in treating a number of functional disorders. Individuals with infertility problems, chronic fatigue, digestive disorders, asthma, insomnia, nervousness, and depression have all found help.

PREVENT AND HEAL EXERCISE-INDUCED INJURIES

Many people are also finding pressure point therapy a great help in their sports or exercise programs. A 15-minute self-treatment can be used as a warm-up to prevent injury, as well as a way to relax after a good workout. You can also use it to relieve cramps, stiffness, or pain. Hopefully you won't ever sustain an injury, but if you do, pressure point therapy can definitely help promote healing and reduce pain.

BRING OUT YOUR NATURAL BEAUTY

Another benefit of pressure point therapy is increased natural beauty. Learning to relax, and improving your overall health and vitality, bring out your natural good looks. We all look better when we feel relaxed and alive. You will learn to relax your facial muscles and stimulate some of the key points known to increase circulation and improve complexion. You will also find a pressure point routine for your face that can help prevent wrinkling. But since we're all going to have wrinkles some day, it's most important to be healthy and feel good, whether you have wrinkles or not!

ESTABLISH A BETTER RELATIONSHIP WITH YOUR BODY

Acupressure, Shiatsu, and Reflexology are effective ways to get more tuned in to your body. Largely because of our sedentary lifestyle, many people are quite alienated from their own bodies. Giving it some attention every day can not only make you more sensitive to its changes and needs, but can also be very healing. Just spending a little time gently massaging, releasing tensions, and opening up the flow of energy is a wonderful way to establish a more loving relationship with your body and to generate feelings of gratitude for this friend that does so much for us every day.

PREVENT ILLNESS, PROMOTE GOOD HEALTH

In ancient China, physicians received a fee only as long as their patients remained healthy. Treating someone who is already ill, they taught, is like starting to dig a well after you have become thirsty. We can learn from them to care for our own future health by eating well, exercising appropriately, and learning to calm the mind and body with relaxation and meditation. Adding a program of touch therapy can provide the extra boost that will keep you strong and prevent slight imbalances from turning into significant health problems.

If you think about it, prevention is the most practical method of health care. "A stitch in time saves nine." "An ounce of prevention is worth a pound of cure." These folk sayings reflect the natural laws of life. Why wait until you become really sick and uncomfortable before seeking out health care that is likely to be expensive and possibly have negative side effects?

Using pressure point therapy is one way to begin taking charge of your own health. You may begin to notice, for example, how habituated you have become to tension, stiffness, or pain. The more heightened your body awareness becomes, the more quickly you will notice tension in your neck, shoulders, or wherever it starts to collect. Now you will be able to dissolve it almost immediately, before it has a chance to develop into something more serious.

It's only common sense to make use of every available option to maximize good health. This includes both conventional Western medicine as well as traditional medicines such as Shiatsu, Acupressure, Ayurveda, and other natural healing systems. The ideal is to maintain good health through natural means, and as much as possible to avoid unnecessary medical services and drugs with side effects. By using pressure point therapy to manage minor ailments and imbalances before they develop into major problems, you will be able to save money, prevent pain and disability, and maintain good health.

So find yourself a comfortable space and set aside some time, with the desire to give your full attention to your body. Whether you spend 15 minutes a day for prevention, or work on specific points when you feel tense, tired, stiff, or achey, please make use of this knowledge!

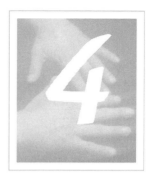

Getting Acquainted with the Pressure Point Therapies

ACUPRESSURE

By now you've become familiar with some of the principles of pressure point therapy and you've learned about some of the benefits. Terms like *Ch'i*, *yin* and *yang*, meridians, and pressure points are no longer unfamiliar. You've also become comfortable—and, we hope, excited—about the notion that our bodies are energy systems, and that finger pressure therapies work with this energy to maintain and restore health and balance.

The terms we have been using, and the basic principles we have been discussing, derive from Acupressure, the oldest of the Far Eastern therapies, originating in China. In this chapter you will learn more about the other systems of pressure point therapy—Shiatsu from Japan, Yoga from India, and Reflexology, which was developed in Europe and America.

The actual origins of Acupressure (as well as Shiatsu and Yoga), are hidden deep within at least 5,000 years of history. They may have a common root in the Indian system of Ayurveda, known in India as "The Mother of all Healing." Wherever they began, we know that these healing practices have been used effectively for thousands of years, and that their revival is helping millions of people today.

SHIATSU

The word *Shiatsu* means thumb or finger pressure, but in actual practice, a variety of other techniques are used too. If you visit a Shiatsu practitioner for a treatment, you may find that the therapist uses his or her palms, knuckles, elbows, fists, or even feet in order to apply pressure in the optimum way for the points and meridians being treated. In this book we won't be using our feet or elbows, but you will learn a variety of ways to relax or enliven various points and channels.

A HOLISTIC APPROACH

Shiatsu, like the other finger pressure therapies, is part of a holistic approach to health. Blockages in energy flow, and imbalances in the system, are often a consequence of personal habits in diet and activity, as well as our perceptions, thoughts, and emotional reactions. Age, lifestyle, even the weather, all play a part.

Because of the interconnectedness of so many factors, it is important not to use pressure point therapy in the typical way many people today use medicines: popping a pill to relieve symptoms rather than finding out why they have the problem and correcting the underlying cause. For example, a stomach ache may be relieved by an antacid, but the cause was probably over-eating, or eating foods that are too heavy, too greasy, or too spicy for you.

That doesn't mean it is wrong to seek symptom relief when something hurts or is out of balance. But it *is* a mistake to rely entirely on the "magic bullet" approach rather than seeking out and correcting the cause, because the same problem, or related ones, will repeatedly arise until you amend your lifestyle.

A Japanese modification of Chinese Acupressure, Shiatsu was probably brought to Japan by Buddhist monks in the 6th century. The principles of energy, meridians, and points are essentially the same as in Chinese Acupressure, but with different names. In Japan, the Life Energy is called *Ki* instead of *Ch'i*, and the points are known as *tsubos*. Tsubos are thought of as vortexes of energy, points where the energy gathers. They are sometimes compared to volcanoes, where energy deep within the earth's core rises to the surface. At these points, energy is particularly active and can be most easily released and balanced.

The main difference in the Japanese approach is that pressure is applied more vigorously. Shiatsu practitioners use their thumbs whenever possible in order to apply firmer, stronger, rhythmic pressure. They also tend to pay more attention to entire meridians, and less to individual points, while most Acupressure practitioners do the reverse.

Shiatsu has been practiced in Japan for about 1,500 years. Japanese families have used it at home for centuries, both as a preventative, and to release pain or fatigue. More advanced practitioners successfully treat particular organs and ailments. Blind people were especially valued as Shiatsu therapists, because their sense of touch became more acute as a compensation for their lost visual abilities.

After World War II, with the introduction of Western allopathic medicine, Shiatsu practice began to wane. General MacArthur, head of the Allied occupying forces after the war, attempted to completely ban it. But Helen Keller was instrumental in reinstating Shiatsu as an honored occupation for many Japanese workers who were blind. Eventually, word of its effectiveness spread among Westerners. Celebrities, including Joe DiMaggio, Marilyn Monroe, and later, Henry Kissinger, were particularly instrumental in calling attention to it. In recent years thousands of Americans have learned it and many have set up practices.

HARA

A unique aspect of Shiatsu is its emphasis on hara. An energy center in the abdominal area about 2-$\frac{1}{2}$ inches below the navel, hara is considered to be the nucleus of our vital energy. It is also a very vulnerable area. All energy, emotion, and physical movement are said to be formed and generated out of the hara, and many points and zones for healing all parts of the body are located here.

Working with *hara* is considered an especially subtle art that takes years to learn, so we will not offer any *hara* exercises or treatments here. If you are fascinated, you might wish to consult a trained Shiatsu practitioner.

REFLEXOLOGY

Like practitioners of Acupressure and Shiatsu, Reflexologists also work with the energy of life, though they restrict their healing work primarily to the feet, with a secondary emphasis on the hands. The hands and feet are seen as microcosms or miniatures of the entire body. The organs, glands, and various parts of our physical structure, are laid out in a pattern similar to the body's.

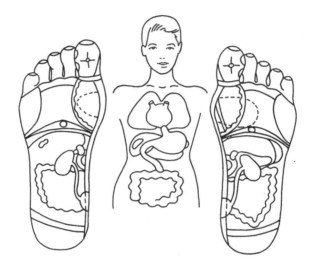

Fig. 7—Correspondence of the Feet and Body

According to this approach, by giving your feet a thorough workout, you can invigorate and/or relax your entire body.

The main focus of a Reflexology treatment is on "reflex zones," which are somewhat more generalized areas than the very specific points used in Shiatsu and Acupressure. Yet many of the meridians do run through the feet. This may be one reason Reflexology is so effective.

Foot massage is a universal and time-honored practice. Pictographs from ancient Egypt and artifacts from the Incas as well as old Europe show people giving and receiving foot massage. Reflexology itself may have roots in the ancient Asian pressure point systems, though it was rediscovered and redeveloped in the late 19th and early 20th centuries. A Connecticut physician named William Fitzgerald discovered that he could do minor surgeries using pressure on points on the hand to prevent pain. Eventually he identified what he named the "reflex zones" of the body, and called his work "zone therapy."

According to this understanding, ten zones run vertically from the top of your head down to the soles of your feet, five on the right side and five on the left, each ending at one of your toes. Every organ, gland, or bodily structure is located within one of these zones, and has a related reflex zone on the bottom of your foot. These reflex zones are the gateways to the energy and organ systems of your body.

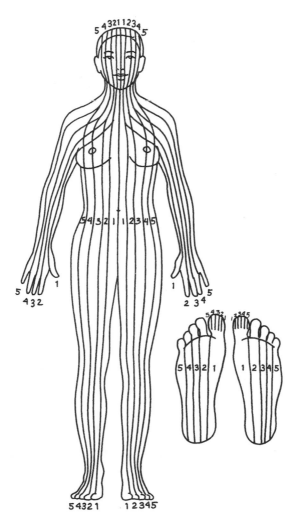

Fig. 8—The Reflex Zones

An American physical therapist, Eunice Ingham, worked with a physician who used zone therapy in his practice, largely on the hands. Following her intuition, she discovered that the feet were more highly responsive, and over 40 years she charted the effects of the reflex zones on the feet, creating the first "maps" showing exactly where to press. Her nephew, Dwight Byers, continued her pioneering work; he is director of the International Institute of Reflexology in St. Petersburg, Florida, author of *Better Health with Foot Reflexology*, and teacher of some of the most prominent and successful Reflexologists working today.

There are over 25,000 trained and certified Reflexology practitioners throughout the world. Reflexology is the number one alternative health modality in Denmark, and is used by the royal family of Britain. "Most of us find that just a simple foot rub feels so soothing," says Byers. "Working with reflex zones takes it to a whole new level."

One reason Reflexologists focus on the feet is that they contain about 7,200 nerve endings, extensively connected through the spinal cord and brain with all areas of the body. Not only are the feet an ideal place to begin relaxing the entire system, but also, because these nerve endings have connections with all of our organs, stimulating the feet can help activate sluggish glands and organs.

The nerve endings in our feet may be important in another way. Native American healers say that our feet are our contact with the earth and the energies that flow through it; by having our feet upon the earth, our Spirit is connected to the universe. Eunice Ingham formulated the same idea: "The nerves of our body may be likened to an electrical system. There is a flow of electricity between the earth and our feet. Reflexology unblocks the pathways in our feet and allows energy to flow freely."

During a Reflexology treatment, tiny mineral deposits (sometimes described as "crystals") in the feet are broken up. These deposits settle throughout the body, but especially in the feet. Because our feet are so far from our pumping heart, the blood tends to stagnate. The increased circulation stimulated by Reflexology removes toxins, breaks up the congestion caused by the crystals, and brings a fresh influx of Life Energy. One of Eunice Ingham's favorite sayings was, "Circulation is life; Stagnation is death." The *Tao Te Ching* of China contains a similar expression, "In Life all things are flowing and bending, in death dry, hard, and brittle."

So create a habit of spending at least five to ten minutes every evening with your feet. You can even do it while watching television, though it's better to pay attention to what you're doing.

OTHER METHODS

Finger pressure practitioners have developed a number of new therapies, such as *Do-in*, *Jin Shin Jyutsu* and others, which are essentially offshoots of the main tree. One system that is different, however, and which we will refer to from time to time, is Yoga.

Yoga comes to us from ancient India. It is connected with the traditional Indian system of health and healing known as Ayurveda, which means literally, "The Science of Life." Ayurveda is probably the oldest system of medicine in the world.

Like traditional Chinese medicine, Ayurveda emphasizes a lifestyle in harmony with the laws of nature. Both systems are products of civilizations that were deeply rooted in Mother Nature, and in these cultures the words "health" and "harmony" are truly synonymous.

The word *yoga* means literally to yoke or join—a union. But a union of what? Not just a meeting of your fingers and your toes! In Hatha Yoga, the branch of Yoga from which the postures come, union means a harmony or balance of one's body, mind, and spirit or consciousness. This harmony or balance is health.

Why is Hatha Yoga included in a book of pressure point therapies? Because many key Acupressure points are automatically pressed or massaged when you hold or get in and out of various Yoga postures.

Michael Reed Gach, Director of the Acupressure Institute in Berkeley and a teacher of both Yoga and Acupressure, has unfolded this knowledge in his teaching of what he calls "AcuYoga." He points out that some very beneficial points would be difficult or impossible to reach with your own fingers, but that with a Yoga *asana* (posture) you can easily apply the needed pressure to these hard-to-reach areas.

Actually, you can achieve even more pressure, as you've got the weight of your body working for you. Plus, you add the benefit of an internal massage to your organs and glands that takes place as you bend and stretch. On a subtler level, the pressure points and meridians are enlivened, promoting the balance and flow of Life Energy, which in Sanskrit, the ancient language of India, is called *Prana*.

Like the Chinese concept of *Ch'i*, *Prana* is understood to be more refined than the physical breath, and yet it is connected with the breath. *Prana* serves as a bridge or link between the physical world of matter and the Consciousness or Energy that is the basis of life itself. In the words of Swami Vishnudevananda, author of *The Complete Illustrated Book of Yoga*:

According to Yoga philosophy, there is no lifeless matter, for everything is consciousness itself. Scientists tell us that inside the tiniest particles of atoms is incredible movement. If there is movement, there must be some kind of energy to cause it, and that energy is the basis of life itself.

Yoga philosophy teaches that this Life Energy circulates throughout the body in a system of subtle channels known as *nadis*. There are subtle channels connecting every cell in the body as well as the organs and glands. In India, just as in China, 14 of these channels are considered to be the most important. World renowned Yoga expert and teacher B.K.S. Iyengar writes:

> . . . the *nadis* penetrate the body from the soles of the feet to the crown of the head. In them is *Prana*, the breath of life. *Prana* is the energy permeating the universe at all levels. It is physical, mental, intellectual, sexual, spiritual, and cosmic energy. It is the prime mover of all activity. It is energy which creates, protects, and destroys. Vigor, power, vitality, life are all forms of *Prana*.

When the energy in these subtle channels of the body flows smoothly, one feels healthy and happy.

In Hatha Yoga, much emphasis is placed on stretching the spine, the central pathway through which our Life Energy flows, and along which lie the body's major energy centers, known as the seven *chakras. (*See Fig. 9 on page 31.) (Minor chakras are located in the wrists, elbows, ankles, and knees.) These chakras are subtle energy centers that are said to regulate the flow of *Prana* through the body.

By balancing these centers and channels, you will be enhancing the flow of Life Energy and promoting your health and well-being.

Many scientific studies have documented the effectiveness of Yoga postures for reducing stress and anxiety and lowering high blood pressure. Other studies have shown improved memory, relief from pain, and help with respiratory problems, thyroid disorders, menstrual difficulties, allergies, and more. Yoga has also been proven helpful in recovery from addictions.

In this book, we will recommend some poses known to benefit particular health conditions. If you want to learn more, we strongly suggest that you take a class with a qualified Yoga teacher or Yoga therapist, who can observe your practice and suggest an individualized program for you.

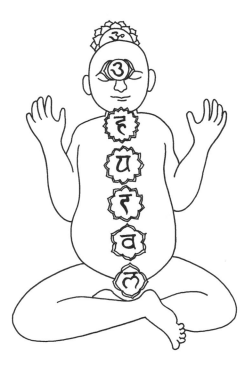

Fig. 9—The 7 Chakras

Now you are just about ready to start putting this knowledge to work. Here's the plan for the rest of the book.

Part Two consists of four chapters:

- Chapter 5 contains illustrations of the Acupressure meridians and key points, as well as the reflex zones of the hands and feet. Use these for reference.

- Chapters 6, 7, and 8 explain the techniques for applying pressure.

- Throughout Part Three you will be directed to specific points and zones to press, to facilitate healing of various ailments and to enhance your energy and immunity.

part two

WHAT YOU NEED TO KNOW

Illustrations

This chapter contains the following illustrations:

- Acupressure points on the head and body
- Reflex zones on the hands and feet
- The meridian system

We hope that you will look these illustrations over now, just for orientation, and that you will return to them when you're working on a particular health concern in Part Three of the book, to help you determine how and where to press.

The final section of this chapter contains 10 key Acupressure points that we refer to frequently in the book.

Note that the drawings in this chapter from pages 36–48 have letters (A to R). Illustrations throughout the rest of the book are numbered.

ACUPRESSURE

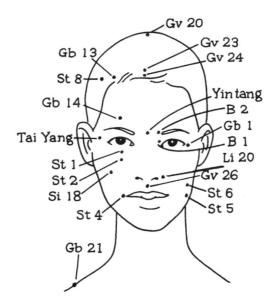

Fig. A—Head, Front View

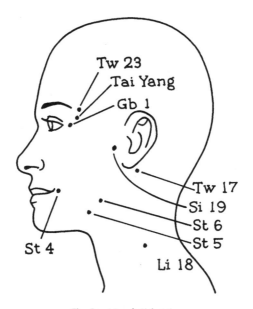

Fig. B—Head, Side View

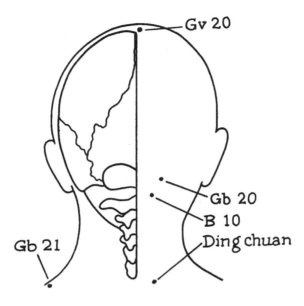

Fig. C—Head and Shoulders, Back View

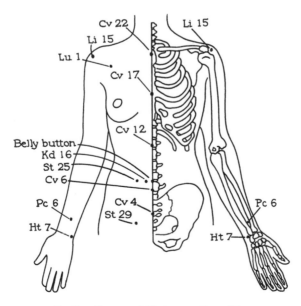

Fig. D—Chest and Abdomen, Front View

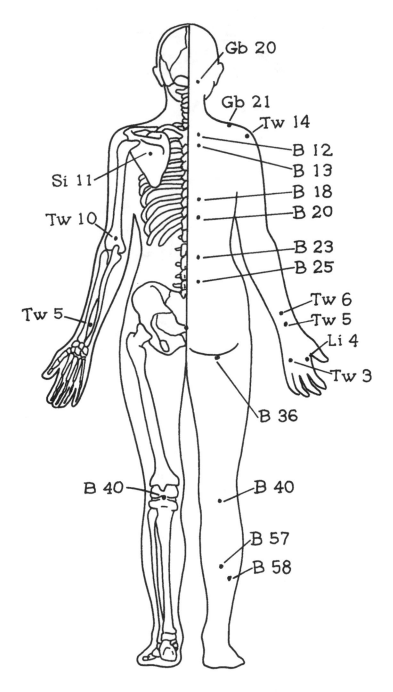

Fig. E—Full Body, Back View

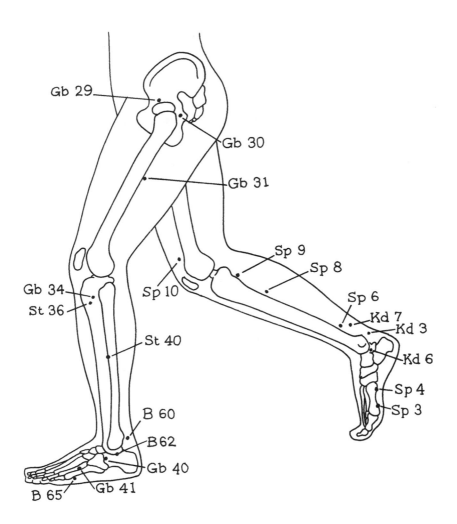

Fig. F—Lower Body, Side View

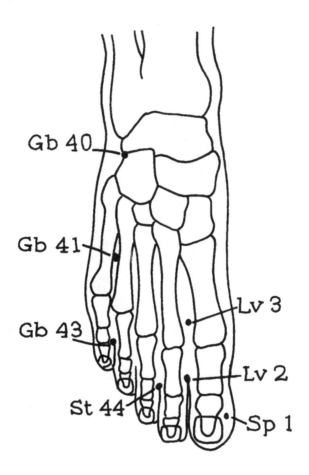

Fig. G—Foot, Top View

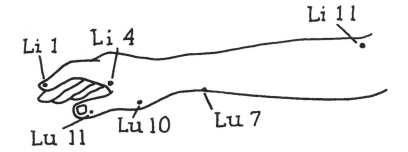

Fig. H—Arm

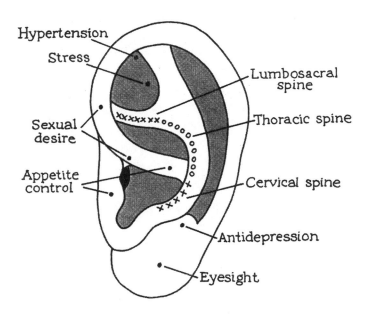

Fig. I—Ear Points

SHIATSU

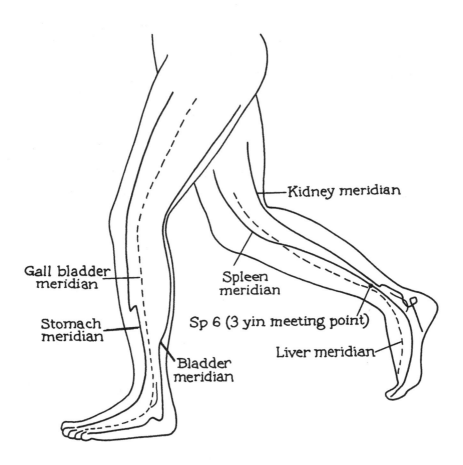

Fig. J—Legs Striding (waist to feet) Showing Meridians

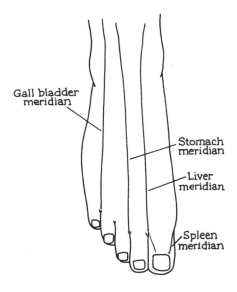

Fig. K—Top of Foot Showing Meridians

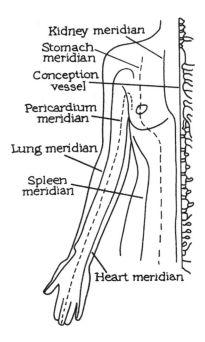

Fig. L—Chest and Arm Showing Meridians

REFLEXOLOGY

Foot Reflexology Key

1. Brain	19. Gallbladder
2. Ears/Eyes/Sinuses	20. Adrenals
3. Neck/Helper to Eyes and Ears	21. Spleen
4. Temple	22. Kidney
5. Pineal/Hypothalamus	23. Pancreas
6. Pituitary	24. Duodenum
7. Spine (Cervical)	25. Spine (Lumbar)
8. Side of Neck	26. Ureter Tube
9. Shoulder/Arm	27. Small Intestine
10. Thyroid	28. Appendix and Ileocecal Valve
11. Thyroid/Bronchial Helper	29. Ascending Colon
12. Chest/Lung	30. Transverse Colon
13. Heart	31. Descending Colon
14. Spine (Thoracic)	32. Sigmoid Colon
15. Solar Plexus	33. Bladder
16. Diaphragm	34. Sciatic Nerve
17. Liver	35. Sacral Spine and Coccyx
18. Stomach	

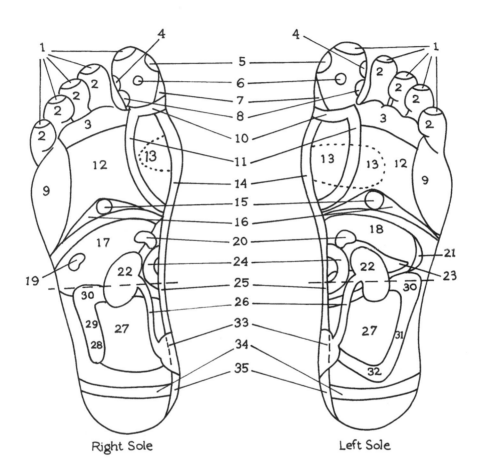

Right Sole   Left Sole

Fig. M—Feet, Bottoms of Right and Left

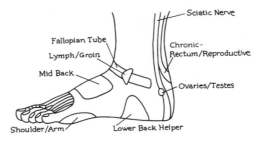

Fig. N—Foot, Outside View

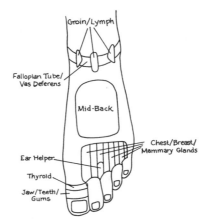

Fig. O—Foot, Top View

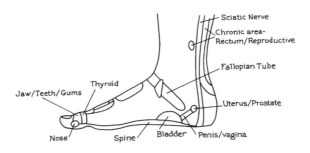

Fig. P—Foot, Inside View

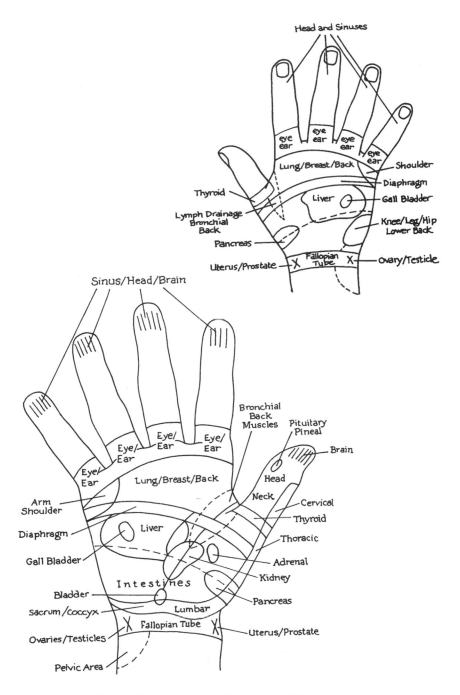

Fig. Q—Right Hand, Large Palm Up, Small Palm Down

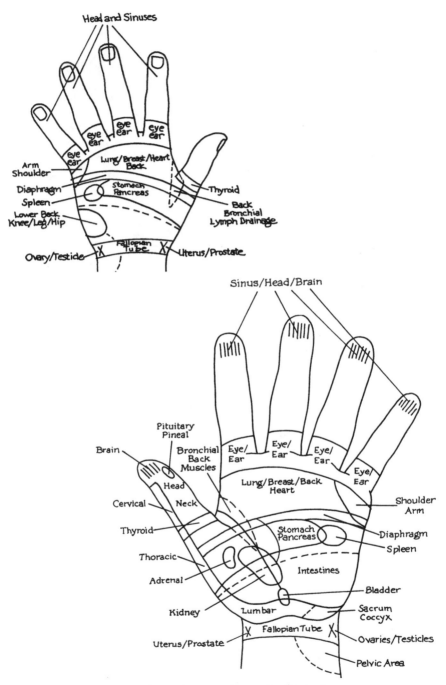

Fig. R—Left Hand, Large Palm Up, Small Palm Down

TEN MASTER PRESSURE POINTS

The following ten points are among the most helpful and most frequently prescribed in Acupuncture and Acupressure. We recommend them many times throughout the book. Whenever we suggest using one of these points, we will refer you to this section for a description and illustration of its location and how to press it.

10 Master Pressure Points

1. (Li 4, Adjoining Valley) Hold your left hand palm down, fingers out straight, and squeeze your thumb against the other fingers. This important point is located in the middle of the fleshy mound that pops up between the thumb and index finger. Release the pressure and, with your left hand still facing down, use your right hand (thumb on top, index finger underneath) to take hold of the webbing between your left thumb and index finger. Squeeze in the center of the webbing, pressing toward the bone of the index finger. Hold one minute, and repeat with the other hand.

One of the most important points in Acupuncture and Acupressure, Li 4 relieves headaches and other pain, relaxes muscular tension, and helps to balance the flow of energy between the upper and lower parts of the body. It is also used to clear excess heat and to promote healthy functioning of the bowels. **Caution:** Pregnant women should not press on this point.

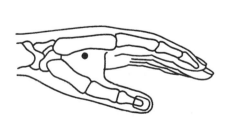

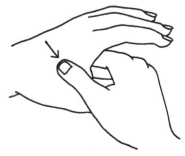

Fig. 10a—Li 4, Anatomical   Fig. 10b—Li 4, Hand position

2. (Li 11, Pool at the Crook) The name of this point refers to its location in the elbow crease. Hold your arm in front of your chest, as if holding a cup in your hand. The point is at the outside end of the crease on your arm at the elbow joint. Another way to find it is to note the length of your thumb from the tip to the first joint, then move this distance up from the outside tip of the elbow bone toward the crease lines at the elbow joint. Hold your left hand close to your chest and use firm pressure with your right thumb; press for about a minute, then switch arms. This point is used to clear excess heat and damp from the body and to relieve pain in the arm, elbow, and shoulder. It also helps regulate intestinal activity.

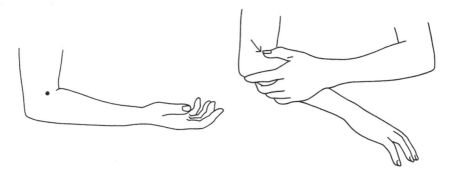

Fig. 11a—Li 11, Anatomical   Fig. 11b—Li 11, Hand position

3. (Sp 6, Three Yin Meeting) This point is located on the inside portion of your leg, above the ankle bone. From the center of the ankle bone, slide up four finger widths. The point is just off the bone, toward the back of the leg. When you find it, press with your thumb or knuckle. Increase pressure until you are pressing quite firmly, hold about a minute, and gradually release.

Located at the crossing point of the three yin meridians of the leg, this is one of the most important Acupressure points. It can nourish the overall yin of the body by simultaneously strengthening the yin of the Spleen, Liver, and Kidney meridians. It also helps move the Liver *ch'i* throughout the body and is considered a master point for healing and regulating the female organs, hence its usefulness in regulating menstruation, relieving cramps, easing menopause, etc. Sp 6 is often used in combination with St 36; the two together tonify both *ch'i* and blood and bring vitality. **Caution:** Pregnant women should not press on this point.

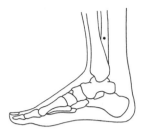

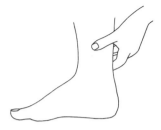

Fig. 12a—Sp 6, Anatomical   Fig. 12b—Sp 6, Hand position

4. (St 36, Three Mile Foot) This point is located four finger widths below the lower border of the kneecap and one finger width off the shin bone to the outside. You've found the point correctly if you feel the muscle move under your fingers when you flex your foot up and down. Using moderate to firm pressure, hold for about one minute. This point, as well as Sp 6 (above), can be stimulated either with the heel of your opposite foot, or with your fingers.

St 36 is the most powerful point for revitalizing the *ch'i* and blood of the entire body.

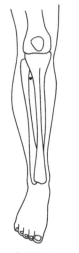

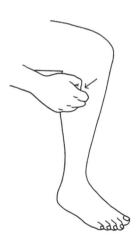

Fig. 13a—St 36, Anatomical   Fig. 13b—St 36, Hand position

5. (Lv 3, Bigger Rushing) This point is on the top of your foot, between the big toe and second toe. Start at the web margin of skin between the two toes, and slide your index finger up between the bones until you feel a depression about ½ inch up. Still using your index finger, press between

the bones (in the direction of the root of the second toe). Start with light pressure, as this point can be sensitive, and increase as much as you can until you are using moderate to firm pressure. Press for about 1 minute.

Press both feet simultaneously if you can reach them comfortably. If you have trouble bending down and/or reaching your feet, try rubbing the area on your left foot with your right heel, and vice versa. Lv 3 prevents *ch'i* stagnation in the body and is the most important point for combating stress.

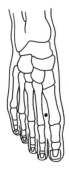   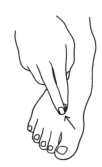

Fig. 14a—Lv 3, Anatomical   Fig. 14b—Lv 3, Hand Position

6. (Kd 3, Supreme Stream) On the inside of the ankle (big toe side), Kd 3 is located halfway between the ankle bone and the Achilles tendon on the back edge of the ankle. Place your thumb on the prominence of the ankle bone, and let it slide down toward the Achilles tendon. Kd 3 is in the depression, approximately half way between the bone and the back of the ankle. Press with your thumb using medium to firm pressure, for about a minute.

The importance of the Kidney energy in Chinese medicine cannot be overstated. It is said to be the root of the *yin* and *yang* of the entire body. Kd 3 is considered to be the "source point" for the Kidney meridian, and thus exerts a powerful tonifying effect on the meridian and the entire body.

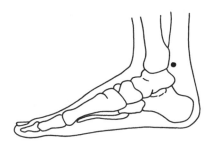   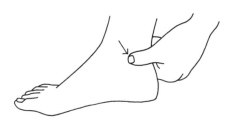

Fig. 15a—Kd 3, Anatomical   Fig. 15b—Kd 3, Hand Position

7. (B 23, Associated Point of Kidney) This point is located approximately 1-½ inches on either side of the spine, just above the level of your belly button and below the center of the back. Even if you have long and flexible arms, the best way you can stimulate these points on your own is to lie on your back on the floor with a tennis ball behind you. Slowly roll up and down on the ball, first on one side then on the other. Or you can put two balls in a sock and do both sides at the same time. There are other valuable points right next to the spine on both sides that you will stimulate with this technique.

Spend several minutes pressing the points on each side. This point in combination with Kd 3 (on page 52) strongly tonifies the Kidney *ch'i*.

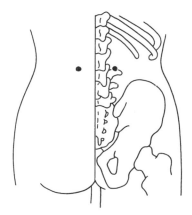

Fig. 16—B 23, Anatomical

8. (Gb 20, Wind Pool) Place your thumbs on your earlobes. Now slide them back toward the center of your neck. You should be approximately one thumb width above the hairline of the neck. Your thumbs will fall into a depression on either side of the vertebra of your neck, at the base of the skull. The depressions may be more evident if you slowly bend your head forward and then back again. Gb 20 is located in these depressions. It is easiest to use the thumbs to apply Acupressure on these points. Use medium to firm pressure, and hold for a minute or even more, remembering to breathe deeply and to build up and release pressure gradually. This point is helpful in relieving headaches and colds, neck stiffness and pain, and helps to regulate the internal movement of energy.

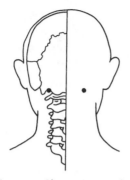
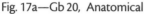
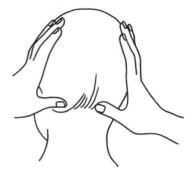

Fig. 17a—Gb 20, Anatomical   Fig. 17b—Gb 20, Hand Position

9. (Sp 10, Sea of Blood) About 2 thumb widths above the top edge of the knee you will feel a bulge in your thigh muscles. It's on the top of your leg, toward the inside. Press firmly for a minute with your thumb or the knuckle of your middle finger. This point helps to prevent stagnation in the blood, especially in the lower abdominal region. It is also healing and nourishing for the skin.

10. (St 40, Abundant Splendor) You will find this point half way between the ankle bone on the outside of the foot and the center of the kneecap. At the half way point, find the shin bone (tibia) and then go 2 thumb widths off the bone to the outside. Press firmly. You may find it easier to use your thumb (with fingers around your leg) or your middle finger. Do what is most comfortable. This point is very useful for reducing mucus and congestion.

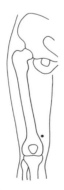
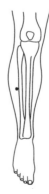

Fig. 18—Sp 10, Anatomical   Fig. 19—St 40, Anatomical

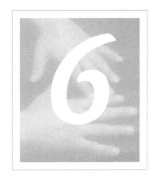

Getting Started—
Acupressure and Shiatsu

As we have explained, Acupressure and Shiatsu both use the same meridians and pressure points. Both come from the same theoretical background. There are some differences in the techniques used by skilled practitioners, such as how long or how hard to press on a point, and these will be reflected in the self-treatment suggestions we offer in Part Three. If you are interested in looking more deeply into these systems, see the Bibliography at the end of the book, take some classes, or see a professional practitioner.

PREPARING FOR YOUR PRESSURE POINT SESSION

The following suggestions are for an ideal session, at home, where it is peaceful and you can settle in for an extended period of time. However, once you've understood the basic techniques and learned the location of points helpful to you, whether for headaches, asthma, arthritis pain, menstrual cramps, or whatever problem you may have, you can press these points almost anywhere you happen to be, at your desk at work, on a plane or train, at the movies.

It is easiest to locate the points on the bare skin, so you can see and feel exactly where they are, and we recommend that you do so the first time you use any of them. Once you know where to press, some light clothing is no obstacle.

For an ideal session, the first step is simply to set aside a time and place where you can be warm, comfortable, and uninterrupted. You may choose to unwind with a warm bath and some soothing music beforehand. Also, it's best not to do finger pressure work on a full stomach. A light snack is okay, but if you have eaten a full meal, wait at least an hour before beginning. (You will be more sensitive as to where to press, and more alert if your energy isn't all tied up with digesting.)

For comfort, get rid of tight clothing, belts, jewelry, and shoes; change into some loose, natural fiber clothing. Wearing shorts and a tee shirt will make most of the points you'll be using easily accessible directly on the skin. Unplug your phone or turn the volume off on your answering machine so you won't be tempted to jump up and take "just this one call." This is a time for *you*, set aside for your inner harmony and health.

You might want to play some mellow background music, or a tape or CD of soothing natural sounds such as flowing water, leaves rustling in the wind, or the songs of birds. Or you may prefer silence. Experiment and choose what helps you relax most easily.

Soft lighting, and perhaps some mild incense or aromatherapy oil if you like a fragrance in the air, may also help you settle into your pressure point session. Sandalwood fragrance would be a good choice, as it helps elicit a calm or meditative mood.

A mat on the floor, or a blanket folded in half will provide a good place for you to sit. Or you may sit on a chair or bench. Sit cross-legged if you are comfortable that way. And, for now, let go of your worries and plans.

START WITH RELAXATION—QUICK WARM-UP

The best way to begin is to relax your body and mind. This can be done in just a few minutes using the Quick Warm-Up on the opposite page.

BREATHE DEEPLY FOR EXTRA RELAXATION

Once your body begins to relax, you can continue by quieting your mind with an easy breathing exercise. There is an old Yoga saying that "the mind rides on the breath." When your breathing slows down and becomes calmer and deeper, your mind will follow and also settle down.

You may even have noticed that as you began to relax your body, your breathing also naturally began to change. Now sit comfortably or lie on your back, and continue to notice your breathing. Keep your breaths full and deep. But don't strain. Breathing involves taking in not only oxygen, but also, on a

QUICK WARM-UP

Most people carry stress and strain in their faces, necks, and shoulders. This is partly due to a high level of mental activity, sedentary jobs, and sitting in front of computers for long periods of time. So start your warm-up by massaging your head, neck, and shoulders, using both hands to lightly rub your head and neck; a little more firmly, rub and knead your shoulders. Use slow strokes now and throughout this mini massage.

Then, use your right hand to rub and massage your left hand (starting with the fingers) and move up your left arm to the shoulder. Use your left hand to massage your right hand and arm. Move to your abdomen and again lightly rub, moving up to the chest around the heart. Reach around behind your waist, and rub up the sides of your body, again toward the heart. You can rub a little vigorously over the solid ribs. Women, be sure to rub only lightly on your breasts.

Then begin at your feet. Take one foot in both hands and rub it. Massage the bottom of your foot for a few seconds. Make circles with your palm against the sole. Move up to the ankle, then up the leg to the thigh and continue up toward the heart. Repeat with your other foot and leg. Spend three to five minutes on this relaxing self-massage. And remember, this is not intended to be invigorating; don't rub vigorously or quickly, but gently and slowly.

more subtle level, *Prana* or *Ch'i*. With long and deep breaths the cells of your body get lots of oxygen, which helps release pain and tension. Deep breathing also encourages the flow of blood and the circulation of energy.

Proper breathing can contribute a lot of power to your pressure point work. A little later, when we discuss visualization, you will learn how to consciously direct your breath to facilitate the flow of *Ch'i*.

Here is a simple exercise to make your breathing calm and regular:

1. Sit comfortably or lie down on your back. You may wish to close your eyes for deeper relaxation.

2. Place your hands on your abdomen below your navel.

3. Breathe in deeply to the count of 4. Be aware of your abdomen rising or expanding. (You will feel your hand moving.) Your breath should feel as though it is first filling your abdomen, then your diaphragm, then finally your lungs. Most people do shallow chest-breaths rather than this full, diaphragmatic breathing. Deep breathing, however, oxygenates the lower lobes of the lungs and brings far more vitality than shallow breathing.

4. Now, retain this deep breath (if you can comfortably do so) for a count of 4.

5. Slowly release your breath, starting with a count of 4 and eventually (over some weeks) working up to a count of 8. Observe your abdomen fall or contract as you release the breath.

6. Repeat steps 3–5 four times at first, building up to eight over a few weeks.

FOUR BASIC PRESSURE POINT TECHNIQUES

FIRM PRESSURE: Use your thumbs, fingers, palms, the side of your hand, or your knuckles to apply steady pressure directly on a point. Most commonly, you will use either the outside edge of your thumb, or your middle finger. In some places, such as on the strong, ropy muscles on the back of your neck, you may have more success pressing with your index, middle, and ring fingers all together.

For relaxation or pain relief, apply pressure steadily for 1 to 3 minutes. *Always* start with light pressure for 5 to 10 seconds and gradually build up, and always end gradually, taking another 10 to 15 seconds to completely release.

For a stimulating, energizing effect, and to relieve muscle spasms, press several times for about 3 to 7 seconds each. This pressure should also start on the lighter side. Increase; hold at its peak, then gradually release.

Variation: Once you have established firm pressure on a point, you can slowly rotate your thumb or finger on the point with a small circular movement.

Note: Be sure to keep your fingernails clipped short so you don't injure the skin when you press.

RUBBING: Using your thumb, finger, or palm, lightly and briskly rub the skin to create warmth and increase circulation. This helps relieve chills and numbness, nourishes the nerves, and tonifies the skin.

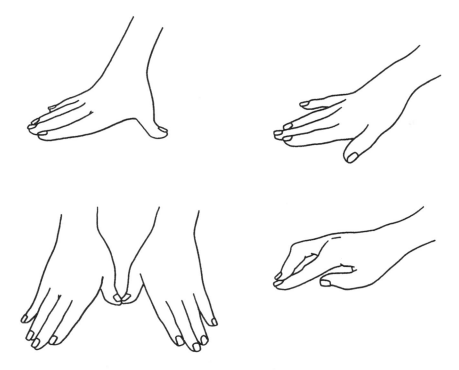

Fig. 20—Four Ways to Apply Pressure

Variation: Place your palm on a large area of the body, such as the abdomen or the lower back over the kidneys. Press lightly on the skin and vibrate back and forth for 15 to 30 seconds. These vibrations penetrate to the internal organs and create a pleasant, healing sensation. Another variation is to place your palm flat on the skin and rotate it in a circular motion, *without* moving the hand over the surface of skin.

KNEADING: This is a massage-like technique in which you use the thumb and fingers, along with the heel of your hand, to squeeze large muscled areas such as the shoulders, calves, and thighs. This technique is helpful for relieving stiffness and tension.

TAPPING: Quick, light tapping stimulates *Ch'i* and improves functioning of the nerves. Tap lightly with your fingertips on sensitive areas such as the face; use a loose fist or the palm of your hand on larger, tougher areas such as the legs, arms, back, and chest. Remember: tap *lightly.*

HOW TO APPLY PRESSURE

Various techniques, rhythms, and amounts of pressure will be suggested at different times, but the basic guideline is to apply firm, strong pressure. The place or places you press will often be tender and may hurt somewhat under the pressure of your fingers. That is okay, but don't press to the point of real pain; this is a healing process, not self-torture! Ordinarily, use some strength, and press firmly unless we mention using lighter or medium pressure. But tune in and listen to yourself: if the pressure starts to become uncomfortable, lighten up.

Here is the general procedure for using the pressure point techniques described on pages 58 and 59:

1. Carefully locate your points. This is obviously crucial! Consult the appropriate diagram and take some time to find the points on your body. They will usually feel more tender and sensitive than the surrounding area. Be patient, as the points may sometimes be a bit hard to find. They are not always in the *exact* same position on everyone, so persevere and explore the area within about an inch of where the point is shown on the illustration.

2. Use your thumb, index, or middle finger to apply pressure. Begin gently, and gradually deepen the pressure. Your thumb is stronger, but not as sensitive as your fingers. Of your fingers, the middle one is the strongest, and in most cases is best suited to apply self-Acupressure. With practice your fingers will become more and more sensitive to the exact location to press, and to the energy, which you may begin to feel.

3. When you have located the spot and decided how you are going to press (using thumb or fingers) position your fingers right on the spot and press at a 90 degree angle from the surface of the skin, so that you are pressing straight down on the pressure point, not at an angle.

4. Begin gently, increase pressure over 5–15 seconds, then hold firmly for about 30 seconds. Sometimes, depending on the location and the desired effect, we will recommend using a series of short, firm pressures of 3 to 7 seconds; other times, a longer time period—up to 2 or 3 minutes—may be suggested. Be sure to read the instructions carefully each time.

Use light pressure where there is acute pain or swelling, if you are weak or tired, or if there are complications such as high blood pressure.

Never use force or an abrupt motion. Apply pressure gradually and stop if pain becomes intense. Too much pressure is counter-productive.

5. When you are ready to release the pressure, gradually reduce the finger pressure (take another 5–15 seconds) and conclude with about 15 seconds of light touch. This gradual application and release gives your body time to respond to the healing.

6. The more conscious attention you give to your finger pressure, the more effective your treatment will be. According to Michael Reed Gach, director of the Acupressure Institute of America, "Consciously and gradually direct the pressure into the center of the part of the body you are working on. . . . The better your concentration as you move your fingers slowly into and out of the point, the more effective the treatment will be."

In some cases, you will be asked to repeat the press/release procedure several times for maximum effect.

7. When possible, press on the corresponding, symmetrical points on both sides of the body simultaneously. If you can't manage to press both at the same time because of their location, be sure to work on them sequentially. *It's important to work on the points on both sides of the body in order to keep the balance of energy.*

The obvious exceptions to this rule are points along the Governor Vessel and the Conception Vessel, the two main meridians that are not bilateral (that is, there is only one, not a matching pair).

8. Work *gently* rather than firmly on sensitive parts of the body such as your face and abdomen, and where there is very little flesh between skin and bone, such as the top of your head.

9. Keep your pressure at a maximum of 15 lbs. (You can teach yourself what 15 lbs. feels like by pressing on a bathroom scale with your thumb or fingers.)

10. If your hand starts to feel tired, take a break. Finish working on the point you are pressing by gradually releasing, then gently shake your hands a few times and breathe a couple of deep, relaxing breaths.

11. When you've completed your treatment, take time to rest and allow your body to integrate the experience. Give yourself 5 to 10 minutes to do absolutely nothing. Close your eyes and lie flat on your back in the Yoga rest posture known as *savasana*, feet slightly apart, arms a few inches from the sides of your body. Be aware of your body, and of the energy flowing through you. You may feel some warmth, or some tingling. Just be there and enjoy it. Then, get up slowly and resume your activities of the day.

KEEP IN MIND . . .

Follow your common sense and see your health care practitioner when necessary. Pressure point therapy should not be considered a substitute for medical supervision or treatment.

Never press in an abrupt or overly forceful way. The most pressure to use is 15 lbs. Again, practice on a bathroom scale to see how much force to exert to register 15 lbs.

Do not practice finger pressure therapy on a wounded or inflamed area. Never practice on unhealed fractures, burns, or scars, or on varicose veins or areas that are hot, red, or swollen. Also avoid pressure directly on lymph glands.

It is best not to do finger pressure therapy right before eating or on a full stomach, unless you are pressing one or two points to relieve indigestion or hiccups or you are trying to stimulate your digestion.

It is usually not wise to practice when you have a fever, unless you are pressing points to relieve it.

If you have brittle bones, such as from osteoporosis, it may be better not to use pressure point therapy at all. Consult your doctor or a qualified practitioner for advice.

Persons with high blood pressure, heart problems, cancer, or other serious or life-threatening conditions should be sure to contact their physician for guidance before using pressure point therapy.

If you are pregnant, there are several points you should not press. This will be mentioned whenever the points are recommended. In particular, keep in mind not to use LI 4, in the webbing of your hand between thumb and index finger. We will frequently recommend this point for relief of pain, headaches, constipation, depression, and other ailments. It is a wonderful, healing point, but it can stimulate premature contractions in the uterus, so be wise and don't use it. Also avoid GB 21, Sp 6, B 60, and any points on the abdominal area. Finger pressure on *any* point during pregnancy should be moderate, not firm.

After each pressure point therapy session, take some time to rest. Keep warm. Your body will be more sensitive and vulnerable for a while. The vital energies have been mobilized inwardly for the healing process.

Getting Started—
Reflexology

Reflexology uses thumbs and fingers to gently knead, rub, stroke, and firmly press specific "reflex areas" of the feet. Our feet are very responsive to treatment. And it's not just the soles of the feet that are sensitive; important points are located on the top of the foot, on the ankles, and on the sides of the feet as well.

In Chapter 5, you will find diagrams of the feet, showing where the reflex areas are located. Use these to get oriented and to get "the big picture." Then, when you use the main part of the book to look up your area of concern—for example, headaches—you will find another, simplified drawing showing exactly what zones to work on.

Just as with the Acupressure points, reflex areas can vary according to individuals and may not be *exactly* at the spot illustrated in the diagram. But explore your foot in the locality indicated on the foot "map" and you will find the right place to rub.

In order to practice foot Reflexology on yourself, you have to be limber enough to sit loosely cross-legged, or to lift one foot onto the opposite knee. You may sit on the floor, on a chair, or on the bed with cushions behind you for support.

If you are unable to sit like this, you have an alternative: reflex zones in the hand. These can be used effectively, though most Reflexologists feel that working the feet is usually more effective. The techniques are essentially the same. Please refer to the detailed illustrations of hands and feet in Chapter 5.

Begin your Reflexology self-treatment by bathing your feet. Dry them completely and, if you wish, apply a *small* amount of oil or light, absorbent lotion. Then, sitting comfortably in a quiet place, simply massage your feet with gentle, relaxing strokes for a minute or two—longer if you can spare the time—to prepare them for deeper work. Use the palms of your hands, and be sure to rub not only the bottom but also the sides and tops of your feet, and around the heels and ankles.

RELAXATION TECHNIQUES

Next spend a couple of minutes with these stretching and relaxing moves:

1. *Lung Press* (also called "Metatarsal Kneading")—With your left foot on your right knee, wrap your left hand around the foot just below the base of the toes. Make your right hand into a fist, and press the fingers of the fist (not the knuckles) into the fleshy part of the foot directly opposite the supporting hand. (This is the area of the foot that corresponds to the chest and lungs.)

Work both hands in a rotating, kneading motion. Relax some of the pressure of your fist, at the same time squeezing with the supporting hand on the top of the foot. Alternate between pressure and squeezing, but keep both hands in contact with your foot. Repeat several times with each foot.

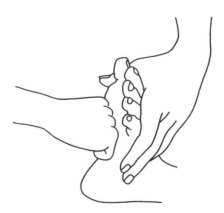

Fig. 21—Lung Press

2. *Ankle Rotation*—Place your hand over the top of your foot (at the ankle) so that the webbing between the thumb and fingers is over the ankle, where the foot joins the leg. Grasp the foot with the other hand and rotate in both directions. Don't forget to repeat with the other foot.

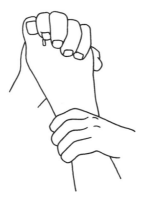

Fig. 22—Ankle Rotation

3. *Toe Rotations*—In this exercise you will stretch and rotate each toe, one at a time. With your left foot balanced on your right knee, use the thumb and index finger of your left hand to hold your foot just below the big toe. With thumb and index finger of your *right* hand, grasp the big toe right down near the base. Then with a slight lifting or pulling motion, gently stretch the toe and rotate it first in one direction several times, then in the opposite direction several times. Repeat with each toe (moving over to hold just below the toe each time) on your left foot, then switch to the right foot.

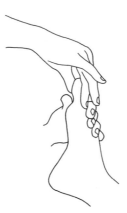

Fig. 23—Toe Rotation

4. *Thumb Press on Solar Plexus Point*—Before you can do this relaxation exercise, you'll have to locate the solar plexus point on your foot. Place one hand over the top of your foot behind the toes, and squeeze gently. You will see a hollow space appear at the center of the sole of your foot. This is the solar plexus point. Release the squeeze, allowing your foot to come back to its natural shape, but remember the location of the hollow point. Then, press your thumb into this point for a few seconds, and release. Repeat, breathing in while you press; hold the breath a few seconds; exhale, slowly releasing the pressure. Rotate the thumb a few times gently on the solar plexus point. Repeat 4 or 5 times, then do the same on your other foot. This is an excellent relaxation exercise that you can do again at the end of your session.

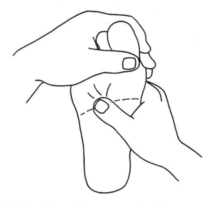

Fig. 24—Thumb Press on Solar Plexus Point

THE BASIC REFLEXOLOGY TECHNIQUES

By the time you have finished the relaxation techniques, the lotion should be gone from your feet. If they are at all slippery, you won't be able to apply pressure properly, so use a little powder and/or wipe with a towel to remove the excess.

Here are the basic techniques you will use:

HOLDING THE FOOT: Although the foot you are working on will be resting on your opposite knee most of the time and will have natural support, you will have better results if you also hold the foot for extra support. When you want to work on your left foot, place it on your right knee. Grasp the top of the left foot with the palm of your left hand. This will enable you to apply pressure to the bottom of the left foot with your right hand. Reverse positions when you work on your right foot.

THUMB WALK: This is the technique you will use most often. You will use your thumb to apply constant steady pressure as you move it forward over the surface of the foot.

Place your hand palm down on a table. Notice the angle of the thumb—about 45°—where it meets the surface. This inside edge will be the working area of your thumb for the thumb walk.

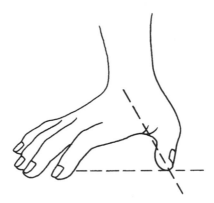

Fig. 25—Position for the Thumb Walk

For your first practice of the thumb walk you may wish to simply move along the table.

Walking the thumb forward involves the following steps:

1. Place your right thumb on the fleshy part of the palm of your left hand or your left foot, with the four other fingers on the back of the left hand or foot for support and leverage.

2. Slightly bend the first joint of the thumb, then straighten it a little so that it moves forward a tiny bit. You will notice that before the forward move, the flesh of the skin is slightly pulled back. This is correct. But the thumb itself never moves backwards; it applies pressure at a point, then moves forward.

3. Repeat Step #2. Maintain constant pressure as the thumb moves forward. Try not to produce an "on and off" feeling. This takes practice!

4. Apply leverage with the other four fingers, which should be directly behind the moving thumb. You will be able to apply more pressure, with less fatigue. Be sure to move the supporting fingers forward to keep pace with your thumb. Don't let them lag too far behind or your hands will get tired.

5. Take very small "bites," moving about ¹⁄₁₆" to ¹⁄₈" with each move forward. (That means 8 to 16 moves per inch!) Beginners almost always move the thumb too far in each bite, so practice making smaller and smaller moves. As Reflexologist Laura Norman says, "You really cannot take steps that are too small."

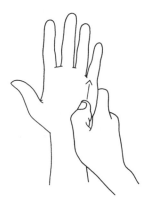

Fig. 26—Using the Thumb Walk

FINGER WALK: This is similar to the thumb walk, except that you will use the inside edge of your index finger instead of your thumb to take "bites" as you move forward. If you can, place your thumb on the other side of the foot you are working on, for leverage. The object is to exert a constant, steady pressure as you move the finger forward in *very small* increments. Again, try to avoid an on-and-off type of pressure. You will master this with practice.

THE "HOOK AND BACK UP" TECHNIQUE: You will use this technique occasionally, to get pin-point accuracy on a single reflex point. (The "walking" techniques apply pressure to many points, over larger reflex areas.) Locate the point you wish to treat. Place your thumb on it, and apply gentle pressure. Then, bend the first joint of the thumb and *slightly* back up, while maintaining steady pressure on the point. Don't slide across the skin or lose contact with the point. Hold for a few seconds, then release.

ROTATION ON A POINT: This is a valuable technique for working on a particularly tender or painful spot. When you come across a very tender area, place your thumb on it with gentle pressure, with the other fingers wrapped around the back of the foot. Then, with your other hand (the holding or supporting hand), grasp your foot and flex it slowly into the thumb. In other words, hold the thumb steady and move the foot. The movement can be in a circular rotation, or it can be a back-and-forth movement. Then shift the pressure thumb from place to place in the area of the painful reflex point and use the same technique—moving the foot—to work on the point.

REFLEXOLOGY WARM-UP

Practice this sequence, which we recommend using every time you treat yourself to a Reflexology session:

- Bathe your feet and dry them. Then, sitting comfortably, massage them with gentle, relaxing strokes for a minute or two. If you wish, you may apply a *small* amount of oil or light, absorbent lotion for the massage.
- Follow with the relaxation techniques described on pages 64–66, including the Lung Press, Ankle Rotation, and Toe Rotation.
- Finish with the Thumb Press on the solar plexus point for 15 to 30 seconds.
- With your supporting hand grasping the toes, thumb walk up each of the 5 zones of one foot starting at the heel in zone 5 (below your little toe), then up the five zones of your other foot. Go all the way from the heel to the tip of the toes. At the heel line, gently bend your toes back with the thumb of your supporting hand. This will expose the tendon in the arch of your foot. Avoid pressing directly on that tendon. (See Fig. 27, on page 70.)
- Wipe off any remaining lotion. You are now ready to begin working on specific reflex areas.

HOW TO USE REFLEXOLOGY FOR PREVENTION AND HEALING

We recommend that you begin each of your Reflexology sessions with the warm-up in the box above. But even if you have no specific complaints or problems to treat, sit down several times a week and give yourself the general treatment outlined below, going over your entire foot. By stimulating the reflex zones of the whole foot, you will be promoting better circulation, removing toxins, relaxing and relieving stress, and enlivening your nervous system, influencing your glands and organs. This is an excellent form of preventive medicine.

1. Spend 3 or 4 minutes on the warm-up and relaxation sequence described in the box on page 69. Do this sequence on each foot. Then, for the rest of the sequence, do one foot completely and then the other.
2. Thumb walk the entire foot, zones 5 through 1, from the heel to the tip of the toes.

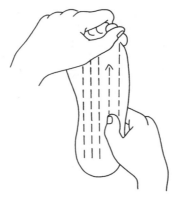

Fig. 27—Thumb Walking the Entire Foot

3. Thumb walk from the diaphragm line (see diagram in Chapter 5) to the base of the toes, zones 5 to 1, both feet. Also work down the top of the foot (finger walk) in this same area.

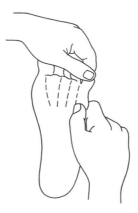

Fig. 28—Up from the Diaphragm Line

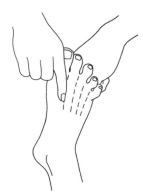

Fig. 29—Finger Walking the Top of the Foot

4. Thumb and finger walk the neck area of the foot, at the base of the toes. Be sure to use your holding hand to pull down on the pad of the foot.

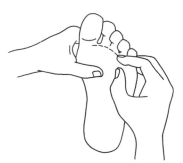

Fig. 30—Walking the Ridge

5. Thumb walk up the bottom of all toes, and finger walk down the front (top) of the toes.

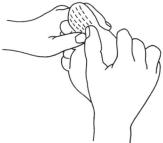

Fig. 31—Thumb Walking Up the Toes

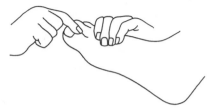

Fig. 32—Finger Walking Down the Toes

6. Work the soft tissue area in the center of the foot, between the diaphragm line and the heel. Thumb walk up, down, and across if you can. This area contains all the body's vital organs and is a key area. Use steady pressure but don't press too hard.

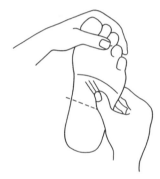

Fig. 33—Working the Vital Organs

7. Thumb walk up and down the spine area, on the inside of the foot, stretching from the base of the heel to the nail of the big toe. Thumb walk across the spine also.

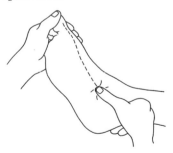

Fig. 34—Thumb Walking the Spine

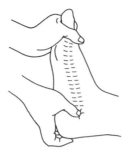

Fig. 35—Thumb Walking Across the Spine

8. Thumb or finger walk up or down the inside of the leg behind the ankle bone, and outside the leg behind the ankle bone (along the Achilles tendon). Positioning for these will be a little difficult, especially the outside of the leg, but do your best. You might be more successful working this area with your fingers rather than your thumbs. You can reach around with your fingers and walk them together, especially your third and ring fingers.

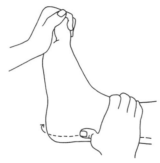

Fig. 36—Walking along the Achilles Tendon

9. Important reflexes near the ankle bone affect the uterus or prostate (on the inside or big toe side of the foot) and the ovaries or testes (on the outside). To locate them, draw an imaginary line between the high point on the ankle bone, and the back/bottom of the heel. The reflex point is halfway in between. To work these points, press with your index or middle finger. Use your thumb if you can't get enough leverage with your fingers, but as these points are very specific and usually quite sensitive, a finger is better. Regarding the uterus/prostate reflex, Dwight Byers points out that "many ankles have a small indentation in this reflex area so look for it as a guidelines?"

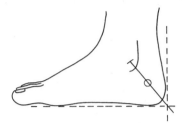

Fig. 37—The Uterus/Prostate Reflex

10. Finish with a few minutes of relaxation exercises, such as the Lung Press (Fig. 21) or the Thumb Press on the Solar Plexus Point. (Fig. 24)

This entire procedure can be done in 10–15 minutes, if you go over each area only once, or you can work some or all areas more thoroughly and take half an hour or more.

After you finish this general session, focus on specific areas needing attention. You will know which areas these are either because you have a health problem you want to treat (then you can look up the recommended procedure in Part Three), or because you encountered tender spots as you worked on your feet.

When you do encounter tender areas, pay special attention to them, as they probably correspond to parts of the body where there is an imbalance. Go over a sensitive spot four or five times, then let it rest. Don't overwork it; this will only add stress and prove counterproductive. Be sure to give the same treatment to both feet. It may take a number of sessions for the tenderness to disappear.

If you feel a really deep pain (when you press) and it doesn't improve after a few sessions, we urge you to consult a certified Reflexologist, who may be able to understand the organic origin of the pain and refer you to a medical doctor. Reflexologists occasionally work on people who have a great deal of tenderness in the area corresponding to a particular organ; when the person has that organ checked out, they have sometimes discovered a serious condition—often early enough to remedy it.

After you have completed your treatment, take a few minutes to totally relax, allowing your body to adjust to the changes in energy flow and integrate them. You might want to lie down on your back in the yogic rest pose, arms at your sides, feet slightly apart, and focus on your breathing.

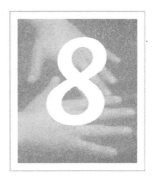

Helpful Hints to Maximize Your Results

INCREASE YOUR BENEFITS WITH VISUALIZATION AND CONSCIOUS ATTENTION

For best results, don't treat pressure point therapy as just a mechanical process, in which you push a button and out pops the desired result. You *will* derive some benefit from that approach (if you push the correct buttons in the correct way!), but you will get the most from these practices if you give your attention to what you are doing. Treat yourself to the same loving, comforting, supportive touch that you would give to a dear friend who needed consolation, or to a crying child.

Your conscious awareness is very powerful; use it to make your finger pressure session more effective. Mentally direct the Life Energy for strengthening and healing.

LISTEN TO YOUR PAIN

Pain is the body's way of seeking attention. So, when pain exists, listen to it and give your body the attention it requires. With these techniques you will be giving attention to healing the pain not only through touch, but with your breath and with your mind.

Your *attention* and your *intention* are both important. Don't let your hands alone be involved, while your mind is off somewhere else. Instead, direct the flow of your breath and attention to the point or area you are treating.

One way to do this is *visualization*. Try visualizing light flowing into an area as you press, or light being "awakened" in the area by your touch. You might also visualize a stream of healing light flowing through your fingers to the point you are pressing.

If, as is frequently the case, the point you are pressing is not the area you are treating (perhaps it is on the same meridian or in the same reflex zone), send light from the point you are pressing to the area you want to help. Remember, this is not purely imagination; *energy is already flowing through your body.* You are simply helping to strengthen and direct it.

A powerful variation is to coordinate your breath along with the visualization. Visualize the Light/Energy being sent to the point or area with your inhalation. Then, when you exhale, visualize the pain or energy block being released and dissolved.

MAKE IT A HABIT

Create a self-care habit by committing 20 to 30 minutes a day to pressure point therapy. But remember, that's the ideal! Even five or ten minutes of Reflexology, Shiatsu, Yoga, or Acupressure feels great and can be healing and refreshing.

"The journey of 1,000 miles begins with a single step." If you start with just five minutes a day, soon you will be looking forward to longer sessions. And you can also practice whenever you have a free moment—while waiting in line, or even while watching tv. Once you create a habit and incorporate this knowledge and these practices into your life, then, whenever you do experience a problem, you'll be more likely to apply what you've learned.

REMINDER: Self-treatment obviously has its limits. There are times to consult your health care practitioner for full diagnosis and treatment. Be wise and get help when you need it.

FOR BEST RESULTS: TAKE A HOLISTIC APPROACH TO YOUR HEALTH

Never forget that your life is a whole, and if you have a health problem, you need to address not just the symptoms, but the whole story of your life.

Everything in this universe is interconnected, and this is equally true of our own lives. Your job, daily routine, relationships, diet, exercise or lack of it—these and many other factors influence your health. To truly remedy your health problems, or to prevent future illnesses from arising, take a good look at your life and do the best you can to live according to the laws of nature and the best advice you can find.

Here are 11 simple, universal guidelines for good health:

1. "Early to bed and early to rise makes a man healthy, wealthy, and wise." This advice is good for women, too!

2. "An ounce of prevention is worth a pound of cure." Some attention to staying healthy is a lot more painless, economical, and rewarding than trying to cure diseases once they arise. Take care of yourself!

3. Get enough rest. This may sound like an impossibility in today's world, but it is very important. Rest is the basis of activity. You can never perform at your best when you are tired. And you are placing a strain on your heart and other vital organs. If you can't get enough sleep at night, take a nap in the afternoon. Pushing yourself eventually wears down the body and creates the fertile ground for disease.

4. Get enough exercise. Everyone needs some exercise every day. For most people, half an hour of walking—not strolling!—every day will take care of it. More vigorous aerobic exercise is fine if you are fit and inclined in that direction. If you have a serious health concern (such as a heart condition) you still need exercise, but be sure to consult with your doctor before undertaking any program. Exercise will make everyone feel more clear-minded and energetic, and is a definite mood-booster.

5. Eat your largest meal at mid-day, and take some time to eat it in a relaxed manner. This goes against the current American lifestyle, but it is extremely helpful. At mid-day our "digestive fires" are strongest. If you eat a large meal late at night it will take a long time to digest, will probably disturb your sleep, and may create heartburn; chances are you will wake up feeling stiff and sluggish.

   So eat lightly for supper. Have a salad, some fruit, some soup, a dish of pasta, or a light grain such as a bowl of hot cereal. Once you make the switch, you will be amazed at how much better you feel.

6. Restrict your fat intake. Studies have shown without any doubt that fat is a major contributor—probably *the* major factor—in heart disease, and probably in many cancers as well. Most Americans get 40%

or more of their calories from fat. Standard advice these days is to restrict that to 30%, but leading-edge researchers such as Dean Ornish suggest that if you could keep your calories from fat to about 10% of your daily caloric intake, you would virtually eliminate all danger of heart disease and cancer. A vegetarian or almost-vegetarian diet, with plenty of fresh fruit and vegetables and lots of whole grains such as rice, oats, and whole wheat and only a little bit of chicken, fish, or turkey, is an ideal low-fat, high-fiber diet.

7. Whenever possible, eat fresh, natural food. Stay away from packaged, frozen, and canned food. They are full of chemical additives and have lost their Life Energy. Leftovers likewise have little life in them.

8. Minimize or eliminate your use of stimulants and drugs. Coffee, tea, alcohol, cigarettes, and other drugs are harmful to the body's vital organs. Cigarettes ravage the heart and lungs; caffeine weakens the kidneys; alcohol gradually destroys the liver.

9. Manage stress. Practice some form of meditation or relaxation, such as Progressive Relaxation, Transcendental Meditation, the Relaxation Response, visualization, or anything that helps you deeply relax and reduce stress. Experts say that at least 70% of all health problems are caused or complicated by stress.

10. Dissolve Negative Emotions. Anger, worry, anxiety, disappointment, grief, depression, and other negative feelings and reactions are emotional forms of stress which take a toll on our nervous systems. Mind-body medicine has clearly shown that our mental state influences our physical health, and that negative feelings generate health problems.

    The Oriental approach to these negative emotions is to observe them, without judgment, and simply allow them to be. When you do this, you will find that these feelings simply quiet down and dissolve away.

11. Be Happy. Make a conscious choice to be as happy as you can. As the title of a recent book proclaims: "Don't sweat the small stuff: and it's all small stuff." In the long run, most difficulties tend to work out; bad feelings dissolve; a solution to problems is found. So get plenty of exercise, listen to music, dance, sing, visit friends, meditate—take some time every day to do whatever it takes to make yourself happier. As a bonus you will be healthier and you will have more to give to the people around you.

part three

PRESSURE POINT HEALING— AN "A" TO "Z" GUIDE

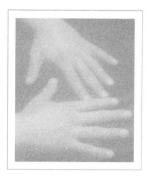

Where to Find
What You Need

To make best use of this "A" to "Z" healing guide:

- Review the descriptions and illustrations of the Acupressure and Shiatsu techniques in Chapter 6, "Getting Started—Acupressure and Shiatsu," starting on page 55.
- Reflexology techniques are explained and illustrated in Chapter 7, "Getting Started—Reflexology," starting on page 63.
- In addition to the illustrations provided with each condition, consult the "master" illustrations in Chapter 5 to help you locate pressure points, meridians, and reflex zones on the hands and feet.

Acne

Acne usually occurs during adolescence and the late teens, but in some individuals it may continue into adulthood. Western medicine attributes acne to a number of causes, including hormonal imbalances or monthly changes, bacterial infection, and an over-production of natural oil (sebum) trapped inside the pores of the skin. Stress, excessive exposure to the sun, and some types of make-up (especially oil-based cosmetics, which may clog the pores) may also contribute, as may certain birth control pills. Some research suggests there is a genetic factor as well.

Chinese medicine classifies acne as a condition of excessive damp heat; treatment seeks to dispel these qualities and restore balance. The major meridians involved here are the Large Intestine and Stomach channels, both of which run along the front of the face.

ACUPRESSURE

For the first three points below, please see "Ten Master Pressure Points" starting on page 49 for descriptions, illustrations, and instructions for pressing them most effectively.

1. (Li 4, Adjoining Valley) Li 4 is useful to treat acne because of its heat-clearing ability, and because it is considered a command point for the face.
2. (Li 11, Pool at the Crook) Li 11 is one of the best points for clearing damp heat, and is widely used in many skin conditions.
3. (Sp 6, Three Yin Meeting) Sp 6 strengthens both *ch'i* and blood. Here it is being used mainly for its ability to regulate dampness and for its calming effect. **Caution:** This point should not be used by pregnant women.

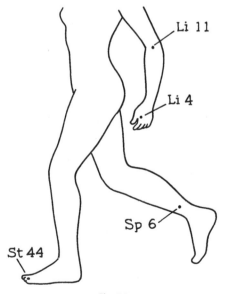

Fig. 38

4. (St 44, Inner Courtyard) This point is located on the top of the foot, in the web margin between the 2nd and 3rd toes. It is right in the center of the web. Use your thumb, and with firm pressure angle into the 'V.' Or, put your thumb underneath your foot, your middle finger on the point. Apply moderate to firm pressure by squeezing the thumb and finger together. This is the most powerful point on the Stomach meridian to clear heat from the body.

REFLEXOLOGY

Before you treat any specific reflex areas for acne, begin with the Reflexology Warm-Up on page 69. This is an important step that helps you relax, tones the energy of the whole body, and prepares your feet to be worked on; please don't skip it!

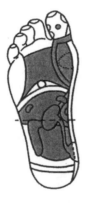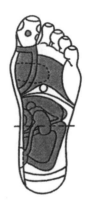

Fig. 39

1. To aid in relaxation and to facilitate deeper breathing, thumb walk the chest and lung reflex zones on the ball of the foot (between the diaphragm line and the base of the toes). You can also finger walk the chest and lymph gland reflexes on the top of the foot, to encourage removal of toxins from the body.
2. To stimulate more balanced and healthy activity of the thyroid gland, work the reflex zone for the thyroid (all around the base of the big toe) by rubbing and pressing. The finger or thumb walk technique is best here.

3. Work on the reflex for the pituitary gland, located in the center of the pad of the big toe, to further regulate metabolism and promote balanced hormonal activity. This "master gland" governs the secretion of hormones, controls body temperature, metabolism, and energy level. To press on this point, it is best to use the "hook and back up" technique described on page 68.

4. To encourage purification of the blood and efficient metabolism of fat, press the liver reflex on the bottom of your right foot. To stimulate the small intestines, stomach, and other internal organs along with the liver, work the entire area in the arch of your foot, from the pelvic line up to the diaphragm line. Use the thumb walk to thoroughly cover this area, moving up, down, and/or diagonally.

5. Next work the kidneys and adrenals. These reflex areas are in the center of the foot, above and below the waistline and on the inside of the large tendon running up the foot. Use the thumb walk.

6. Finally, work on the colon reflexes. In Fig. M (page 45), you'll see that the reflexes for various parts of the colon are divided between the two feet. Work these reflexes thoroughly and carefully using the thumb walk.

SHIATSU

In this Shiatsu procedure you will stimulate the Stomach, Liver, and Large Intestine meridians.

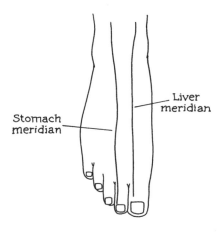

Fig. 40

1. The first procedure stimulates the Stomach and Liver channels. Use the press and release technique (press for 6–7 seconds with your thumb, release, move a short way along the meridian, and press again). Start in the middle of the top of your left foot, and start working slowly— moving only a fraction of an inch with each press—toward the toes. As you get closer to the toes, be sure to be in the channel between the 2nd and 3rd toe. Work down to the web margin. From there, go along the side of the 2nd toe as far as the nail. Repeat with the right foot.

Now go back to the top of one foot, but this time in line with the space between the big toe and 2nd toe. Again using the press and release technique, work down the channel, stop at the web margin, and repeat on the other foot.

2. Next work on the Large Intestine meridian. This channel begins at the tip of the index finger and runs along the thumb side of the finger bone to the wrist, up the forearm to the elbow, and then continues on. (see page 131.) Start at the tip of your left index finger (on the thumb side) and use the press and release technique. Use firm pressure with your thumb.

When you come to the knuckles, press just under the bone on one side of the knuckle and then the other; it's better not to press on the knuckle itself. Follow the channel as it moves upward, close to the side of the finger bone in the hand up to Li 4 in the center of the web margin between the thumb and the index finger. Keep following it with the press and release technique.

From here the meridian follows a virtually straight line up the outside (back) of your arm, to the outer edge of the elbow crease. To be sure you are on the right line, position your arm in front of you with the palm facing your stomach about 4–5 inches away from your body. Imagine the line drawn on your arm in this position. Press and release along the entire length of your forearm to the elbow. Stop at the elbow crease. Be sure to do both arms.

ADDITIONAL SUGGESTIONS

WATCH YOUR DIET.   In Chinese medicine, excess dampness is said to be caused by sweet and greasy foods. Cut back on excess sugar, as well as fried foods. Though Western medicine currently says eating chocolate is not a factor, it is certainly sweet and fatty, so you might try eliminating it from your diet, or at least cutting down, and observe any results. Indian

Ayurvedic medicine says that acne is a condition of excess "pitta"—almost a one-to-one correspondence to "moist heat"—and recommends cutting down on spicy foods and citrus fruits, as well as fats, meats, and sweets.

TRY MELON—ON YOUR SKIN.   The Ayurvedic physician, Vasant Lad, recommends rubbing some melon on your skin at night for a cooling, soothing, healing effect. "It also makes your skin soft," he says.

RELAX.   Stress is increasingly implicated as a causal or complicating factor in acne, so we urge you to unwind with long walks, soothing music, meditation, or any stress management program you find helpful. See the "Additional Suggestions" starting on page 104 in the section on Anxiety for meditation tips.

KEEP CLEAN.   Wash your face regularly to remove excess oil, bacteria, and dead skin cells, but wash gently and use a mild soap. Be sure to get all your make-up off. Also, keep your colon clean; eat plenty of high-fiber foods (fresh fruits and vegetables, and whole grains) to prevent constipation.

AVOID TOO MUCH SUN.   Since acne is caused by excess heat in the system, a lot of sunshine is not helpful.

Allergies

Allergies are sensitivities to various substances, such as foods, pollens, chemicals, dust, mold, pet hair, and certain types of cloth. "Hay fever" is an allergic reaction to certain pollens or grasses. The immune system mobilizes against this perceived invader, usually by releasing a flood of histamine, a chemical that causes runny noses, bloodshot eyes, sinus headaches, sneezing, etc. Even a tiny particle can provoke an allergic reaction, which may go beyond a runny nose to include dizziness, difficulty breathing, stomach cramps, fever, and hives.

Pressure point therapy can provide a great deal of symptom relief, and can also strengthen your system to help prevent future allergic reactions.

ACUPRESSURE

For quick relief, use one or both of these points.

1. (Li 4, Adjoining Valley) Please see, beginning on, page 49, "Ten Master Pressure Points," for a description and illustration of the location of this point and how to press it. **Important:** Pregnant women should NOT use this point, as it may stimulate contractions in the uterus.

2. (B 2, Gathered Bamboo) Locate the point at the inner end of your eye sockets, near the bridge of your nose, where there is a small indentation. Use the thumbs of both hands to press on this point for 1 minute. Close your eyes and breathe deeply as you press. You may allow your head to lean forward into your fingers. This point is good for relieving headaches, sinus congestion, and allergy symptoms.

3. (B 10, Celestial Pillar) About ½ inch below the base of the skull and ½ inch outward from the spine, there is a powerful point on the neck muscles that can help relieve headache, swollen eyes, and other allergy symptoms. It is about ½ inch within the hairline of the neck. Use your index and middle finger together to press directly on this point. Or, interlace your fingers behind your head, grasp the neck, and press firmly for about 1 minute.

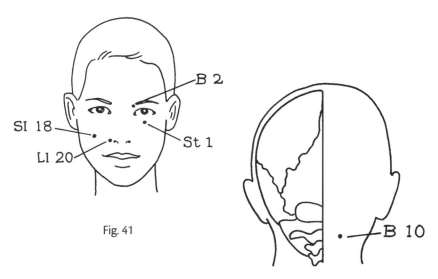

Fig. 41

Fig. 42

4. (Li 20, Welcome Fragrance)—This is an excellent point for any kind of nasal symptoms common to allergies, especially stuffy nose and sinus headaches. Place your index or middle finger on either side of each nostril, in the groove right next to the nostril. Press on these points, directing the pressure upward. Build pressure gradually, hold about a minute, and release.

5. (Si 18, Cheek Bone Crevice) Drop straight down from the outside edge of the eye socket, until you are on the lower border of the cheek bone. You'll find the point in a natural depression there. Use medium pressure and hold for about a minute before releasing.

If you have more time, the following two points may also be helpful. Illustrations and detailed descriptions of their locations and how to press them begin on page 49, "Master Pressure Points."

6. (Lv 3, Bigger Rushing)
7. (St 36, Three Mile Foot)

REFLEXOLOGY

Before you begin to treat specific reflex areas for your allergies, please be sure to begin with the Reflexology Warm-Up in the box on page 69. Don't skip this important step!

To relieve allergy symptoms, you will work primarily on three areas: 1) the reflex areas in the arch of the foot for most of the internal organs; 2) the area on the ball of the foot that affects the lungs and chest; and 3) the toes, to affect the sinuses, throat, and nose.

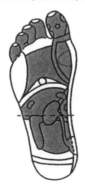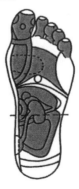

Fig. 43

1. To stimulate the liver, small intestines, stomach, and other internal organs, work the entire area in the arch of your foot from the pelvic line up to the diaphragm line. Use the thumb walk to thoroughly cover this area, moving up, down, and diagonally.

2. Work the kidney and adrenal reflexes (also in the soft center of the foot) using the thumb walk.

3. Work on the thyroid gland (around the base of the big toe) by rubbing and pressing. The finger walk technique may be helpful here.

4. Thumb walk the chest and lung reflex zones on the ball of the foot (between the diaphragm line and the base of the toes). You can also finger walk the chest and lymph gland reflexes on the top of the foot, in the troughs between the toes. Work up from the webbing toward your ankle.

5. Press the sinus reflexes on the bottom of the toes, and the pituitary gland in the center of the big toe, using the "hook and back up" technique. (See page 68.)

Don't forget you can work the same reflex areas in the hands and fingers. Refer to the hand diagrams on pages 47–48.

SHIATSU

Shiatsu instructor Pamela Ferguson offers the following procedure, using pressure along the lung meridian to help clear the congestion of allergies.

1. Slide both hands under your opposite armpits, leaving the thumbs protruding. Now use your thumb to press and release in a circle, between your shoulder and collarbone. Press firmly for 7 to 10 seconds in several spots.

2. Stretch out your left arm, palm up. With your right hand, press along a line (the lung meridian) that reaches from the circle (#1 above) all the way to the tip of your left thumb. The line does not run down the center of the arm, but slightly to the outside.

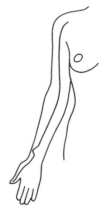

Fig. 44

ADDITIONAL SUGGESTIONS

AVOID THE CAUSE.   The easiest way to prevent allergic reactions is to avoid any substance you know you are allergic to. Dust, mold, synthetic fibers and fabrics such as polyester, cat or dog hair, certain perfumes, and chemicals such as in cleaning supplies, are fairly easy to avoid. Stay indoors and use an air conditioner, if possible, when the pollen count is high.

FIND YOUR FOOD ALLERGY.   If you have food allergies and you don't know for sure what you're allergic to, experiment. Common foods that provoke allergic reactions include dairy products such as milk, yogurt and cheese; eggs; wheat; hot, spicy dishes; citrus or sour fruits; soybeans; tomatoes; potatoes; eggplant. Quite a number of people are also allergic to peanuts and shellfish. Try these in isolation and see if any of them upset your system. If they do: don't eat them!

HERBAL SOLUTIONS.   Burdock root is an excellent blood purifier and can help relieve many allergy symptoms. You can obtain burdock in bulk in most natural food stores. Make a tea using about ½ teaspoon of the herb per cup of hot water. Steep for about 10 minutes and drink. Echinacea (readily available in tincture form in dropper bottles) may also be helpful.

QUIT SMOKING.   Smoking weakens the lungs and reduces immunity, making the smoker more susceptible to allergens.

YOGA POSTURES.   Doing Yoga postures regularly can help open up your breathing and increase immunity. A full set of postures is always most helpful, and/or use the Sun Salutation. Include the Plow and Lion poses in your routine.

Anemia

Anemia may be due to a variety of causes, including iron deficiency; low red blood cell count; insufficient hemoglobin; blood loss due to injury, excessive menstruation, or hemorrhoids; and vitamin B-12 deficiency. Successfully treating anemia generally requires nutritional supplementation, such as iron, vitamin B-12, and/or folic acid. But some help can be provided by pressure point therapy.

ACUPRESSURE

For the three points below, please see "Ten Master Pressure Points" beginning on page 49 for descriptions, illustrations, and instructions for pressing them most effectively.

1. (St 36, Three Mile Foot) This is the major point to tonify the *ch'i* and blood of the body. In combination with Sp 6 (below) it strongly revitalizes the entire body.
2. (Sp 6, Three Yin Meeting) In combination with St 36, this point nourishes the *ch'i* and blood and brings vitality. **Caution:** pregnant women should not press on Sp 6.
3. (Lv 3, Bigger Rushing)

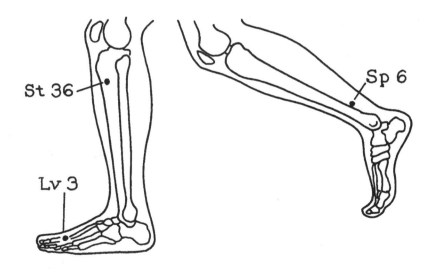

Fig. 45

These points will be more effective if combined with the Shiatsu sequence described on page 93.

REFLEXOLOGY

The most important reflex zones for treating anemia are the spleen area on the bottom of the left foot and the liver area on the right foot. The spleen serves as a storehouse for iron needed in the blood, and filters out broken-down red cells. A healthy spleen is necessary for healthy blood. Similarly, the liver constantly filters the blood and supplies some of the substances required for blood creation.

Locate the liver and spleen areas on the bottom of your feet using the foot map on page 45. These are the reflex zones you will be focusing on. A reminder:

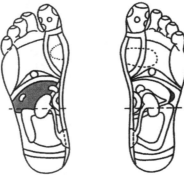

Fig. 46

1. It's helpful to begin with a brief treatment to your whole foot. For this, use the Reflexology Warm-Up in the box on page 69. Please don't skip this step!

2. Begin specific treatment by working the reflex zones for your spleen, located on the bottom of your left foot. It is on the outer edge (below your two smaller toes), and in the center of the arch, between the waistline and diaphragm line. If you are indeed anemic, you will probably find the reflex points for the spleen quite tender. Don't press too hard and hurt yourself, but keep working the area for a few minutes, using alternating deeper and lighter pressure.

3. Another area that will almost certainly be tender in individuals who are anemic is the liver reflex area. To stimulate the liver, work the liver reflex zone (almost the entire arch of your right foot, from the pelvic line up to the diaphragm line). Use the thumb walk to thoroughly cover this area. You might want to criss-cross the area from several directions.

4. If you cannot conveniently get to your feet, you can, as usual, work the same reflex points on your hands. You can do this even during a spare moment at work, or while watching television, though a more attentive, conscious style of working is recommended. The reflex areas for the spleen and liver are located in areas of the hand corresponding directly to the points on the feet. Work them with the thumb.

SHIATSU

To help you combat the fatigue that almost invariably accompanies anemia, here is a quick, all-natural Shiatsu pick-me-up for generating more energy.

1. Rub your hands (palms facing each other) briskly for 5–10 seconds.

2. Rub your warmed-up palms briskly up and down on your cheeks for 5–10 seconds. Then rub your palms across the back of your neck for 5–10 seconds. Next place your palms on your cheeks next to your ears, thumb on one side of the ear, the four fingers on the other. Rub 5–10 seconds. End by squeezing your ears. Start at the earlobe and work up and around to the top, squeezing with moderate pressure. Now work your way back down. Your ears will tingle for several minutes afterwards.

3. *Gently* tap the top of your head with the flat of your hands for 5–10 seconds.

4. Cup your hands in a loose fist, and tap up and down the inside and outside of each arm. Go up and down each arm 3 times. With the same loose fist, go up and down your legs. Start at the inside of the ankles, come up the inside of the leg and thigh, cross over to your buttocks, then start down the outside of the legs. (In this way you will be following the natural energy flow of the meridians.)

5. Place your thumb in the hollow at the base of your skull (at midline of the back of the neck, where the head sits on the spinal column). Press in slowly and then hold for 30 seconds. Slowly release.

Please remember that even though this sequence of pressure points and mini-massages will temporarily boost your energy, it does not heal the underlying condition of anemia. For that, you should see your doctor.

Caution: Although iron deficiency anemia is one common form of anemia, particularly affecting women of menstruating age, an *excess* of iron can also be toxic to the body and can cause serious health problems. Very few men suffer from iron deficiency anemia. So don't just take iron supplements without first consulting your health practitioner to discover the cause of your anemic condition. You might be doing more harm than good.

Angina

See also "Heart Tune-Up"

Angina—attacks of chest pain caused by a decrease in oxygen supply to the heart—are due to blockages or spasms in the arteries leading to the heart. The pain often radiates to the shoulder and left arm, sometimes all the way to the tip of the little finger.

The causes of angina are many. At the top of the list is a fatty diet which builds plaque in the arteries (atherosclerosis), thus narrowing the blood vessels and limiting the amount of oxygen-rich blood that can reach the heart. Smoking is at least equally to blame, as it increases carbon monoxide levels in the blood, displacing the life-giving oxygen and starving the heart. Lack of exercise, and outbursts of anger, are also prime causes of angina attacks.

Here are some ways to relieve angina with pressure point therapy. For further suggestions for maintaining a healthy heart, please see "Heart Tune-Up."

Please note that if you have just had your first attack of angina and you are not already under the care of a physician for a heart condition, please seek medical attention immediately. Angina is a warning sign that should not be ignored. Studies have shown that people who receive prompt medical attention have a much better chance for recovery than those who delay even a few hours.

ACUPRESSURE

1. (Pc 6, Inner Gate) You will locate this point on the palm side of your wrist, two thumb widths above the wrist crease in the center of the

arm. This point regulates *ch'i* as well as blood in the chest. It's the point of choice for any pain or discomfort of the chest. Use medium pressure; build up gradually, hold about a minute, and gradually release. Be sure to do both wrists.

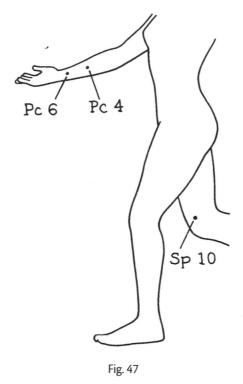

Fig. 47

2. (Pc 4, Cleft Gate) This point is also on the palm side of your wrist. Locate the midpoint between the wrist crease and elbow crease. From this point, go down one thumb width toward the wrist. Pc 4 is right in the center. This point is very powerful for any discomfort in the chest area; it is the point to use first when the pain is intense or acute. In Chinese medicine, this point is also used for heart palpitations and arrhythmia. Use medium pressure for about a minute. You may repeat the pressure several times if pain is acute. Be sure to work on both arms.

3. (Sp 10, Sea of Blood) About 2 thumb widths above the top edge of the knee you will feel a bulge in your thigh muscles. It's on the top of your leg, toward the inside. Press firmly for a minute with your thumb or the knuckle of your middle finger.

REFLEXOLOGY

To help relieve acute angina pain immediately, grasp the tip of the little finger of your left hand (the area above the first joint) with your right thumb and forefinger, and hold it tightly. (In Acupuncture and Shiatsu, the little finger is at the end of the Heart meridian.) Grasping the little toe in the same way also helps.

Then use the thumb walk to work on the heart reflex area in either your left hand or left foot. Authorities differ on the precise location of this reflex on the foot, but all agree that it is on the sole of the left foot between the diaphragm line and the base of the toes. Some feel it is more on the inside of the foot, toward the big toe; others place it more in the direction of the little toe. For safety, work the entire area, thumb walking up, down, and across. You can even use double thumb action. Take plenty of time to work this area thoroughly.

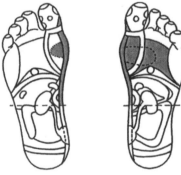

Fig. 48

If you have more time, it is always good to give a brief treatment to your whole foot. Start by simply massaging your feet for a few minutes, and use the relaxation techniques described in the Reflexology Warm-Up on page 69. You will find these very helpful.

Following the warm up, begin specific treatment by working the reflex zones for your heart, as described above. Work the entire area from the diaphragm line to the base of the toes of the left foot. Also work on zones 1 and 2 (below the big toe and first toe) of the *right* foot, using the thumb walk.

You can work the corresponding areas on the palm of your left and right hands, instead of working your feet, or in addition.

It is also helpful to work the spine reflex, especially the upper spine. (See Fig. 34 on page 72.)

SHIATSU

Angina pain follows the path defined in Oriental medicine as the Heart Meridian, which goes from the armpit down the arm to the tip of the little finger.

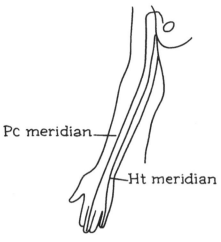

Fig. 49

One way to immediately relieve angina is to simply apply pressure to points along the route of the pain. You will probably find that points along this meridian are quite tender and painful when pressed.

1. Search out sore or tender areas in the chest above the nipple line. Press for a few seconds, using a slightly vibrating, rotating pressure once you have settled in on the spot. (Women, don't press on the breasts; press only on points above or below.)

2. Feel under the left armpit for more tender spots, and use gentle repeated pressure of 5–10 seconds duration.

3. With the palm of your left hand facing up, use your right hand to follow the line of the heart meridian from the armpit down to the little finger, tracing along the inside of the upper arm and forearm to the hand. When you find tender spots, press and vibrate the sore areas until they feel eased.

Then start again at the top of your arm and trace the same line again, except move an inch or so closer to the top of the bicep, which will be the Heart

Protector or Pericardium meridian. Look for and press any tender spots. When you reach the elbow crease, press a few extra times on the point just to the inside of the biceps tendon, which is located in the center of the crease. Remember, your palm is still facing up. Continue tracing down the center of the forearm across the palm to the little finger. Give the area on the lower half of your forearm some extra attention, as this area is rich with beneficial points.

After working your left arm, switch and do your right. Remember, all the meridians (except the Conception Vessel and Governing Vessel) are bilateral.

ADDITIONAL SUGGESTIONS

1. For current care of your heart and prevention of future problems, we recommend that you take a careful look at the 11 Guidelines for Good Health starting on page 77, and begin putting them into practice. Four of these are particularly crucial for you. They are:

- *Low fat diet*—To lower your risk of painful angina attacks, as well as of heart disease and heart attacks, trim the fat from your diet. Cutting down to 30 percent of calories consumed is not good enough: research has documented tremendous improvement in heart patients who stuck to a diet containing only 10 percent of calories from fat. Increase your daily intake of fresh fruit and fresh vegetables, and eat more whole grains such as whole wheat, rice, and oats.

- *Reduce your stress level*—Sudden stress, whether from exertion or emotional excitement, can bring on an attack of painful angina. So every day, spend at least 15 to 20 minutes practicing some form of meditation or relaxation. (See "Anxiety" section for tips on meditation.)

- *Exercise*—Angina attacks commonly occur during exertion, so angina patients sometimes shy away from exercising. This is a mistake, as the following story shows. A group of seriously ill cardiac patients who were awaiting heart transplants were put on an exercise program, to build up their strength for the surgery. After participating in the program for several months, half the patients' hearts improved so much that they no longer needed the surgery!

  A suitable exercise program is essential to maintain a healthy heart. But—especially if you are a heart patient or are over 40 and have not been a regular exerciser—consult with your doctor before beginning any exercise program.

- *Quit smoking*—This may be the best thing you can do for your heart. Studies have found that angina patients who quit smoking cut their death rate in half compared to those who continue to smoke.

2. *Try Herbs*—Many people have found hawthorn berry very helpful. It acts as an antioxidant for the cardiac tissue. This herb is used in both Chinese and Western herbology to benefit the heart.

3. *Yoga*—Some gentle Yoga stretching can improve circulation to the heart, thus helping to reduce the cause of angina. Unless you have acute pain, you can do the Sun Salutation every day (slowly), as well as the Cobra and Locust poses (which will help stretch the coronary arteries and increase blood supply to the heart). A gentle Spinal Twist will also be effective. But, as mentioned above, please consult your doctor before starting any exercise program, including Yoga postures. You can always do the Savasana (yogic rest pose) for relaxation.

Anxiety

Everybody feels nervous, worried, or anxious at least once in a while. Too many difficult decisions to make, too many responsibilities, uncertainty about the future, worries about children or aging parents, economic woes, health concerns, relationship problems that won't go away—our lives are filled with potential sources of anxiety. Then there are all the smaller opportunities to be on edge: job interviews, exams, public speaking requirements, first dates—these and a host of other common occurrences can give us butterflies, sweaty palms, and sleepless nights.

Most of these worries come to an end, when the exam is past, the speech given, the interview over. When anxiety continues on for a long time and begins to interfere with normal social or occupational functioning, you may need to see a doctor for help. This is especially true if your anxiety is very intense and associated with panic attacks, phobias (strong fears of things like heights, open spaces, enclosed spaces, or certain social situations), or persistent, obsessive thoughts and/or repetitive behaviors.

Most of our everyday worries and anxieties can easily be managed at home, using pressure point therapy and some simple, natural remedies we will describe at the end of this section. With a little attention and the knowledge you will gain in the next few pages, you can definitely get a grip on your nervousness and tension.

ACUPRESSURE

Try some of these pressure points for reducing anxiety and restoring balance.

1. (Ht 7, Mind Door) The first point is on your hand, at the "wrist crease." It is on the heart meridian and is very effective for reducing anxiety, nervousness, and fear. Find the bony knob on the outside of your left wrist (the little finger side). The point is next to that, in a small indentation directly below your little finger, in the crease. Press for 30 seconds with your thumb; release gradually; switch hands.

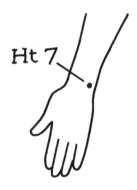

Fig. 50

2. (Gb 21, Shoulder Well) Place your right hand on your left shoulder. Midway between the neck and the outer edge of the shoulder, on the highest point of the shoulder, is Gb 21. (See Fig. C on page 37.) Don't be surprised if this point is quite tender. Use your middle finger to press firmly on the point. Or, you can press both shoulders at the same time by curving the left hand over the left shoulder and right over the right. Increase pressure gradually, then press quite firmly for up to 2 minutes and gradually release. Remember to take slow, deep breaths as you do this and the other techniques. This point helps restore normal flow of *ch'i* in the lungs. **Caution:** Don't press this point if you are pregnant.

3. (Gb 41, Falling Tears) This point is on the top of your foot in the channel between the little toe and the 4th toe. It's a little less than half way between the ankle bone and the web margin between the toes, a little closer to the toes. (See Fig. G, on page 40.) Once you locate the point, press firmly for about a minute with your index or middle finger. Gb 41 is effective in restoring the smooth flow of *ch'i* which can be interrupted by stress, worry, and anxiety.

4. (Gb 13, Mind Root) Just inside the hairline directly above the outer edge of the eye socket. (If your hair is receding, locate the point where your hair used to be. It should be approximately 4 finger widths above the eyebrows.) This point has a powerful effect on calming the mind and relieving anxiety. Press firmly for about a minute. You may use your index or middle finger, whichever is more comfortable.

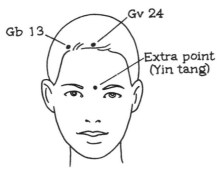

Fig. 51

5. (Gv 24, Mind Courtyard) This point is also just inside the hairline of the forehead (or what used to be your hairline!) directly above the nose. Pressing here has a powerful calming effect on the mind. Use medium to firm pressure and hold for about a minute. Remember to always increase and decrease pressure gradually, not suddenly.

6. (Cv 17, Chest Center) This point is on the Conception Vessel meridian, which is powerfully *yin* or female in nature (see Fig. 58 on page 113). Pressing this point is very soothing and healing. It is located right in the center of the chest, on the breastbone. Traditionally it is said to be "even with the nipples" and men will easily locate it that way. It is about 3 finger widths up from the bottom of the breastbone, "at the level of the heart." Hold your index, middle, and ring finger together and press on this point for about 1 minute with your middle finger, with your eyes closed. Use medium pressure. Remember to breathe slowly and deeply.

Keeping your eyes closed always helps, but particularly in this sequence of relaxing points.

7. ("Extra Point") Finally, press on your "third eye" point (in the indentation between the eyebrows) for a full minute. You can use your thumb or middle finger (use light to medium pressure).

REFLEXOLOGY

When you are suffering from stress and anxiety, the most important thing you can do is relax, and for this, there's nothing like a good foot rub, even one you give to yourself! So start your Reflexology session by spending a little extra time with the relaxation techniques in the Reflexology Warm-Up, which you will find in the box on page 69.

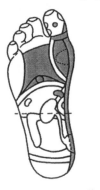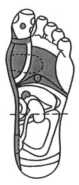

Fig. 52

1. Return to the solar plexus point and press for a full minute, keeping your eyes closed and breathing deeply for extra relaxation. Then follow by thumb walking across the diaphragm line.

2. Work the entire chest area (including the lungs and heart) to help regulate breathing and heart rate, which both get out of balance when we are anxious. Use the thumb walk technique in this area.

3. Next, work on the spine reflexes. These reflexes are located on the inside edge of both feet (zone 1), extending from the heel nearly to the top of the large toe, opposite the root of the toenail.

When you work the spinal reflexes, work slowly up the foot using the thumb walk technique. You will need a little extra strength on the thick skin of the heel area.

Thumb walk all the way *down* the spinal reflex area, and then take some time to walk across small areas horizontally, moving up the foot from the heel to the big toe.

4. Look at the master chart of the foot in Chapter 5 and spend a little time working some of the key endocrine glands, including the pituitary (in the center of the bottom of the big toe), the thyroid (at the base of the big toe), and the adrenals (between the waist line and the diaphragm line, toward the inside of the foot). Working these areas will promote balance in the body and nervous system and help relieve your anxiety.

SHIATSU

1. The first Shiatsu technique to calm anxiety is to press on the point just above the "third eye" point, in the center of your forehead just above the eyebrows. You will find a small indentation in the bone. Place your index finger on the point, and then put your middle finger on top of the index finger. Press firmly for 5 to 7 seconds, 3 to 5 times.

2. Bend your left arm to locate the elbow crease, then unbend it. This point is at the lower end of the crease (toward your fingers) and opposite the thumb side of the hand, slightly to the inside of center. Hold for 30 seconds and release gradually, then switch arms. This point will help relieve heart palpitations, which sometimes accompany acute anxiety.

3. If you have more time, use the following sequence of points recommended by Shiatsu expert and educator Toru Namikoshi. It will help relieve anxiety, worry, and insomnia and will be very balancing.

- Using medium to firm 3-finger pressure, press along the midline of your head (as if your hair were parted in the middle), from the hairline in front, over the top, all the way to the edge of the hairline in back, moving about ½ inch after each press. Press for 5 seconds at each stopping point. Repeat the sequence twice.

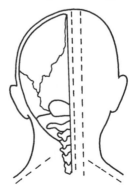

Fig. 53

- Press with your thumb in the indentation at the back of the neck, in the middle, at the base of the skull. Press quite firmly for 5 to 7 seconds and repeat twice.
- Press along the top of your shoulder (slightly to the back, about ½ inch). Use 3-finger pressure. Repeat twice. Press firmly.

ADDITIONAL SUGGESTIONS

In their book, *Ayurvedic Secrets to Longevity and Total Health*, Peter Anselmo and psychiatrist James S. Brooks, M.D. offer a number of helpful suggestions to alleviate anxiety:

MEDITATE.   To quiet the mind and relax the body, practice some form of meditation or relaxation, such as Progressive Relaxation, Transcendental Meditation (TM), the Relaxation Response, visualization, or whatever you have found that helps you relieve stress. (In an important study comparing methods of relaxation and meditation, TM was found twice as effective as any other method for reducing anxiety.)

It is better to have meditation instruction from a qualified teacher. To help you right now, however, try this: Sit with eyes closed and mentally "watch" your breathing. Notice the cool air coming in through the nostrils, and how your chest or belly expands; notice the exhalation, the warmer air against your nostrils, your chest and belly settling. Just sit quietly and maintain your awareness like this, bringing it quietly back whenever you drift off. Do this for 10 to 15 minutes. Twice a day is best.

TRY A MASSAGE.   If you can afford it, get a full body massage from a trained professional. This is one of the best ways to relax and let go of stress and tension.

You can give yourself a very soothing massage at home in just a few minutes. *Slightly* warm up 2 or 3 ounces of oil (sesame, sunflower, or coconut are good), and apply to your entire body. Rub some oil into your scalp with your palms, rub across your forehead and along your cheekbones. Rub along the long bones of your body (arms, legs), and use a circular motion on elbows, knees, shoulders. Rub your chest and abdomen, and as far around on your back as you can reach. Just use the flat of your palms; kneading the muscles is not essential. Then massage your feet, especially the soles. Follow with a hot bath or shower, and see how relaxed you feel! **Tip:** If you don't have time for the entire massage, rub a little oil into your scalp and the soles of your feet.

TRY SOME YOGA POSTURES.   Yoga can help relieve tension and anxiety. If you have time, do an entire set of postures. If you have only a few minutes, the Shoulder Stand and Forward Bend will be soothing.

DO SOME ALTERNATE NOSTRIL BREATHING.   Here is a very simple, soothing breathing exercise:

- Sit comfortably, either in a chair, or with your legs crossed, on the floor or wherever you are comfortable. Keep your back in an upright position.
- Bend your left arm so that it is against your belly, palm up. Rest your right elbow in your left hand, so that your right hand can be up around your face.
- Inhale normally. Then close your right nostril by pressing it with your right thumb, and exhale through the left nostril.
- Inhale normally through the left nostril. When the inhalation is complete, close the left nostril with the middle or ring finger of the right hand and open the right nostril; exhale comfortably.
- Continue repeating this cycle for 5 minutes, switching nostrils after each *inhalation.* If it feels comfortable, you might want to make your breaths a little deeper and slower than usual, but don't strain.

Your relaxation will be deeper if you do this breathing exercise with closed eyes.

CUT DOWN ON STIMULANTS.   Coffee, tea, colas, and other sources of caffeine are just the opposite of what you need if you want to sleep well and reduce your anxiety. Cut back gradually, but try to eliminate caffeine from your diet.

GET PLENTY OF EXERCISE.   Regular daily exercise will help you reduce your anxiety level. All most people need is a daily walk for about half an hour, but if you like to play tennis, jog, swim, dance, etc., go ahead! The key is regularity. But don't overdo it. Overexertion can be worse than non-activity. If you are over 40, consult your doctor before starting an exercise program.

These suggestions for relieving anxiety are very effective. Please try them.

Arthritis

Arthritis is believed to be one of the oldest ailments on earth. Extremely common, it may afflict as many as 40 million Americans. The pain, stiffness, and swelling of arthritis range from slight to severe and even crippling. Arthritis comes in many varieties and can start at any age, even in childhood. Of the two main types, rheumatoid arthritis (which affects about 2 million of us) is the more serious, as it may affect the entire body. It usually begins between the ages of 20 and 50. Rheumatoid arthritis is generally considered to be an autoimmune disease.

The other main type is osteoarthritis, also called degenerative joint disease. It involves chronic breakdown of cartilage in the joints, leading to pain, stiffness, and swelling. Extremely common, osteoarthritis affects millions of Americans, most over the age of 45. By age 65, whether we feel pain or not, as many as 75 percent of us show x-ray evidence of this condition in our hands, feet, knees, or hips.

Millions of prescriptions a year are written to help relieve the pain and swelling of arthritic joints. But through pressure point therapy and other natural means, you may find remarkable healing. The mobility of your joints may increase, your pain may be considerably reduced or even eliminated, and joint deterioration may be halted. But you will need to use these techniques every day, perhaps twice or three times, in order to gain the benefits.

ACUPRESSURE

We will offer suggestions first for treating rheumatoid arthritis, and then for osteoarthritis. Remember that you do not have to use all these points; just using 1 or 2, when you have a chance, can be effective.

To Treat Rheumatoid Arthritis

1. (Li 4, Adjoining Valley) Li 4 helps relieve pain and inflammation in the hand, wrist, elbow, shoulder, and neck. See page 49 for the beginning of "Ten Master Pressure Points," for a description and illustration of the point and how to press it. **Important:** Pregnant women should not press this point, as it can stimulate uterine contractions.

2. (Lv 2, Moving Between) This point is located in the web margin between the big toe and second toe. Use medium pressure with your index fingers, pressing on both feet at the same time if that is comfortable, otherwise one at a time.

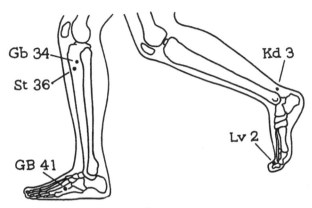

Fig. 54

3. (Gb 41, Falling Tears) This point is on the top of the foot, in the channel between the little toe and the 4th toe, slightly less than halfway between the ankle bone and the web margin between the toes (closer to the toes). The pain and discomfort of rheumatoid arthritis, and the emotional response to that pain, can constrict the circulation of *ch'i*. This point is effective in restoring the flow. Press with your index or middle finger, using firm pressure. Remember to start with light pressure, build up, hold, and gradually release.

4. (Gb 34, Yang Hill Spring) At the lower border of the kneecap, slide your finger off the shinbone toward the outside (little toe side). Two bones come together here. Press in the soft tissue area between them, using your index or index and middle fingers together. This is a major point in Acupuncture and Acupressure for nourishing the tendons and joints. It also has a strong effect on promoting the smooth flow of *ch'i* throughout the body. Obstruction to the smooth flow of *ch'i* causes pain and discomfort.

The following points on the palm of your hand are excellent for joint pain in general, and are also specific for rheumatoid arthritis. They have been popularized by Richard Tan, a prominent Acupuncturist in San Diego.

On your palm, locate the area about one thumb width above the wrist crease, and about one finger width on either side of the midline of the palm. Find the points in this area that are the most tender. Press with the thumb or the knuckles of the opposite hand. Use strong pressure. If the pain is worse on the left side of your body, use the points on the right hand for relief, and vice versa.

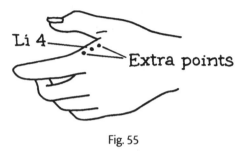

Fig. 55

To treat arthritis pain in specific parts of your body, please turn to "Pain," for self-treatment suggestions for pain in the wrist, arm, shoulder, and other areas.

Note: It might interest you to know that in Oriental medicine, rheumatoid arthritis, which is a hot, inflammatory type of disorder, is often associated with repressed anger and resentment.

To Treat Osteoarthritis

Please see page 49 for the beginning of "Ten Master Pressure Points," for a complete description and illustration of the points listed below, and suggestions on how to press them most effectively.

1. (Li 4, Adjoining Valley) This is one of the most important points in Acupuncture and Acupressure. We are recommending it here for its ability to relieve pain and circulate the *ch'i*. **Important:** Please remember that pregnant women should not press this point.

2. (St 36, Three Mile Foot).

3. (Kd 3, Supreme Stream) Disorders of the bone and cartilage are related to the Kidney energy in traditional Chinese medicine. That's why, for osteoarthritis (which is a degenerative condition), it is beneficial to strengthen the Kidney energy. Kd 3 is considered the source point of the Kidney meridian.

4. (B 23, Associated point of Kidney) This point in combination with Kd 3 (above) greatly strengthens Kidney *ch'i*.

REFLEXOLOGY

Cortisone is commonly used for relief of arthritis pain. According to New York Reflexologist Laura Norman, author of *Feet First*, stimulating the reflex areas for the adrenal glands often helps people with arthritis cut down (or even eliminate) their cortisone dependence. Mildred Carter, author of *Healing Yourself with Foot Reflexology*, supports that view. She says pressing certain reflex areas stimulates the body to produce natural cortisone. However, *Do not suddenly stop taking your cortisone!* If you feel that you could reduce your dosage, consult your doctor and discuss it. Sudden reduction of cortisone can have serious negative effects.

The main theme of treatment in this section will be using reflex areas on the hands and feet to stimulate the adrenal glands. However, you may also gain relief from working zones corresponding to the painful areas of your body.

1. Before you start to treat specific reflex areas for your arthritis, please be sure to begin with the Reflexology Warm-Up in the box on page 69. Don't skip this step!

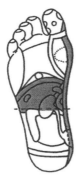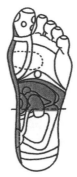

Fig. 56

2. To increase flexibility throughout the body and facilitate the flow of healing energy, thumb walk up, down, and then across the spine reflexes on the inside of your feet. These reflexes are located on the inside edge of both feet (zone 1) and extend from the heel nearly to the top of the big toe.

3. Work the entire area of the arch of the foot, from the "midline" to the "diaphragm line." Use the thumb walk to go up, down, and back and forth in this area. This will naturally stimulate the adrenal glands in a balanced way, along with working the kidneys, liver, and other internal organs.

ADDITIONAL SUGGESTIONS

EAT CAREFULLY.   Certain foods seem to aggravate arthritic conditions. Many experts recommend that you avoid the nightshades (tomato, white potatoes, eggplant, and peppers), greatly reduce or eliminate dairy products, and stop eating red meat. Try a vegetarian or largely vegetarian diet. If your arthritis tends toward inflammation (not all types get inflamed) and is very painful, avoiding spicy foods and citrus fruits may help.

RX FOR GOUT.   For gout—a type of arthritic condition involving an excess of uric acid in the blood—it is important to stay away from organ meats such as liver, as well as shellfish, strong aged cheeses, and port wine.

MASSAGE.   A gentle massage with some warm oil over the affected joints once or twice each day for a few minutes can help relieve pain and reduce inflammation. Just a little warmed up sesame oil is ideal. Rub gently, mostly with your fingertips.

TRY VITAMIN C.   Some experts believe vitamin C can help heal arthritis. Try taking about 500 mg. over the course of the day for a week or so, preferably not on an empty stomach, and see if it helps. If you feel it might be aggravating your condition, discontinue.

GLUCOSAMINE SULFATE.   For osteoarthritis, you might wish to try glucosamine sulfate, a precursor building block for joint cartilage. Research is suggesting that it can be very helpful. The current recommended therapeutic dose is 500 mg. 3 times a day. We suggest checking with your doctor about whether you should try glucosamine sulfate, and the optimal dosage for you.

RELAX.   Pain tends to worsen with tension. Just as women in childbirth can reduce their pain by using relaxation and deep breathing techniques, most pain can be lessened by relaxing. Sit with eyes closed and take five slow, deep breaths. Keep your eyes closed and allow your breathing to return to normal, but follow it with your attention, "watching" the inhalation and exhalation. Sit quietly watching the breath for 10 to 20 minutes. Open your eyes but sit another minute or two before standing up; you may be more settled and relaxed than you think!

Asthma

Asthma affects at least 12 million Americans and is becoming increasingly common, especially in highly polluted cities like Los Angeles where large numbers of children are falling prey to it. The bronchial passages contract, breathing becomes difficult, the chest feels tight, and the person often coughs or begins to wheeze.

The majority of asthmatic conditions are caused by allergies or pollutants, such as pollens from grasses, trees, and flowers; animal dander; dust; mold; and air pollution. For older people (middle aged or older) asthma is equally likely to be triggered from within, by emphysema or another lung disorder. Emotional factors, such as fear and anxiety, or a feeling of constriction or suffocation by a relationship or situation, often cause or complicate asthma.

We all take thousands of breaths every day and most of us never think about it. Severe asthma, one of the most frightening health conditions, in which a person struggles just to get a little air, can remind us how precious air is to our lives.

Asthma can be effectively treated with modern medicines, such as bronchodilators, which relax the bronchial muscles and make breathing easier. However, such drugs are very powerful and can have serious negative side effects, such as rapid heart rate, which itself can become life-threatening!

Pressure point therapies can offer a great deal of relief from asthma. Combined with changes in your diet and some appropriate exercise, these therapies can help you control asthma and may allow you to reduce or eliminate any medications you may be taking. Of course, never stop taking your prescription medications without the approval of your doctor.

ACUPRESSURE

Chinese medicine classifies asthma as either acute or chronic. Asthma is acute when the person is right in the midst of an attack, or has frequent attacks with difficult breathing and wheezing. Asthma is in a chronic phase for someone who is prone to attacks, but is currently either not experiencing them or has them only infrequently or with minor symptoms. Treatment is quite different. For the acute phase, the goal is symptom relief. In the chronic phase, emphasis is on strengthening the respiratory system and building resistance to future attacks.

Respiration is understood to depend on the smooth functioning of Lung and Kidney *ch'i*. Therefore, points that energize these meridians are included in the pressure point prescription.

Acupressure is effective for asthma sufferers of any age. However, it is especially helpful for children or young adults. Be diligent and you will see good results. Acupressure will not conflict with the use of inhalers. If you currently use an inhaler, once you start using Acupressure we suggest monitoring your usage (in conjunction with your doctor if possible) as a way to chart your progress.

Treatment for Acute Asthma (For symptom relief)

1. ("Extra Point") Locate the vertebra on the back of your neck that sticks out as your head bends forward. Place your hands on your shoulders next to the neck (your elbows will be out in front of you) and use your middle fingers (or if it's easier, use your index, middle, and ring fingers together) to press firmly on the points on either side of the protruding vertebra. Press for 30 seconds. This is the primary point for wheezing and asthma. Repeat several times as needed.

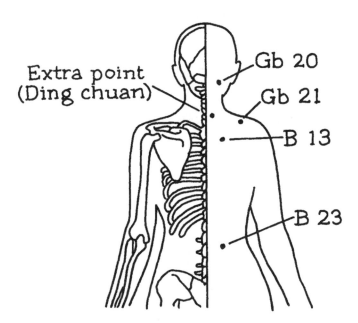

Fig. 57

2. (Gb 21, Shoulder Well) Place your right hand on your left shoulder. Midway between the neck and the outer edge of the shoulder, on the highest point of the shoulder, is Gb 21. Don't be surprised if this point is quite tender. Use your middle finger to press firmly on the point. Or, you can press both shoulders at the same time by curving the left hand over the left shoulder and right over the right. Increase pressure gradually, then press quite firmly for up to 2 minutes and gradually release. Remember to take slow, deep breaths as you do this and the other techniques. This point helps restore normal flow of *ch'i* in the lungs.

Caution: Don't use this point if you are pregnant.

3. (Lu 1, Central Residence) This is the first point on the Lung meridian. It helps to stop wheezing and coughing, tones the lungs, and is helpful for relieving asthma and all kinds of breathing difficulties, as well as for reducing tension and congestion in the chest.

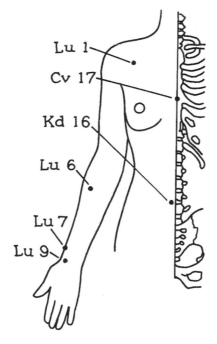

Fig. 58

Be patient as you look for this point, as it is a little difficult to pinpoint without experience. It is located in the groove between the chest muscle (pecs) and the deltoid at the level of the space between the 1st and 2nd rib.

Another way to find it is to go 3 finger widths, or about 2 inches, below the collarbone and 1 finger width, or about 1 inch, inward from the armpit.

Cross your arms in front of your chest and use the index, middle, and ring fingers of the right hand to press on the left side, and vice versa. Alternatively, you can put your hands on your chest, fingers toward the breastbone, and press these points with your thumbs. Use only moderate pressure; this point may be painful. Hold for about 1 minute.

4. (Lu 6, Biggest Hole) Hold one arm with the palm up. Imagine a line drawn from the center of the elbow crease to the wrist crease on the thumb side. Divide this distance in half and then move one thumb width closer to the elbow. Use medium to firm pressure, and hold for about a minute. Then repeat with your other arm. This point is very useful in any acute conditions involving the lungs.

5. (Lu 7, Broken Sequence) Hold one hand out in front of you with the palm facing down. Start from the V shape formed by your thumb and index finger. Use the index finger of the other hand to trace along the top of the thumb to the wrist. Your finger will fall into a natural depression where the base of your thumb joins the wrist. Keep going another inch and a half and you will be on Lu 7. It is used here for its powerful effect on the lungs. Maintain firm pressure (you can use your thumb or index finger) for about a minute, then switch hands.

Optional: If you have time, add:

6. (Gb 20, Wind Pool) Please see page 49 for the beginning of "Ten Master Pressure Points," for a description and illustration of this point and how to press it.

Treatment for Chronic Asthma

1. (Cv 17, Chest Center) This point is also known as the "Upper Sea of *Ch'i*." It strengthens and circulates *ch'i*, especially the *ch'i* of the chest which is derived from the air we breathe. The point is directly on the breast bone, at the level of the space between the 4th and 5th ribs. For a man, this is at the level of the nipples. For women, using the level of the nipples may not be accurate due to the wide variation in the shape of the female breast from individual to individual. You will find it about 3 finger widths up from the bottom of the breast bone.

Use the tips of three fingers to press. This point is often tender. Hold for about a minute.

Try stimulating this point at the same time you stimulate the points on your back. (See B 13 below.)

2. (B 13, Lung-Back Associated Point) Lie on your back with a tennis ball next to your spine, about 3 to 4 inches below the top of your shoulder. Roll across the ball slowly (up and down rather than from left to right) to stimulate this area and the area a few inches above and below it. To work the points on both sides of the spine that energize the Lung function, put two balls in a sock, one ball on either side of the spine. (Instead of tennis balls you can also use tightly rolled up socks.)

3. (Kd 16, Vital Transporting Point) These points are located half an inch on either side of the belly button. They have both a calming and a tonifying effect. Put your hands on your sides, and press with your middle fingers. Use firm pressure. *Don't press these points—or any points on the abdomen—if you are pregnant.*

4. (Kd 3, Supreme Stream) On the inside of the ankle (big toe side), Kd 3 is located half way between the ankle bone and the Achilles tendon. (See Fig. 54, on page 107.) Place your thumb on the prominence of the ankle bone, and let it slide down toward the Achilles tendon on the back edge of the ankle. Kd 3 is in the depression approximately half way between the bone and the back edge of the ankle. Pressing it nourishes the Kidney energy. Press with your thumb using medium to firm pressure, for about a minute.

5. (Lu 9, Greater Abyss) This point is on the palm side of the wrist crease under the thumb. Find the pulse in your wrist at the wrist crease. The point is on the thumb side of the artery that you feel. Lu 9 is the most important point to strengthen the Lung meridian.

Optional: The following points will also be helpful if you have time. If you only have time to add one, alternate them: use different ones for different sessions. (Please see page 49 for the beginning of "Ten Master Pressure Points," for a description and illustration of the points and how to press them.)

6. (B 23, Associated point of Kidney).

7. (St 36, Three Mile Foot).

8. (St 40, Abundant Splendor).

REFLEXOLOGY

In using Reflexology to treat asthma, you will primarily be working on the lung and bronchial reflexes on the top and bottom of both feet. Your lungs take up a lot of space in the chest cavity; similarly, the lung reflexes occupy a large area of the hand and foot.

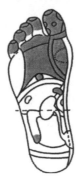 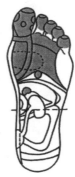

Fig. 59

You will also be working on the adrenal glands, the solar plexus/diaphragm point, and the sinus reflexes on the toes and fingers. Here is a helpful sequence:

1. Begin with the Reflexology Warm-Up in the box on page 69. This is an important step that helps you relax, tones the energy of the whole body, and prepares your feet to be worked on; please don't skip it!

2. Use the thumb press on the solar plexus point on each foot for 15 to 30 seconds. (See Fig. 24 on page 66.)

3. Now work the lung area in the center of the ball of the foot. Cover the whole pad under your toes. Thumb walk up, down, and diagonally across this area, going right up under the base of the large toe.

4. Finger walk the chest area on the top of the foot. Work up from the webbing toward your ankle, in the troughs between the toes. Start at the base of the big toe, in zone 1, and go up about 2 inches. Continue working each zone, ending in zone 5 near the outside edge of your foot. Work this area with your index finger, using the finger walk.

5. Use thumb or index finger to walk across the ridge at the base of the toes. (See Fig. 30 on page 71.) This will help free up the flow of energy in the shoulders, neck, and head. To work this area properly, pull the thick pad of the foot downward with your holding hand.

6. Work all the toes, especially the top two joints, to treat the sinus cavities and nasal passages for better breathing. Walk up the bottom of the toes and down the top, or just give them a good rubbing.

7. Thumb walk the adrenal reflex zones in the central portion of the sole, approximately under the second toe.

8. Finally, spend a minute on the reflex for the ileocecal valve, which helps regulate mucus in the body. This area is on your right foot only.

9. After all this work on your feet, you might want to finish with a simple brisk foot rub, or relax by pressing on the diaphragm/solar plexus point, as in #2 on page 116.

SHIATSU

The Shiatsu sequences in this section will help relieve neck muscles strained by asthmatic coughing, and help to open up the chest and facilitate easier breathing.

To relax tense neck muscles, do the following 3 steps. Be careful: the neck is delicate, so start with light pressure and gradually increase it.

1. With your 4 fingers, rub the back of your neck. Rub in long strokes along the thick muscles, and also use your fingers to push and pull across the muscles. Work for 3 to 5 minutes on one side and then switch.

2. Locate the point in the center of the back of your neck, in the indentation below your skull. Use your thumb to press upward firmly on this point for 5 seconds, then release. Repeat 3 times.

3. With your hands behind your head, lace your fingers together. With palms against the neck, squeeze and release several times. Don't pull forward, just squeeze.

This next Shiatsu sequence is good for the lungs and chest and can relieve asthma.

1. Use 3 fingers (index, middle, and ring finger) of both hands to press on a sequence of points between your ribs. Spread the fingers and place them so that they are between the ribs. Start close to the breastbone, at the top of the rib cage, below the collar bone, and move out-

ward. Then move down to the next row of points. Apply pressure for 5 seconds at each place. **Women:** don't apply pressure directly on the breasts; press only above, around, and below the breasts where you can work directly over the ribs.

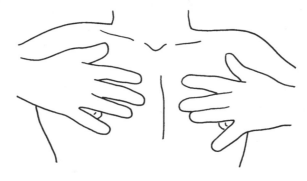

Fig. 60

2. Again using 3-finger pressure, press the points of the breastbone in the center of the chest, working downward. Press for 7 to 10 seconds; move down about ½ inch and press again, and so on, pressing in about 6 or 7 places. Don't press on the cartilage extending off the bottom of the bone. Repeat twice.

3. Place both palms on your chest, fingers pointing slightly downward and toward each other. Pressing firmly, rotate your hands in opposite directions, going upward toward the outside and downward as you move toward the center of the chest. Make 10 circles. **Women:** apply pressure only above the breasts.

ADDITIONAL SUGGESTIONS

YOGA.   A number of Yoga postures are helpful for relieving asthma. Some of the best are the Locust, Cobra, and Bow poses, which stretch and open the chest, the Head-to-Knee posture, and the inverted poses including Shoulder Stand and Plow.

AVOID AGGRAVATING FOODS.   One of the most important actions you can take to curtail asthma is to avoid foods which may aggravate or bring on asthmatic attacks. For most people these include dairy products, such as milk, yogurt, ice cream, and all cheeses. Also avoid red meat and most fermented and salty foods. You might experiment and see if abstaining from wheat, or minimizing wheat consumption (in the form of bread and pastas as well as cookies and cake) helps you feel better. Some people also need to avoid mushrooms, peanuts, walnuts and other nuts, and yeast.

DRINK PLENTY OF WATER.   One of the problems with asthma (and other pulmonary conditions such as pneumonia and bronchitis) is the gummy, stringy mucus which can plug up the bronchial tubes and literally choke us. Although many drugs have been devised to liquefy this thick mucus (they are often called "expectorants"), the best way to thin and liquefy it is plain old water. Increase your water intake to between 6 and 8 glasses a day. And don't drink it iced. Room temperature, warm, or hot (perhaps as herbal tea) will be better for your condition. Try a cup of hot water with a spoonful of lemon juice and a spoonful of honey.

TRY THESE HERBAL REMEDIES.   The following herbal remedies will help reduce mucus congestion and relieve asthma and difficult breathing.

Drink ginger tea. Use ½ teaspoon of ginger powder or a few thin slices of fresh ginger per cup of boiling water.

For immediate relief of acute asthma, the Ayurvedic physician, Dr. Vasant Lad, recommends squeezing an onion and drinking ¼ cup of the onion juice mixed with 1 teaspoon honey and ⅛ teaspoon black pepper.

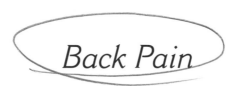

Back Pain

Low back pain is said to be the largest single medical complaint in the United States, afflicting millions of people and costing billions of dollars in lost work and medical bills. For this reason, we are going to allot considerable space to methods you can use both to relieve pain and to prevent future recurrences.

Experts say that 80 percent of us—four out of five—will experience back pain at some time in our lives. Women suffer more from back problems than men do, probably because of the more pronounced lumbar curve in their backs, and the stresses of childbearing. Pain in the lower back is quite common during pregnancy, particularly in the last months.

If you are one of the unlucky ones who have experienced back pain, you know that it can be not only disabling, but excruciatingly painful. You also may have been suffering from recurring back pain for years—even decades—despite treatments and advice from doctors of all kinds, and you may have had to resign yourself to periodic bouts of pain and disability.

Low back pain, says Dwight Byers, author of *Better Health with Foot Reflexology*, "is an international plague. Many back pain sufferers attribute low back pain to a slipped disk. Most of the time, however, low back pain has other origins, such as weak muscles, asymmetrical posture, and overweight." Lack of exercise, and muscle tension caused by stress, also contribute.

Fortunately, remedies for all these causal factors can be found in daily life. Specific exercises can strengthen back muscles and/or develop greater flexibility. Meditation and relaxation techniques can help you overcome stress. Poor posture can usually be corrected just by repeatedly reminding yourself to sit or stand up straight.

It's a fact that most back pain heals without medical care; it just goes away by itself, given enough time. But the healing may often take weeks. The remedies in this chapter can help speed your healing, and some of the Additional Suggestions at the end of the chapter should help you prevent future recurrences.

ACUPRESSURE

The ancient Chinese who formulated the theory behind the pressure point therapies believed that in order for us to be healthy, the Life Energy (*Ch'i*) in the body had to circulate freely through the energy meridians. If there is a break or an obstruction in the flow, pain or illness would result. Backache is said to be caused by blocks of the *Ch'i* in the bladder meridian, which has dozens of points along the back, and we will show you ways to work on those points. But first try these more accessible places:

1. (Li 4, Adjoining Valley) Please see page 49 for the beginning of "Ten Master Pressure Points," for a description and illustration of this powerful point and how to press it. Li 4 is recommended here for its ability to relieve pain and to circulate the *ch'i*. **Important:** Pregnant women should NOT press this point; it may stimulate premature contractions in the uterus.

2. ("Extra Points") Just above and below Li 4 are two more points that are remarkably effective for relieving back pain. From Li 4, slide up about half an inch toward the knuckle of the index finger. You are still in

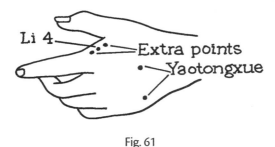

Fig. 61

the webbing between your thumb and index finger but you're closer to the knuckle than Li 4. Apply strong pressure with your thumb.

Now return to Li 4 and this time slide past it about half an inch up toward the wrist. You are still in the web margin portion of the hand, but close to where the thumb and index finger come together. Again, apply strong pressure with your thumb. For better leverage when applying pressure, you can grip the flesh of the webbing with your thumb on top and your index and middle finger underneath the hand.

These points have been popularized by Richard Tan, a prominent Acupuncturist in San Diego. Use the points on the hand opposite to the side of the pain: if the pain is worse on the right side, use the points on the left hand and vice versa.

3. ("Extra Points") Two more highly effective points for low back pain are located on the back of each hand, one between the 2nd and 3rd and the other between the 4th and 5th finger bones. Find a natural depression approximately halfway between the knuckles and the wrist. There should be flesh, not bone underneath your fingers. To stimulate these points, press with the tip of your thumb or index finger. Apply strong pressure to the point of mild discomfort and hold for about a minute.

You can increase the effectiveness of these points by slowly moving your back at the same time you stimulate the points. Depending on how much pain you feel, try to include back to front bending, side to side bending, and left and right rotations.

This sequence of hand points (starting with Li 4) is very powerful for relieving back pain. If you find that they bring you pain relief, but after some time you find the pain returning, repeat the sequence. With regular sessions, the intervals of pain relief will get longer, with the pain steadily diminishing.

In addition to the hand points, add the following if you have time.

4. (B 40, Middle of the Crook) A very helpful point for relieving lower back pain is located in the back of your knee, in the crease that forms when you bend the knee, and right in the center between the two large tendons. You can use your thumbs or middle fingers to press that point while you are sitting up. Or, follow this inventive suggestion by Michael Reed Gach, author of several helpful books on Acupressure. Lie on your back; raise your legs by bending your knees; place your fingers on these points on both legs; use your arm muscles to rock your legs back and forth for about a minute. Then let your feet rest on the floor, with knees bent. This point exerts a powerful influence on the back and is known as the command point for all low back problems.

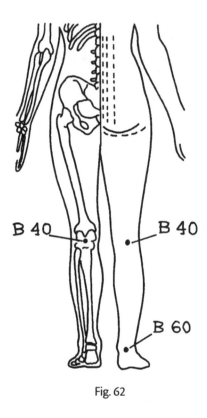

B 40   B 40

B 60

Fig. 62

5. (B 60, Kunlun Mountains) Put your right thumb on the right ankle bone (on the little toe side of the foot). Let your thumb slide into the depression between the bone and the Achilles tendon, located on the back side of the ankle. If you feel bone under your fingers you are too close to the ankle. This point is helpful for relieving chronic or longstanding pain.

Because it has an effect on the entire course of the bladder meridian, it can be used for upper as well as lower back pain or neck pain.

After using the points starting on page 120, add some of the following exercises if you have the time. The points pressed in these routines are a little hard to get to, but they can be very helpful in alleviating back pain so they're worth the effort. Most are on your back, so you will not be able to press them easily yourself, and it also may be difficult to figure out exactly where to press. Here are several creative ways of applying pressure.

- Use three fingers (index, middle, and ring) and press in the general vicinity.
- Make a fist and rub or press with your knuckles behind your back, along both sides of the spine. For comfort, use only light pressure directly on the spine.
- Put a couple of tennis balls in a sock, put this on the floor, sit down, and lie back on it, with one of the balls on each side of your spine at the lower back. You can then position the sock a little higher and/or a little lower, or roll up and down, in order to reach all the important pressure points.
- Wooden rollers, designed to stimulate the points along the spine, are available in many natural food stores and "new age" bookstores, or can be ordered by mail. Ads for them often appear in Yoga magazines.
- Finally, you can lie on the floor and simply roll or rock over the points in your lower back. A number of helpful points along the spine, and in the hips and buttocks, will be worked this way.

Now here are the exercises:

1. Kneel on a comfortable surface, or sit on a firm bench or on a chair facing the back of the chair. Reach both hands behind your back as high as you can go, with your fingers pointed forward and wrapped around your sides, and your thumbs on the ropy muscles on either side of the spine. Press with your thumbs in a line down both sides of the spine, keeping the thumbs even with one another.

Press in one spot for about 30 seconds, starting lightly, building up to as firm a pressure as you can use without causing discomfort. If your back is hurting a lot, you may only be able to press very lightly in some spots. That is okay. Release gradually. Then move downward about ½ inch, and press again. Continue in this way until you reach the level of your hips.

Then, move back up your back, and work down again, but this time about 1 inch farther out from the spine, at the outer edge of those strong ropy muscles. Again, continue down to your hips, pressing and releasing.

If this procedure seems to be effective, you can repeat the process one more time, about another ½ to 1 inch out from the spine.

If it feels better just to lightly massage along these vertical lines, rather than pressing, that will also be helpful. Try the deeper pressure when the pain in your back has started to diminish.

2. Next, with your hands on your hips, thumbs still pointing toward the back, locate the ridge at the top of your hip bones. Press down toward that ridge, into the soft tissue. Start in the center and work along the ridge to the sides of your back. Press for about 30 seconds at each point.

If your hands and arms are getting a little tired from working in this unaccustomed position, rest them a minute or two before proceeding.

3. Again with your hands on your hips and thumbs in the center, move onto the sacrum, the bony triangle at the base of the spinal column. Or, you might find it easier to work this area using your index, middle, and ring fingers instead of your thumb. (The fingers would be pointing down, with your thumbs around the outside of your hips.) Start at the top, in the center, and work downward. Wherever you find an indentation, press there, but don't restrict yourself to those areas. Then, as in Step 1 above, work down another vertical line, out from the center.

In his book, *Acupressure's Potent Points*, Michael Reed Gach suggests an ingenious way of working this area:

Lie on the floor on your back, knees bent, with your hands underneath your buttocks, palms down. Rock your knees slowly from side to side for a couple of minutes. Reposition your hands once or twice to put pressure on different muscles. Also, try pulling your knees toward your chest so that your feet come up off the floor, and continue the side to side movements. Move slowly, and allow the weight to rest on one side for a few seconds before going back to the other side, so pressure can go a little deeper on each point.

REFLEXOLOGY

Self-reflexology for a bad back in its acute stage (when it hurts badly) has to focus primarily on using the reflex zones in the hand. Why? As anyone who has suffered from back problems knows, when your back is in pain, it is pretty close to impossible to lift your foot high enough, or bend forward far enough, to work the reflexes on the bottom of your feet. When your back starts to feel better, working the foot reflexes will help speed your recovery and prevent future problems.

Reflexologists differ on the most effective way to treat the back via the hands. For the following suggestions, please refer to Figures Q and R in Chapter 5:

1. Hold your left hand palm up. Before getting started, use your right thumb to lightly trace along the outside edge of your left thumb, from the tip, along the bone down the side of your hand, to the wrist; turn "inland" and keep going across the bottom of the hand (above the wrist) till you reach the little finger side of the hand. This is the reflex area for the spine. Now use the thumb walk, or simply press and massage along this entire area. Give more attention to sore spots, but don't work them too hard. Repeat on the other hand.

2. Turn your left hand over so that the palm is facing down. Focus on the line running along the inside edge of your index finger (next to the thumb) all the way to the wrist. Some Reflexologists also consider this a reflex zone for the spine. You will probably find it easier to work this area with your index finger. Don't forget to also work the other hand.

Most back pain is caused by tension in the muscles surrounding the spine. When a muscle in the back becomes strained, due to stress and emotional tension, poor posture, wrong lifting, overwork, or for any other reason, it tends to tighten and pull on specific vertebrae, causing the spine to be pulled out of alignment. The Reflexology solution to back problems, once you are able to work on your feet, lies primarily in alleviating the tension and working the reflexes of the spine.

3. For tension reduction, massage your feet and relax them with the techniques described in the Reflexology Warm-Up in the box on page 69.

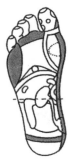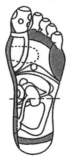

Fig. 63

4. Now you are ready to begin work directly on the spinal reflexes, which run up the inside edge of your feet (in zone 1), extending from the heel all the way up to the toenail of your large toe.

Use the thumb walk technique to work your way slowly up the foot. You will need to apply extra strength on the thick skin of the heel area. You will also have to switch your hand position a few times to get the right angle.

When you have worked all the way up, then turn around and thumb walk down the spinal reflex area.

Reflexologists believe that curves in the foot correspond directly to the curves in the spine. Thus, to work on a low backache, for example, you need to pay special attention to the arch of the foot, where the reflexes corresponding to the lower back are located. When you work on those areas, one Reflexologist says, "you are stimulating a renewed life force into the part of the spine that for some reasons is not getting a full supply of energy."

But always be sure to work the entire spine, not just the problematic area. It's also helpful to work on the neck (along the ridge at the base of the toes) and shoulders (on the edge of the sole below the little toe) to release tensions there. Also press on the sciatic nerve reflexes on the bottom of the foot close to the heel, and along the Achilles tendon.

SHIATSU

Shiatsu expert Pamela Ferguson suggests the following procedures in her book, *The Self-Shiatsu Handbook*.

1. Make a fist with both hands. Use the knuckles to work your way down both sides of your spine and buttocks, pressing at intervals.

2. Use your knuckles to work points on your sacrum and buttocks.

You may find it helpful, and less painful if your back is hurting, to do steps 1 and 2 kneeling in the Yoga posture known as the Pose of the Child. Kneel down, knees close together, and bend forward till your head touches the floor (or is close to it). With hands behind your back, work the points on the low back and buttocks as above.

3. Using your knuckles or three fingers (index, middle, and ring) press points between your buttocks and thighs on the back of both legs. Or try this by simply sitting on your knuckles (palms down). Make sure they are underneath the creases between buttock and thigh.

4. Place your right foot on the edge of a chair or stool. Hold the Achilles tendon between thumb and fingers, and squeeze it in several places, for a few seconds at each point, as you raise and lower your foot. (Keeping the toes on the chair, raise the heel; keeping the heel stationary, raise the toes.) Repeat with the other foot.

5. Place your hands on your hips, fingers pointing forward. With your thumbs lined up even with your navel, press them into your back at the edge of the spine (but don't press directly on the spine).

ADDITIONAL SUGGESTIONS

REST.   When your back goes out, immediately lie down and rest. Lie on your side in a fetal position, all curled up. This is almost always easiest on the spine. You will also find it comfortable to sleep this way.

However, researchers have found that *prolonged* rest is not the best way to heal. For decades, doctors put back pain sufferers to bed for days, sometimes even weeks. Although it is important to give the muscles a time-out, too much rest can be just as bad; bed rest for more than two or three days can actually make the problem worse. Try to find the balance between rest and activity that works for you. After some amount of rest, start to move slowly and carefully, and gradually progress to more vigorous activity.

YOGA.   Yoga stretching is an excellent way to increase strength and flexibility and help prevent back problems. The traditional postures stretch the muscles, massage the meridians, and help to release tension and restore the harmonious flow of energy.

Most of the basic postures should be safe and helpful for most people with chronic back problems, provided you do them comfortably, without strain. (It is always safer to consult your doctor or a certified Yoga instructor.) Many people have excellent results by regularly performing the Sun Salutation (slowly is best). When your back hurts, don't do any Yoga without expert guidance.

BACK EXERCISES.   In addition to the Yoga postures recommended above, a number of other stretching and strengthening exercises can help you prevent future back pain. You may be able to do some of these even when your back is "out," but be very careful. For most, you'll have to wait until the pain starts to diminish.

- Lying on the floor with knees bent, locate the curve in your back above your buttocks, and press it toward the floor. You will feel your abdominal muscles tighten. Hold for a few seconds; release; repeat 6 to 8 times.

- Lying on your back on a hard surface, do leg lifts: lift your right leg up, keeping the knee straight, until the leg is at a 90 degree angle. Probably you won't be able to lift it that high at first, but just lift as high as you can. What matters is the stretch and the strengthening, not the perfect position. Repeat twice more with the right leg, then switch and do three repetitions on the left side.

TRY SWIMMING.   Swimming, which takes pressure off the body, is an excellent exercise for low back pain.

RELAX YOUR SHOULDERS.   Tight shoulders, pulled up around your ears, stretch all the muscles in your back and can result not only in shoulder and neck stiffness, but lower back pain as well. Try pulling your shoulders up high and tight as you inhale, hold your breath for a few seconds as you tense your shoulders in that raised position, then exhale as you let your shoulders fall. Repeat at least 3 or 4 times, and do this several times a day.

You can also relax your shoulders with a little self massage. Reach back over your right shoulder with your right hand and, starting close to the neck, squeeze firmly, hold, and release your trapezius muscles (the large muscles at the top of your shoulders). Move outward away from the spine.

Next, raise your elbows a little so you can reach farther down your back, and continue to massage, from the spine out to your sides.

Lightly slap the area you have just massaged, with an open palm, then rub the area with a few light, smoothing strokes.

Repeat this sequence on the left side.

DO THE CRUNCH.   To do these modified sit-ups, lie on your back with your knees bent and your feet flat on the floor. Cross your arms, resting your hands on your opposite shoulder. Raise your head and shoulders off the floor as high as you can (don't worry if it's only a few inches) while keeping your lower back on the floor. Hold for just a second or two, and repeat up to 10 times.

SLEEP COMFORTABLY.   Experts recommend two sleeping positions for back pain. First, lie on your back, with a pillow or two under your head, and another under your knees. Alternatively, lie on your side in the curled up fetal position. If this is better for you, you might benefit by putting a pillow between your knees to keep your top leg from moving forward and rotating your hips.

LIFT WITH YOUR KNEES—NOT WITH YOUR BACK.   Don't forget this standard advice if you want to prevent back pain.

DON'T WEAR HIGH HEELS.   You may not want to hear this, but wearing high heeled shoes can easily throw your back out of alignment and result in back pain.

DRINK PLENTY OF WATER.   But don't drink too much. Lower back pain is often associated with kidney problems, which can be caused by drinking too much or too little liquid. Depending on your own individual body, 6 to 8 cups of liquid per day is about right.

MODERATE YOUR SEXUAL ACTIVITY.   Excessive sex can strain back muscles and put your back "out," as well as aggravating an existing back problem. Be careful.

Bad Breath

See also, "Indigestion"

A temporary case of bad breath is probably due to something simple, such as not drinking enough water, eating some strong-tasting food such as garlic or aged cheese, or a case of indigestion. Persistent bad breath is usually due either to chronic indigestion leading to toxicity in the colon and intestinal tract, or poor oral hygiene, which has resulted in plaque and/or gum disease.

Pressure point therapies are not aimed at oral hygiene. (Talk to your dentist about this, and see some of our "Additional Suggestions" on page

132.) But they can help very much to improve digestion and remove the toxicity. When digestion is weak or sluggish, the food you eat may undergo fermentation and putrefaction in the gastro-intestinal tract, resulting in bad breath.

In traditional Chinese medicine, the primary cause of persistent bad breath is excess heat in the stomach meridian. The following four points help correct this imbalance by draining heat from the stomach.

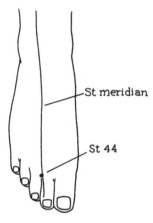

Fig. 64

1. (St 44, Inner Courtyard) This point is located on the top of the foot, in the web margin between the 2nd and 3rd toes. It is right in the center of the web. Use your thumb, and with firm pressure angle into the 'V.' This is the most powerful point on the Stomach meridian to clear heat in the Stomach channel.

For thorough descriptions and illustrations of the next three points, and instructions for pressing, please see page 49 for the beginning of "Ten Master Pressure Points."

2. (Li 4, Adjoining Valley) Here, this powerful and versatile point is being used for its heat-clearing properties.

3. (Li 11, Pool at the Crook).

4. (St 36, Three Mile Foot) This is a major point to nourish the *ch'i* and blood; we recommend it here for its beneficial effects on the digestive system.

SHIATSU

The following Shiatsu routine works first the Large Intestine (LI) and then the Stomach (St) meridian.

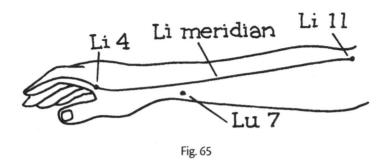

Fig. 65

1. The large intestine channel begins at the tip of the index finger and runs along the thumb side of the finger bone to the wrist, up the forearm to the elbow, and then continues on. Start at the tip of your left index finger (on the thumb side) and use the press and release technique. Press for 6 or 7 seconds; release; move a little way along the channel; and press again. Use firm pressure with your thumb.

When you come to the knuckles, press just under the bone on both sides of the knuckle, not on the knuckle itself. Follow the channel as it moves upward, close to the side of the finger bone in the hand up to Li 4 in the center of the web margin between the thumb and the index finger. Keep following it with the press and release technique.

From here the meridian follows a virtually straight line to the outer edge of the elbow crease. To be sure you are on the right line, position your arm in front of you with the palm facing your stomach about 4–5 inches away from your body. Imagine the line drawn on your arm in this position. Press and release along the entire length of your forearm to the elbow. Stop at the elbow crease. Be sure to do both arms.

2. To press the Stomach meridian (see Fig. 64 on the previous page) start at the tip of your second toe, slightly on the little toe side, and move upward using the press and release technique to move along in small increments. The meridian runs over the top of the foot between the 2nd and 3rd toes, and up the front of the ankle. From the ankle it continues along the front of the leg about 1 finger breadth to the little toe side of the shin bone. Stop just below the knee. Use firm pressure.

ADDITIONAL SUGGESTIONS

Here are some suggestions in the realms of diet, exercise, and oral hygiene which may help with the problem.

DRINK ENOUGH WATER.   And drink primarily water. All alcoholic beverages leave their traces behind, as does coffee. As an alternative, try peppermint tea. It has a fresh taste and smell.

AVOID FOODS THAT LEAVE A STRONG RESIDUE,   such as garlic, onions, aged cheeses, and spicy meats such as pepperoni or salami. Avoid heavy meals, and don't drink ice cold drinks, which slow down digestion. Also stay away from ice cream, cheese, and yogurt.

EAT PARSLEY.   This little green leafy vegetable not only cleans your breath, but contains large amounts of vitamins and minerals.

EAT MORE FRUITS AND VEGETABLES.   These high-fiber foods help to keep your intestinal tract clean. Fresh is best (rather than frozen or canned).

CHEW FENNEL SEEDS.   After meals, chew about 1 teaspoonful of roasted fennel seeds. Roast an ounce or two on a dry frying pan for just a minute or so; be careful not to burn them! Store in a jar and chew a small handful after meals to improve digestion and sweeten the breath.

TAKE CARE OF YOUR TEETH AND GUMS.   Try to clean your teeth after each meal, and floss once a day. Many cases of bad breath are due to gum disease. An excellent way to help heal receding or infected gums is to use tea tree oil, a natural antiseptic available in most natural food stores. Either place a few drops on your floss, or place a drop or two on your (clean, washed) index finger and massage your gums. Rinse out the residue; don't swallow it.

GET ENOUGH EXERCISE.   There's nothing like exercise to stimulate a sluggish digestive system and clear toxins from the body. Be sure to get at least ½ hour of exercise every day, either a good walk or something more vigorous if you're in shape for it.

TRY YOGA.   Yoga postures which give the abdominal organs a good pressure point massage, may improve digestion and elimination. The Fish,

Locust, and Cobra stretch the abdominal area; the Forward Bend puts gentle pressure on the internal organs. The Lion Pose opens circulation in the mouth and throat.

Beauty Secrets

Beauty has many facets. There is no doubt that cosmetics, clothing, and even surgical procedures may enhance and bring out one's natural beauty. But there is also little doubt that beauty comes largely from within, in the form of radiant health. A person with lackluster eyes, blotchy skin, or dull hair is a person who is not healthy. When vibrant health returns, the skin clears, the hair shines, and the eyes become luminous. Thus the main beauty secret we wish to convey is the secret of maintaining and improving your health: the topic of our entire book!

In this section, we will offer you a natural and effective non-surgical pressure point facelift, as well as some dietary and herbal suggestions to enhance the beauty of hair and skin.

ACUPRESSURE FACE LIFT

Millions of dollars are spent every year in the United States on surgical facelifts. But the quest for a youthful look is not just a Western obsession. In China, facelifts are also common, but with a difference. They use Acupuncture to stimulate natural toning in the muscles of the face. With more muscle tone, the facial skin is naturally lifted and tightened to a more youthful appearance.

The good news is that Acupressure can achieve the same results, without the needles. The bad news is that it doesn't happen overnight. However, facial rejuvenation can be accomplished with a consistent Acupressure program. You will be amazed at the results.

The following facelift formula is from Mercedes Martine, a gifted Acupuncturist in the Los Angeles area who is rapidly developing a reputation for her successful beauty treatments. The results gained by her patients speak volumes for the success of this treatment. Use this treatment every day, and you will soon see results. For some people, improvements may appear in a few days to a week; if it takes longer, persevere. It works.

Press the following points with firm pressure for one minute each. With the exception of the first and last point (Li 4 and Cv 24), press the points on both sides of the body at the same time.

1. (Li 4, Adjoining Valley) For a complete description of the location of this very important point, and illustrations to show you how to press, please see page 49 for the beginning of "Ten Master Pressure Points." In addition to many other functions, this point is considered the command point for the face and head. We're using it at the beginning of our self-treatment to open the flow of energy to the entire face and head area. It makes the rest of the treatment more effective. **Caution:** Pregnant women should NOT use Li 4. It can cause premature uterine contractions.

Now that we have opened the flow of energy to the face, the next set of points focuses on rejuvenating the muscles around the eyes, lifting the eyebrows and eyelids, and diminishing wrinkles.

2. (B 2, Gathered Bamboo) Locate the point at the *inner* end of your eyebrow, near the bridge of your nose, where there is a small indentation. Press upward with the middle finger of each hand, or use both thumbs to press on these points for about 1 minute. Remember to begin with light pressure, build up, and hold; then gradually release. Close your eyes and breathe deeply as you press. You may allow your head to lean forward into your fingers.

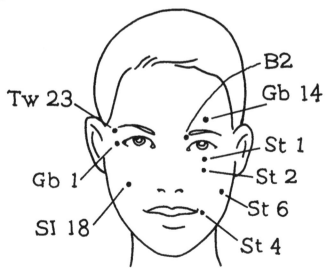

Fig. 66

3. (Gb 14, Whiteness of Yang) This point is one thumb width above your eyebrow, in line with the midpoint of the pupil when your eyes are looking straight in front of you. Push upward with the middle finger of each hand for about a minute.

4. (Tw 23, Silken Bamboo Hollow) This point is located at the *outer* edge of the eyebrow, right on the eyebrow line. Feel for a natural depression. Again, press for about a minute, on both sides at the same time, with your middle fingers.

5. (Gb 1, Pupil Crevice) From the outside of the eyebrow let your fingers drop down even with the outside of the eye socket. Slowly move the skin over the skull and you will feel a pronounced depression. Press firmly with the middle fingers of each hand. Apply pressure slightly upward and outward.

6. (St 1, Contain Tears) Place your middle finger just below the eye socket, in line with the center of the pupils. Now gently roll up on the pads of your fingers until you feel the ridge of the bone of the eye socket. With gentle sideways movement you should feel a small notch in the bone. St 1 is located at this notch. Press straight in toward the bone. *Use gentle pressure on this point.* (You won't be able to work on this point with long fingernails.)

The next set of points is to tighten and lift the cheeks.

7. (St 2, Four Whites) Located directly beneath the pupil and below St 1 (point 6 above). It is just about at the level of the upper border of the nostrils. Use the middle two fingers of each hand to press straight in.

8. (St 4, Earth Granary) This point is just outside the corner of the lips, in the groove that is formed when you smile. You can press straight in with your index finger.

9. (St 6, Jawbone) To find this point, clench your teeth, and find the center of the muscle that bulges at the jaw. Relax, and press where the center of the bulge was. Press with the index and middle fingers of each hand for about a minute.

10. (Si 18, Cheek Bone Crevice) Drop straight down from the outside edge of the eye socket, until you are on the lower border of the cheek bone. There is a natural depression there. Press straight in with the middle finger of each hand. Use medium pressure and hold for about a minute before releasing.

REFLEXOLOGY

As we've emphasized, beauty is a natural result of a healthy body. Reflexologist Laura Norman writes (in her book, *Feet First*):

> "My clients who look at themselves in the mirror after a session are always pleased at how good they look. Dark circles and puffiness under the eyes disappear or fade. Tension lines and general tiredness are gone. . . . Usually the skin glows. And the reason has nothing to do with magic or miracles. It's really quite simple: a relaxed face looks more beautiful; and when circulation is improved, the skin takes on a healthy glow."

The following Reflexology sequence will help bring out your natural beauty by promoting relaxation and clear, healthy skin.

1. We suggest that you start off with the Reflexology Warm-Up in the box on page 69. This is an important step that helps you relax, tones the energy of the whole body, and prepares your feet to be worked on; please don't skip it!

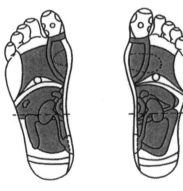

Fig. 67

2. The thyroid regulates metabolism and the building of skin cells. It also affects our energy level. Many people with low thyroid hormones feel tired and sluggish much of the time, and do not exude the vitality we usually associate with beauty. Work the reflex zone for the thyroid gland (it goes in a circle around the base of the big toe) and the thyroid "helper" below it by rubbing and pressing. The finger walk technique may be helpful here.

3. Oxygen is vital not just for energy and metabolism, but for healthy skin. To open up the chest and facilitate deeper breathing, thumb walk the chest and lung reflex zones on the ball of the foot (between the diaphragm line and the base of the toes).

4. Also work the top of your foot, in the solid part of the foot, above the toes. Work up from the webbing toward your leg, in the troughs between the toes. Work this area with your index finger, using the finger walk. This area may be quite tender.

5. To promote healthy digestion and the elimination of toxins, work the entire area on the bottom of your foot from the diaphragm line (across the ball of the foot) to the pelvic line (at the end of the arch and beginning of the heel). Thumb walk up, down, and diagonally. In this way you will stimulate the stomach, liver, kidneys, large and small intestines, adrenals, and gall bladder.

ADDITIONAL SUGGESTIONS

Most beauty problems that appear on the skin have their origins within. Unhealthy diet, inefficient breathing, clogged innards, stress, all contribute. This book contains numerous suggestions for avoiding these problems and unfolding your natural beauty by becoming more vibrantly healthy and free of disease. In particular, please look at the recommendations in the "Daily Health Builder" section; "Skin Problems" (which helps you to avoid and heal them); and the 11 Guidelines for Good Health starting on page 77 (Chapter 8).

Also, please see the Resources section for helpful books on natural beauty treatments from the Oriental and Ayurvedic perspectives.

Here are a few more suggestions:

HERBS TO PURIFY THE BLOOD.   All sorts of skin blemishes are due to impurities in the blood. Good herbal blood purifiers include red clover, burdock root, dandelion root, and gotu kola. These herbs cleanse the blood and promote growth of healthy new skin. You can take capsules or make a tea of any of them and drink two or three times a day.

REDUCE STRESS.   One of the greatest causes of wrinkles and other signs of premature aging is stress. Reduce your stress with regular exercise, meditation or relaxation techniques, getting enough rest, and doing more things that you enjoy, such as listening to or making music, dancing, being out in nature, art projects, and whatever makes you happy. As Letha Hadady, D. Ac. writes in her book, *Asian Health Secrets*, meditation helps to "restore the nerves and clear the emotions. This cultivates an inner calm that leads to beauty. Have you even seen an edgy Buddha, or one with wrinkles?"

CLEAN UP YOUR DIET.   Several kinds of food are almost guaranteed to adversely affect your skin. In particular, a diet rich in fatty and sugary foods increases acidity, clogs the system, and weakens circulation. Heavy foods, such as meats, fried foods, and most dairy products such as cheese, yogurt, butter, and ice cream, weaken digestion and elimination, and promote congestion. Spicy foods may irritate the skin and cause redness or acne.

Breastfeeding Problems

The benefits of breastfeeding are so numerous that countless books have been written about it. Not surprisingly, Mother Nature has set things up so that breastfeeding provides infants with exactly the nutrients they need. Immunity is improved, growth is enhanced, and the likelihood of inheriting family illnesses such as asthma or allergies is reduced. Brain development proceeds normally, resulting in rapid intellectual growth and fewer learning problems. And the psychological benefits of the close nurturing and bonding provided by the nursing experience are still being revealed.

Mom benefits too—not just from the deep emotional bonding, but also from various hormones released during breastfeeding, such as oxytocin which helps the uterus return to its pre-pregnancy shape. Her body's iron stores are conserved, and her chances of developing breast cancer and osteoporosis in later years are significantly reduced.

Several problems can occur when nursing an infant, such as sore or infected nipples. Our focus here will be on the most common problem, which is insufficient lactation. The following pressure points will encourage milk production.

1. (St 18, Breast Root) This key point promotes and regulates lactation. There are 2 easy steps to locating it. First, find the notch at the bottom of the breastbone, in the center of your chest. The "breast root" point is located at this level (between the 5th and 6th ribs), but several inches out from the center of the chest. Second, measure 4 thumb widths on either side of the center of the breast bone. The points are below and underneath the breast. **Caution:** You are pressing below (underneath) the breast, not pressing down through the breast tissue.

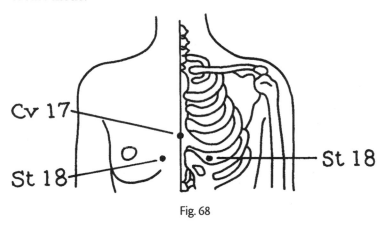

Fig. 68

2. (Cv 17, Chest Center) This point is on the Conception Vessel meridian, which is powerfully *yin* or female in nature. It is located right in the center of the chest, on the breastbone, about 3 finger widths or 2 thumb widths up from the bottom of the bone. Hold your index, middle, and ring finger together and press on this point for about 1 minute. Use medium pressure; this point is often tender. Remember to breathe slowly and deeply.

For the next two points, please see page 49 for the beginning of "Ten Master Pressure Points," for descriptions of the points and instructions for locating and effectively pressing them. Also see Fig. 70 on page 141.

3. (Sp 6, Three Yin Meeting) Located at the crossing point of the three *yin* meridians of the leg (Spleen, Liver, and Kidney), this is one of the most important Acupressure points. Since it strengthens the overall *yin* of the body by simultaneously stimulating the *yin* of the meridians, it is very beneficial in nourishing the body during lactation.

4. (Lv 3, Bigger Rushing) This point helps nourish the fluids of the body. It also has a direct effect on the breasts as the Liver meridian passes through them.

REFLEXOLOGY

Though you will be pressing on specific parts of the foot to enhance milk production and balance your hormones, it will be helpful to begin by massaging your feet and relaxing them (and yourself!) with the Reflexology Warm-Up in the box on page 69. This is an important step that tones the energy of the whole body, and prepares your feet to be worked on; please don't skip it!

The primary focus for this session will be your chest area and the reflex zones for your breasts, as well as the pituitary gland (the body's master gland for hormone regulation) and your kidney reflex, to help regulate the body's water level.

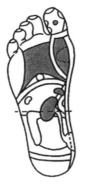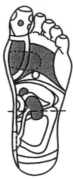

Fig. 69

1. The reflex zone for the chest area is on the ball of your foot (between the diaphragm line and the base of the toes). Pull the toes back with one hand, and work this area with the thumb of the other hand. Use the thumb walk technique. Work slowly up the foot, covering the area well.

2. Specific reflexes for the mammary glands are located on *top* of your foot. Work up from the webbing toward your leg, in the troughs between the toes. Start in zone 1—at the base of the big toe, and go up about 2 inches. Continue working each zone, ending in zone 5 near the outside edge of your foot. Work this area with your index finger, using the finger walk. This area may be quite tender—like the breasts themselves—so don't press too hard.

3. The pituitary gland is of vital importance, as it regulates all the body's hormones as well as the secretion of milk by the mammary glands. The reflex area for the pituitary gland is in the center of the big toe. Use the "hook and back up" technique for pinpoint accuracy on the pituitary reflex. (See page 68.)

4. At the kidney and adrenal reflexes, in the soft center of the foot, use the thumb walk.

SHIATSU

In this sequence, we are going to enliven two channels intimately connected with lactation, the Liver and Spleen meridians. Use the press and release technique. Press for 6–7 seconds, release, move half an inch to an inch along the channel, and press again.

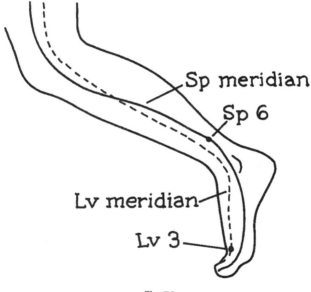

Fig. 70

To stimulate the Liver meridian, start in the center of the top of your big toe. Progress along the toe to the web margin between the big toe and second toe, then move up the channel between the big toe and second toe. From the ankle, the channel proceeds up the inside part of the leg, along the bone. Use only mild to moderate pressure along the bone. About halfway up the leg the meridian comes off the bone and continues up the middle of the inside of the leg. Above the knee, the pathway travels slightly higher than the middle of the inside portion of your thigh. Stop at the groin. On the thigh above the knee, you can use strong pressure.

The Spleen meridian also starts at the big toe. The first point is very close to the nail cuticle at the inside corner of the big toenail. From there, the meridian follows along the side of the big toe bone, at the inside of the foot, up the side of the ankle and the inside of the leg. Along the leg it follows just below the bone. Use the press and release technique from the big toe to just below the knee.

When you are finished with one foot and leg, be sure to repeat the entire procedure on the other side.

ADDITIONAL SUGGESTIONS

GET ENOUGH REST. Even if you are able to stay home with your infant child, your "schedule" will be constantly disrupted by late night feedings and diaper changes. This is exacerbated by job demands and other family responsibilities. Be careful not to burn out. Stress not only reduces lactation, it also changes your body chemistry, which will affect the quality of your milk. So get help from your partner or older children, or from friends and other relatives. Take naps. As much as you can, cut down on your work schedule.

DIET IS CRUCIAL. It is important to eat nourishing food. Avoid junk foods, as well as meat, canned and processed foods, and hot, spicy dishes which can make the milk taste bitter.

AVOID TOXINS. In addition to junk foods, avoid excess sweets, foods high in residues from pesticides, herbicides, and antibiotics (such as meats and fatty dairy products), alcohol, tobacco, and other toxins. Don't forget that what comes out in mother's milk reflects what goes into her mouth.

DRINK A LOT. You need plenty of liquids each day to replace the fluids used in making the milk.

MEDITATE TO MAINTAIN SERENITY. Anxiety and tension tend to reduce milk production. To help you keep calm and relaxed in the midst of all your work and family responsibilities, we strongly recommend that you meditate, close your eyes and listen to soothing music, or use whatever relaxation technique works best for you.

It is best to receive meditation instruction from a qualified teacher. Try to take care of this *before* you are nursing! To help you right now, see the meditation instructions in the Anxiety chapter, under "Additional Suggestions."

LEARN THE BASICS.   Although there is nothing more natural than breastfeeding, doing it right is not instinctive. Every new mother can benefit from advice from an experienced mother, or a doctor, nurse, or other expert about how to hold and position the infant, how to help the child take the nipple, and other subtle aspects of successful nursing. Be sure to learn these *before* you need them!

Caution. If you run a fever or have flu-like symptoms, and if your breast feels inflamed, you may have mastitis, a type of breast infection. You need to see a doctor.

Breathing Difficulties

See "Asthma"

Circulatory Problems

Imagine the difference between a vibrantly rushing stream and one that has been slowed to a crawl by debris cluttering the stream bed. Once the flow is blocked, muddy gunk accumulates and unwanted growth takes root in the sluggish side eddies. Just as the sluggish stream creates a breeding ground for unhealthy conditions, blocked flow of *ch'i* in our body eventually leads to discomfort and disease.

In Oriental medicine, stagnation is considered the cause of most illness. Stress, overwork, lack of sleep, irregular schedule, overeating, and emotional ups and downs all contribute to the disruption of the smooth flow of *ch'i*. Since *ch'i* is the commander of the blood, stagnation of the *ch'i* can easily lead to disruption of blood circulation. Therefore to stimulate better circulation, it is important to remove obstructions to the free flow of *ch'i*. Unblocking the obstructions helps to return the entire system to a state of greater health and better balance.

The following points strongly break up *ch'i* stagnation as well as directly improve circulation of the blood.

ACUPRESSURE

For thorough descriptions and illustrations of the points in this section, as well as instructions for how to press them most effectively, please see page 49 for the beginning of "Ten Master Pressure Points." If you already know how to work with them, here is a pictorial reminder:

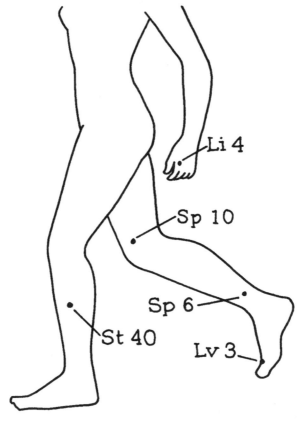

Fig. 71

1. (Lv 3, Bigger Rushing) Don't be surprised if this point is tender. Often, stagnation of any type is reflected here.

Lv 3 is considered to be the source point of the Liver meridian, and is used to help stimulate the Liver energy to do its main job, which is to keep all the *ch'i* in the body flowing smoothly. When the Liver energy goes out of balance, it can cause stagnation and imbalance everywhere else.

This is the most effective point for regulating the flow of *ch'i* throughout the body. It is an important point to include in a daily routine. If you were to choose just one point to stimulate every day, this would be a worthwhile candidate.

2. (Li 4, Adjoining Valley) We are recommending this key point because of its ability to circulate *ch'i* throughout the whole system.

3. (Sp 6, Three Yin Meeting) Located at the crossing point of the three *yin* meridians of the leg (Spleen, Liver, and Kidney), this is one of the most important Acupressure points. It nourishes the overall *yin* of the body by simultaneously nourishing the *yin* of the meridians. It also helps move the liver *ch'i* throughout the body. **Caution:** This point should be avoided by pregnant women.

4. (Sp 10, Sea of Blood) This is the main point in Oriental medicine for breaking up blood stagnation.

5. *Optional.* If you have time, add another point (St 40, Abundant Splendor) also described in the "Ten Master Pressure Points" section beginning on page 49.

SHIATSU

The following exercises will help open the channels through breathing and the stretching of the body along key meridian pathways.

1. Start by standing with your feet shoulder width apart. Let your arms hang loosely at your sides. With deep, slow inhalation, slowly lift your arms over your head, then turn your palms to face the ceiling, with the fingertips pointing together. On the exhalation, lower your arms until they are again loose at your sides. Continue these movements for 3–5 minutes. If your balance is good, raise your heels off the ground as you lift your arms. Stretching the arms above you and standing on the toes helps open the channels and improves circulation of the *ch'i*.

2. Place your right foot in front of you at a 45 degree angle from the left foot. (Your feet should still be shoulder width apart.) Let most of your weight shift forward to the right foot. Stretch your right arm out in line with the right leg, and stretch your left arm out behind you. Your right hand should be level with the top of your head, your left arm stretched down towards the ground.

Now bend your right wrist back as far as you can, with the fingers pointing to the left, not up toward the ceiling. Bend your left wrist at the same time, so that the fingers are pointing down and toward your right foot. Hold this position for 15 to 30 seconds.

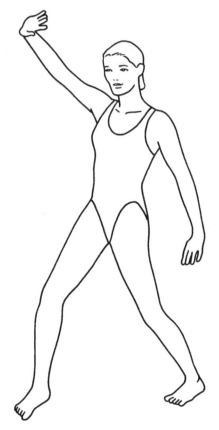

Fig. 72—Shiatsu Standing Stretch

Now switch sides and repeat the exercise, with your left arm lifted and right arm pointing downward.

Breathe evenly throughout the exercise.

Repeat the exercise again, and continue to repeat for a total of 3 to 5 minutes.

This sequence serves multiple functions. Not only does it exercise and strengthen the legs, but it also stimulates the Heart meridian. Since the Heart meridian runs along the little finger side of the arm, it gets stretched and opened by these positions.

If you want a little more active version of the exercise, hold the position for only 5 seconds, then switch to the other arm. Again, make the exercise last at least 3-5 minutes.

ADDITIONAL SUGGESTIONS

HERBAL HELP.   The herb hawthorn berry is used in Chinese medicine to decrease cholesterol levels. If your circulatory problems are due to clogged blood vessels caused by high cholesterol, this herb may help.

GET MOVING.   Exercise is always helpful for improving circulation, which may become more stagnant due to a sedentary lifestyle. Walking for half an hour a day is good for everyone; try more strenuous exercise if you are inclined to do so and are fit for it. If you are over 40 and just about to begin an exercise program, it is wise to consult your physician.

YOGA STRETCHING.   One of the best all-round exercises for improving circulation to all parts of the body is the Sun Salutation. The Shoulder Stand is also helpful.

Colds

That all-too-familiar bout of sneezing, sniffling, runny nose, and coughing attacks all of us sooner or later. So far, medical science has found no cure for the cold virus. The vast array of cold medicines can do little more than reduce your symptoms, and many have undesirable side effects. The following pressure point recommendations, plus the "Additional Suggestions" at the end of the section, may help to relieve your symptoms, without any side effects. Plus, they can help to revitalize your immune system and harmonize the flow of *Ch'i* in your body, helping to speed your recovery.

ACUPRESSURE

Several of the following points (Li 4, Gb 20, Li 11) are among the most powerful (and thus most commonly prescribed) in Acupressure. For thorough descriptions and location illustrations for these points, as well as instructions on how to press them most effectively, please see page 49 for the beginning of "Ten Master Pressure Points."

    1. (Li 4, Adjoining Valley) This point is beneficial for many cold symptoms, including headaches and congestion. **Important:** Pregnant women should NOT press on this point, as it may stimulate contractions in the uterus.

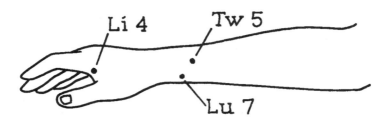

Fig. 73

    2. (Lu 7, Broken Sequence) Hold one hand out in front of you with the palm facing down. Start from the V shape formed by your thumb and index finger. Use the index finger of the other hand to trace along the top of the thumb to the wrist. Your finger will fall into a natural depression where the base of your thumb joins the wrist. Keep going another inch and a half and you will be on Lu 7. It is used here for its powerful effect on the lungs. Maintain firm pressure (you can use your thumb or index finger) for about a minute, then switch hands.

    3. (Gb 20, Wind Pool) Acupuncture and Acupressure practitioners use this key point as part of every prescription for colds.

    4. (B 12, Wind Door) and (B 13, Lung Associated Point) These points are used to help expel the cold in Chinese medicine. Using these points at the very earliest signs of a cold will help prevent it from settling in. The B 13 point also helps energize the Lung *ch'i.*

These two points are located on both sides of the spine, at just about the level of the top of your shoulder blades. First reach over your shoulders and press with your fingers on both sides of your spine about 1-½ inches from the spine. Use firm pressure for about a minute.

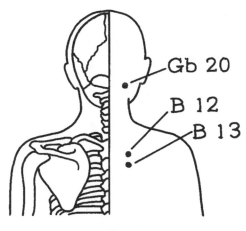

Fig. 74

Next, lie down on a carpeted floor with two tennis balls placed between your shoulder blades and the spine. (If you put them in a sock they'll stay in place and won't roll around.) Hold about 1-½ minutes, then move slightly to redirect the pressure. Relax for another minute and a half. While lying down, put your fingers below your collarbone and press about 2 inches on either side of the breast bone. This point helps stop coughing and soothes the lungs.

What type of cold do you have? Chinese medicine differentiates between two major types of colds, based on whether or not signs of heat are present. Heat signs include fever (as opposed to little or no fever); raw sore throat (as opposed to just an itchy throat); yellow or green colored mucus (as opposed to clear or white mucus); sore and swollen glands; greater-than-normal thirst; and urine that is darker in color than normal. If you think you have a heat-type cold, then add the following two points to help clear away the heat.

5. (Tw 5, Outer Gate) Hold your arm in front of you with the palm down toward the floor. Measure two thumb widths above your wrist. The point is right in the center of the wrist, between the two bones. This point specifically aids in expelling colds of the heat type. Use medium to firm pressure for about a minute.

6. (Li 11, Pool at the Crook) Hold your arm in front of your chest, as if holding a cup in your hand. Li 11 is at the outside end of the crease on your arm at the elbow joint. Hold your left hand close to your chest and use firm pressure with your right thumb; then switch arms. (See page 50.)

REFLEXOLOGY

1. Before you treat specific reflex areas for your cold, begin with the Reflexology Warm-Up in the box on page 69. This sequence of steps helps you relax, tones the energy of the whole body, and prepares your feet to be worked on; please don't skip it!

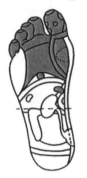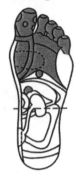

Fig. 75

2. Begin specific treatment for your cold by working the lungs and chest. Slowly thumb walk the chest and lung reflex zones on the ball of both feet (between the diaphragm line and the base of the toes). Then finger walk the chest and lymph gland reflexes on the top of the feet, in the channels between the toe bones.

3. Thumb walk the bronchial area starting between the big and second toe and curving around the ball of the foot.

4. The toes contain the reflex areas for the head, so you will want to spend as much time as you can working the bottom of all the toes, to open up the sinus cavities and nasal passages for better breathing. Thumb walk up and down the bottom of the big toe, being sure to cover the entire area. (It will take several "trips.") Thumb walk down the smaller toes, two or three times for each toe.

5. While you are there, walk across the ridge at the base of the toes, which is the reflex area for the neck, as well as the eyes and ears. To do this successfully, it helps if you pull the pad of the foot downward with your "holding" hand. Then go around the base of the big toe to work on the throat reflex.

6. The pituitary gland located right in the center of the pad of the big toe is a key to health. This "master gland" not only regulates the secretion of hormones, it also controls body temperature and metab-

olism, governs energy level, and has hundreds if not thousands of other functions. To press on this point, it is best to use the "hook and back up" technique described on page 68.

7. Return to the solar plexus point and use the thumb press for another 30 seconds to facilitate relaxation of the chest muscles and easier breathing.

8. Finally, work the lower part of the foot as a whole, thumb walking up and down all 5 zones from the heel to the diaphragm line. This stimulates the internal organs, including digestion and elimination. Pay special attention to the adrenal gland reflexes; the adrenals produce hormones that are natural anti-inflammatories.

SHIATSU

Follow the sequence of pressure points described in the Acupressure section, starting on page 148. When you get to the point where you are lying on your back, stimulating B 12 and B 13 with the tennis balls, add the following:

Place your hands on your ribs. Spread your fingers out so that each finger is in the space between two ribs. Starting from the sides, slowly trace the rib spaces towards the breast bone. Use gentle but steady pressure. Then start at the breast bone and trace outwards.

Next place the fingers of both hands on the breast bone and slide down to about the nipple level. **Caution:** Attached to the lower end of the breast bone is a small piece of bone that feels springy and gives with pressure. Do *not* apply pressure at this spot. Be sure you are feeling the firm bone underneath your fingers before applying pressure.

Finally, trace along the bottom edge of the collar bone on each side.

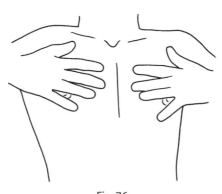

Fig. 76

ADDITIONAL SUGGESTIONS

TRY GINGER.   The best cold remedy is ginger. Drink a cup of hot ginger tea several times a day. Boil a few thin slices of fresh ginger, or use about ⅓ to ½ tsp. of powdered ginger per cup. Adding a little cinnamon will add to the heating quality.

ECHINACEA.   Another useful herb is echinacea, which you can take either as a tea or in tincture form; follow the directions on the bottle. Tablets are okay too.

VITAMIN C.   Vitamin C is generally quite helpful in speeding up recovery from a cold.

REST.   Be sure to get plenty of rest to help your system fight off the cold.

EAT LIGHTLY.   Avoid heavy foods such as meats and fatty foods; stay away from dairy products such as yogurt, cottage cheese, ice cream, and other milk products. Drink some hot or at least warm water several times a day.

YOGA POSTURES.   A few cycles of the Sun Salutation will stimulate circulation of blood and energy in the body and promote elimination of toxins. You might also try the Shoulder Stand and Plow, as well as the Lion pose, which helps relieve sore throat.

KEEP YOUR NECK WARM.   In Oriental medicine, the back of the neck is considered the part of the body most vulnerable to exposure to cold. As a preventative measure in cold or drafty conditions, be sure to use a scarf or turned up collar to keep this area warm.

Constipation

Occasional constipation is not a serious problem, but chronically sluggish bowels, causing infrequent or irregular elimination, may lead to more serious consequences such as fatigue, headaches, depression, and the re-absorption of toxins into the system. Experts generally agree that the main cause of constipation is faulty diet, especially insufficient high-fiber foods such as fruit, vegetables, and whole grains. Inadequate intake of liquids may also contribute. Other causes include insufficient exercise and stress (especially worry and anxiety). A very large number of medications, ranging from antibiotics and antidepressants to antihypertensives, produce constipation as a side effect, so if you are frequently constipated, see if a medication you are taking may be the culprit.

ACUPRESSURE

1. (Cv 6, Sea of *Ch'i*) This point is about one and a half finger widths directly below the navel (see Fig. 80, on page 158, for Cv 6, St 25, and Cv 12). Place the middle finger of both hands there, and press inward with the fingertips of both hands to a depth of about an inch. Use moderate pressure and hold for a minute or two, breathing deeply.

As the name implies, this point nourishes the body's *ch'i* and helps circulate it throughout the body. You might try lying on your back to work this and the next three points. Start by taking a few deep breaths to relax.

Caution: Pregnant women should not use pressure on any abdominal points.

2. (St 25, Heavens Pivot) This point is located two thumb widths to the side of the belly button, on both sides (see Fig. 80). This is the most important point for treating a wide range of intestinal disorders. It is used for both constipation and diarrhea. Press on both sides at the same time, with medium to firm pressure for a minute. Use your middle fingers or thumbs, whichever feels more comfortable and effective.

3. (Cv 12, Middle Stomach) Find a notch at the bottom of your breast bone. Cv 12 is midway between this notch and your belly button (see Fig. 80). Use firm pressure for about a minute here; use thumb, middle finger, or middle on top of index.

The use of Cv 6, Cv 12 and St 25 is a famous combination in Chinese medicine known as the four doors. It can be used for any type of stomach or gastrointestinal distress including constipation or diarrhea.

4. (Tw 6, Branching Ditch) This point is on the back of your forearm. Go up 3 thumb widths from the wrist crease. Tw 6 is in the center, between the bones. Press firmly for about a minute after building up your pressure gradually.

One of the common causes of constipation is excess internal heat. This dries up the stool and makes it hard to pass. If you have some of the following signs this probably applies to you: reddish face, feeling thirsty a lot, dark yellow urine, tendency to irritability, or just feeling warm or hot frequently. If so, add the points below to help clear the excess heat. If not, just stick with the previous points.

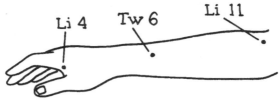

Fig. 77

5. (Lv 2, Moving Between) This point is in the webbing between the big toe and second toe. Use medium pressure with your index fingers, pressing on both feet at the same time if that is comfortable, otherwise one at a time (see Fig. 90 or Fig. G on page 40).

For the next two points, please see page 49 for the beginning of "Ten Master Pressure Points" for thorough descriptions and location illustrations, as well as suggestions on how to press them most effectively,

6. (Li 4, Adjoining Valley) Li 4 has many important functions, one of which is to clear heat.

7. (Li 11, Pool at the Crook) This point on the large intestine meridian clears heat in general from the body and helps regulate activity of the colon.

REFLEXOLOGY

1. Begin with the Reflexology Warm-Up in the box on page 69. This is an important short sequence of steps that helps you relax, tones the energy of the whole body, and prepares your feet to be worked on.

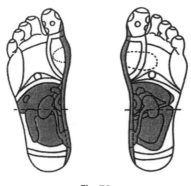

Fig. 78

2. Most of the reflex areas you will want to work on are in the lower part of the foot, between the diaphragm line and the heel. We suggest you spend at least 5 minutes on this area on each foot. Thumb walk up from the heel to the diaphragm line, down, horizontally across, and diagonally, covering the entire area from all directions. In this way you will stimulate the stomach, liver, gall bladder, adrenals, small intestines, and the various aspects of the colon (ascending, descending, transverse), influencing digestion and stimulating peristaltic action.

3. The lower spine contains the nerves that feed into the colon, so we recommend spending some time stimulating the spine reflexes, located on the inside edge of both feet (zone 1). They extend from the heel nearly to the top of the big toe, but our concern here is primarily with the lower spine, up to about the waist line of the foot.

When you work the spinal reflexes, work slowly up and then down the foot using the thumb walk technique. You will need a little extra strength on the thick skin of the heel.

4. You might wish to spend a little extra time working specifically on the colon reflexes. If you study the foot map (pages 45 and 46), you will notice that the reflexes for various aspects of the colon are divided between the two feet. The ascending colon reflex is located in zone 1 of the right foot while the descending colon reflex is in zone 1 of the left foot. The sigmoid colon reflex is on the left foot only, at about zone 3.5 just above the reflex for the sciatic nerve. Work these reflexes (and the transverse colon, which is on both feet just below the waist line) thoroughly and carefully.

SHIATSU

The following Shiatsu sequence is designed to help relieve your constipation by stimulating the Large Intestine (Li) and Stomach (St) meridians.

1. Start with the Li meridian (see Fig. 65 on page 131), at the tip of your index finger on the thumb side. Use the press and release technique: Press for 6–7 seconds, release, move a little way (maybe ½ inch) along the channel and press again. The meridian runs along the thumb side of the index finger bone. At the knuckle, press just under the bone on both sides of the knuckle, not on the knuckle itself.

From here the meridian continues along the side of the bone in the hand to Li 4 in the center of the web margin between the thumb and the index finger. Then it follows a line to the outer edge of the elbow crease.

To be sure you are on the right line, position your arm in front of you with the palm facing your stomach about 4–5 inches away from your body. Imagine the line drawn on your arm in this position. Press and release along the entire length of your forearm to the elbow. Be sure to do both hands and arms.

2. The beginning points of a meridian have a strong effect along the whole course of the channel. Since the Li meridian starts in the index finger, the following finger exercises will enliven the entire channel.

First make a loose fist with both hands. Now extend only your index finger. Trace small circles with your fingers. Start with both fingers moving in toward each other for about 15 seconds. Then reverse directions for another 15 seconds. Now bend the fingers up and down using the top two joints. Start with small movements and gradually increase the range of motion. Continue for 45 to 60 seconds.

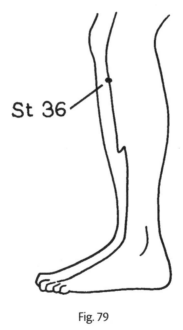

St 36

Fig. 79

3. Now go to your second toe, on the little toe side, and begin to use the press and release technique. The Stomach meridian runs between the 2nd and 3rd toes, across the top of the foot and the front of the ankle. From the ankle it continues up the front of the leg about 1 finger breadth to the little toe side of the shin bone. Stop just below the knee. Be sure to work on both legs.

ADDITIONAL SUGGESTIONS

Constipation can usually be relieved and prevented by using the above procedures and following a few simple guidelines.

DRINK ENOUGH. Make sure to drink enough liquid (6 to 8 glasses a day is best for most people).

EAT ENOUGH FIBER. Consuming sufficient fiber is a high priority. Eat whole grains, such as whole wheat bread, oatmeal, and brown rice. Make sure to have several portions of fresh fruit and vegetables every day. In fact, a high-fiber, largely vegetarian diet is your best dietary bet for constipation relief.

AVOID THESE CLOGGERS. Stay away from processed foods and grains, such as white bread, as much as you can. Eating a lot of meat can also clog you up.

EXERCISE. Get some daily exercise, at least 30 minutes a day. A brisk walk is sufficient for most people. Yoga stretching is helpful, and more dynamic aerobic activity if you are fit for it. The best Yoga for constipation is the Sun Salutation, a series of 12 movements that stretch the abdominal organs and get energy moving throughout the entire system. You can do up to 12 cycles of these postures, but do not strain. The Shoulder Stand, Forward Bend, and Cobra are also recommended.

Cough

See also, "Colds"

In Chinese medicine, coughing is said to occur due to a reversal of lung *ch'i*: Instead of its normal descending action, the lung *ch'i* rebels and moves upward. The two points described below are the best for soothing rebellious *ch'i* of the lungs. If your cough is part of an ordinary cold, please also see the section on "Colds." If you have smoker's cough, see page 159 for suggestions on how to soothe it. Of course, the best thing to do for smoker's cough is to quit smoking before a more serious disease develops.

ACUPRESSURE

1. (Lu 7, Broken Sequence) Hold one hand out in front of you with the palm facing down. Start from the V shape formed by your thumb and index finger. Use the index finger of the other hand to trace along the top of the thumb to the wrist. Your finger will fall into a natural depression where the base of your thumb joins the wrist. Keep going another inch and a half and you will be on Lu 7. Use your thumb to apply pressure. There's not much tissue between the skin and the bone here so mild to moderate pressure is enough. Be sure to switch hands and work the other side.

This point has the strongest effect of any point for descending Lung *ch'i*. It can be used not only for cough but for the common cold, sneezing, and stuffy or runny nose.

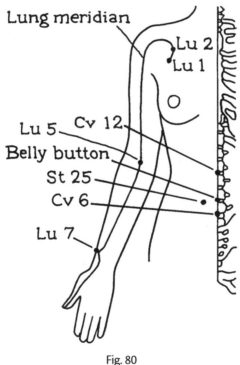

Fig. 80

2. (Cv 22, Heaven Projection) Place your middle or index finger in the "V" at the front of your neck, in the bony notch where the collar bones meet the breastbone. Don't press inward, as you could damage the wind-pipe. Press vertically down toward the bone, with a light pressure. Hold for

10 seconds, then lightly massage the area with downward strokes. This point is commonly used for its effect on descending the Lung *ch'i*. It also helps clear congestion from the throat.

If you have a lot of phlegm and mucus accompanying your cough, adding St 40 (Abundant Splendor) will help clear the congestion. For a description and location illustration of St 40, and guidance on how to press it most effectively, please see page 49 for the beginning of "Ten Master Pressure Points."

If you have smoker's cough, use the following point in addition to Lu 7 and Cv 22.

3. (Lu 5, Cubit Marsh) Let your right arm hang in front of you with the palm up. Put the fingertips of your left hand on the elbow crease (of the right arm). Keep your palm facing up and slowly raise your forearm. Feel for the tendon in the elbow crease that pops out as you raise the forearm. Lu 5 is in the elbow crease on the thumb side (with the palm up) of the tendon. Either the thumb or middle finger works well here. Use moderate to strong pressure. This point helps clear heat and moisten the throat.

REFLEXOLOGY

1. Before you treat specific reflex areas for your cough, begin with the Reflexology Warm-Up in the box on page 69. This is an important step that helps you relax, tones the energy of the whole body, and prepares your feet to be worked on; please don't skip it!

2. For treating coughs, the reflex areas described in the section on "colds" will be very helpful. We suggest that you emphasize the chest/lung area, the bronchial area, the sinus reflexes, and the throat and neck reflexes, as described in the following steps.

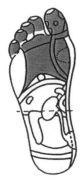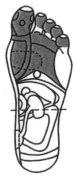

Fig. 81

3. To open up and energize healing in the lung and chest area, thumb walk the chest and lung reflex zones on the ball of the foot (between the diaphragm line and the base of the toes). Also finger walk the chest and lymph gland reflexes on the top of the foot.

4. Thumb walk the bronchial area starting between the big and second toe and curving around the ball of the foot.

5. To encourage drainage and healing in your sinuses, work on the bottom of your toes, especially the pads opposite the nail. Thumb walk up and down the bottom of the big toe, being sure to cover the entire area. (It will take several "trips.") Thumb walk down the smaller toes, two or three times for each toe.

6. Finish by working on the throat reflex, which is at the base of the big toe. Use the thumb walk.

SHIATSU

This procedure will help relieve your coughing by stimulating the Lung meridian. (See Fig. 80) You'll use the press and release technique, which works this way: press with firm pressure, hold for 6–7 seconds, and release. Then move up half an inch to an inch and repeat.

Start at the outside edge of your thumb, next to the cuticle. Move up the outside of the bone to the second knuckle (don't press on the knuckle itself, but only at the edges), and then move "inland," pressing in the fleshy part of the palm between the thumb and wrist. Use the press and release technique until you reach the wrist crease.

At the wrist crease, the meridian is located right where you would feel your pulse, but just off the artery to the thumb side. From this point on the wrist, imagine a straight line drawn up to the center of the elbow crease. The lung meridian follows this line. Continue pressing and releasing.

About 1-½ to 2 inches up from the wrist crease the meridian makes a slight jog to the outside and then comes back to our imaginary line. The slight jog is where Lu 7 is located (see description of point 1 in Acupressure section starting on page 158). Give some extra attention to Lu 7. Then continue pressing and releasing up to the elbow crease.

At the elbow crease, give extra stimulation to Lu 5. It is in the center of the elbow crease, but on the thumb side of the large stringy tendon in the center of the crease.

Continue up towards the top of the shoulder. As you move up the arm you are on the outside of the biceps. If you curve your fingers over the top of the biceps muscle, "make a muscle" and slowly move your arm up and down at the elbow joint, you'll feel a depression below the top of the biceps. Its about ⅓ of the way from the top of the biceps to the back of the arm. Remember, we're on the outside side of the arm. The Lung meridian follows this groove up to the top of the shoulder, then circles back across the top of the shoulder to Lu 1. Lu 1 and Lu 2 are in the crease above the armpit, between the chest muscle (pecs) and the shoulder muscle (deltoid). End with 1–2 minutes of pressure on Lu 1.

ADDITIONAL SUGGESTIONS

1. Most of the recommendations made for colds apply to coughs as well, so please check that section. If your cough persists longer than a week, it would be wise to see a doctor.

2. Yoga postures. Inverted poses help to drain the mucus that is one of the major causes of cough. Try the Shoulder Stand and/or Plow. The Fish is also helpful; it stretches the throat area.

Daily Health Builder

Pressure point therapies are valuable not only as a means to heal existing conditions, but as a preventive measure, to strengthen the body's immunity, reduce stress, and build up vitality and resistance to disease. Use the techniques in this section to gain those results!

ACUPRESSURE

The points we recommend on the next pages will help to move and circulate the *ch'i* and produce an overall strengthening effect on the whole body. Together they stimulate *yin* and *yang*, the *ch'i*, and the blood.

The first four points (Lv 3, Kd 3, Sp 6, and St 36) are among the most powerful and important in Acupuncture and Acupressure. They are thoroughly described starting on page 49, "Ten Master Pressure Points," where you will find illustrations showing the points and how to press them most effectively.

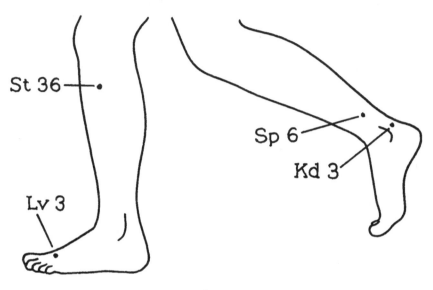

Fig. 82

1. (Lv 3, Bigger Rushing) This is the most powerful point for harmonizing and regulating the flow of *ch'i* throughout the body. It is the source point of the Liver meridian and helps stimulate the Liver energy to do its main job, which is to keep all the *ch'i* in the body flowing smoothly. If you had to choose just one single point to stimulate every day, this would be a worthwhile candidate.

2. (Kd 3, Supreme Stream) The importance of the Kidney energy in Chinese medicine cannot be overstated. It is thought to be the root of the yin and yang of the entire body. Kd 3, as the source point for the Kidney meridian, exerts a powerful strengthening effect, which gives support and nourishment to all the other energy systems of the body.

3. (Sp 6, Three Yin Meeting) Located at the crossing point of the three *yin* meridians of the leg (Spleen, Liver, and Kidney), this powerful

point nourishes the *yin* of the entire body. It also helps move the liver *ch'i* throughout the body and reinforces the effect of Lv 3 (see number 1 of this list). **Caution:** Pregnant women should not press this point.

4. (St 36, Three Mile Foot) This is the most effective point to nourish and strengthen the *ch'i* and blood. Legend has it that soldiers in China relied on this point to sustain themselves when exhausted or weakened by lack of food. In combination with Sp 6 (above), it strongly revitalizes the entire body.

5. (Lu 1, Central Residence) Place 4 fingers on the armpit crease next to the shoulder muscle (deltoid). You will feel a groove between the chest muscle (pecs) and the deltoid. You'll be able to feel this more clearly under your fingers if you slowly raise the shoulder up and down once or twice. The point is in this groove at the level of the space between the 1st and 2nd rib. (See Fig. 80)

Don't worry if you can't tell one rib from another! Because you will be using the middle three fingers to stimulate this area, you can be a little inexact on the point location and still be over the point with one of the three fingers. Apply steady, moderate to strong pressure 1–3 minutes. This point has an energizing effect on the Lung energy. If it is very tender start with less pressure.

REFLEXOLOGY

The best use of Reflexology as a daily health builder is to spend a few minutes working all the major reflex areas. Rather than repeat ourselves, we will simply refer you to the section in Chapter 7 entitled, "How to Use Reflexology for Prevention and Health," beginning on page 69. It provides a detailed, step-by-step program you can use every day (or as often as you like) to build better health.

When you have finished the sequence, we suggest that you make a quiet, reflective inventory of your health and note how you feel. If you have any health problems or concerns, spend a few minutes consulting the "map" of reflex zones and working on the appropriate areas on your feet.

Don't forget that you can also work the corresponding reflex areas on your hands, though most people find working on the feet more effective. Consult the master drawings of the hands on pages 47 and 48.

SHIATSU

The following traditional sequence of techniques can be used either in the morning after waking up, or before going to bed at night. You can use all of them, if you have time, or select the items that seem more attractive or important to you.

1. *Tap your teeth.* With your lips lightly closed, tap your upper and lower teeth together 30 to 40 times.

2. *Rub your hands.* Rub your palms vigorously together. Start slowly and pick up speed. Rub 30 to 40 times until they become quite warm. Immediately proceed to #3.

3. *Touch your face.* With hands still warm, touch your face on the left side, up and across the forehead, and down the right side. Repeat 7 or 8 times. Then go the opposite way 7 or 8 times—up the right side, across the forehead, and down the left side.

4. *Massage your eye sockets.* Using the first knuckle (nearest the fingertip) of the index, middle, and ring fingers, rub across the eye sockets at the eyebrow. Start at the bridge of the nose and move to the outer edge. Repeat 7 or 8 times. Then go the opposite way 7 or 8 times.

5. *Brighten your eyes.* Locate the point on your temples, about ½ to 1 inch from the outer edge of the eye socket, in an indentation. With the middle finger of both hands, massage these points with a rotary motion. Go in one direction 7 or 8 times and then reverse.

6. *Massage your forehead.* Place both middle fingers at the "third eye" point between the eyebrows. Move both fingers outward, toward the temples. Come back to the center, but a little bit higher, and repeat the outward swipe. In this way, slowly move up to the hairline.

7. *Massage your ears.* Place your palms over your ears, with the 4 fingers at the back of your head. Rapidly and rhythmically rotate the palms over the ears 30 to 40 times.

8. *Tap on your skull.* With your hands in the same position (palms firmly over the ears, fingers at the back of the head), begin to tap on the back of the skull with the index and middle fingers of both hands. Tap about 20 times.

9. *Slap your chest.* With palms open, slap your chest with the fingers of both hands. Slap 7 or 8 times. Women, slap the upper chest, above the breasts only.

10. *Rub your sides.* With open palms, and especially with the meaty part of the palm beneath the thumbs, rub both flanks (your sides) from armpit to waist. Rub up and down rapidly about 30 to 40 times.

11. *Massage your abdomen.* Place your left hand on your abdomen, palm over the navel; place your right hand on top of the left. Then push in firmly and rotate in a clockwise direction, 30 to 40 times. (This exercise is good to do sitting on your knees, back straight, if you can do it comfortably.) Don't do this after eating!

12. *Rub your back.* With your hands made into fists, use the knuckles of both hands to rub up and down your lower back on both sides of the spine. Rub rapidly and firmly about 30 to 40 times.

13. *Tap along your spine.* With your hands still in loose fists, use the back of the hand to lightly tap along the edges of the spine, from as high up as you can reach, down to the sacrum. Tap downward and upward 3 or 4 times.

14. *Rub your thighs.* While sitting use both palms to rapidly rub your left thigh 30 or 40 times, then your right thigh.

15. *Grasp your calves.* Sitting cross legged, grasp the calf muscle of your left leg with your hands, and work down from below the knee all the way to the ankle, including the Achilles tendon as you go. Then do the same with your right calf.

16. *Energize.* In Oriental medicine, the kidney is the storehouse of *Ch'i* or Life Energy. The Kidney meridian starts on the bottom of the foot, about one third of the way down from your toes and just about in the center of the sole. With the edge of your palm, rub rapidly and strongly over this point 30 to 40 times, until the center of the foot begins to feel warm. First do the left foot, then the right.

ADDITIONAL SUGGESTIONS

1. *Meditate.* One of the best things you can do on a daily basis to ensure good health is to meditate. It helps you relax, relieve stress, and revitalize from within. For information and simple instructions for meditation, please turn to the "Additional Suggestions" section in the chapter on Anxiety. (Page 104.)

2. Daily Yoga stretching, tai chi, or qi gong will help greatly to create and maintain excellent health. One Yoga exercise that uses all the major

muscles and stimulates all the internal organs, as well as putting pressure on the meridians and dozens of pressure points, is the Sun Salutation. We recommend doing it daily.

3. We also suggest you review the 11 Simple, Universal Guidelines for Good Health at the end of Chapter 8, starting on page 77.

Depression

Just about everyone has the blues sometimes. It's quite normal to feel sad and low for a while after we suffer a loss, or when things don't work out as we hoped and planned. Internal conflicts and indecisions can also sap our strength and lower our mood. Cyclical hormonal patterns can take us on a roller coaster ride, with the lows sometimes quite low.

But clinical depression—when our dark mood lingers for weeks or months—is something different.

When we are truly depressed, life loses its charm. Nothing matters; nothing seems to be working out. Energy is low, decisions are difficult to make, and even simple everyday tasks feel overwhelming. Everything looks flat, bleak, and gray and we tend to focus only on the negative side of things, seeing the worst in ourself, our life, our friends, our accomplishments, our prospects.

According to Western medicine, there are three basic causes of depression.

- *External causes* such as the death of someone close to us, serious financial problems, a prolonged stressful situation, etc.
- *Biological causes,* including chemical imbalances in the brain and nervous system, and/or a genetic predisposition to depression, just like the tendency to develop a physical illness such as diabetes.
- *Psychological causes* such as, in Freud's words, "anger turned inward." If you are frustrated and angry long enough without expressing it, you may turn the anger inward against yourself, and end up depressed.

In Chinese medicine, depression is usually associated with *ch'i* stagnation, especially in the Liver channel. The East has long understood the intimate, reciprocal connection between emotional health and the healthy functioning of the body. Feelings of depression—whatever their origin— cause the vital energy to become stuck, and obstruct its smooth flow. Conversely, lack of smooth flow of the *ch'i* in the meridians can adversely impact the emotions.

We have a similar expression in the West—we refer to someone's emotions as being "stuck." To heal this situation, pressure point therapy aims to move the *ch'i*, to unblock it, and also to raise or lift the *ch'i*. Does the expression "lift your spirits" sound familiar?

ACUPRESSURE

For Acupressure self-treatment, we recommend a combination of points that are excellent for circulating *ch'i* through the entire system, another combination to "lift the spirits," and a final point specific for healing emotional problems.

The first two points (Li 4 and Lv 3) are fully described in the section, "Ten Master Pressure Points" (beginning on page 49) where you will also find pinpoint illustrations of the point locations and suggestions on how to press them for maximum benefit.

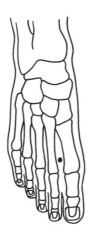

Fig. 83—Lv 3

1. (Li 4, Adjoining Valley) **Important:** Pregnant women should NOT use this point, as it may stimulate premature contractions in the uterus.

2. (Lv 3, Bigger Rushing).

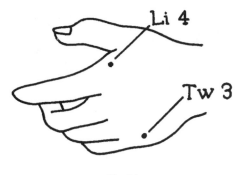

Fig. 84

3. (Tw 3, Middle Islet) This point is on the back of the hand, in the channel between the little finger and 4th finger. To work on your left hand, slide the fingers of your right hand up from the fingers toward the wrist. Find a depression about halfway between the knuckles and the wrist (on some people it will be slightly closer to the fingers) and press with your index finger for about a minute. Then switch hands.

4. (Gv 20, Hundred Meetings) This point gets its name because all the *yang* channels of the body meet here. It is located at the top of the head, midway between the tips of the ears. If you were drawing a "map," one line would go straight up from the center of your ears, the other straight along a line running along the midline of your head from front to back, with the point where the two lines cross. Use medium pressure. Let the middle fingers of each hand meet together at the point, and press with both fingers for 1 to 2 minutes.

REFLEXOLOGY

1. Before you treat specific reflex areas for depression, begin with the Reflexology Warm-Up on page 69. This is an important step that helps you relax, tones the energy of the whole body, and prepares your feet to be worked on; please don't skip it!

Now you are ready to work directly on reflex areas that can help you dissolve your depression.

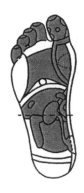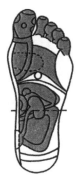

Fig. 85

2. The liver can be a source of stagnant energy leading to feelings of depression. To stimulate the liver, small intestines, stomach, and other internal organs, work the entire area in the arch of your foot, from the pelvic line up to the diaphragm line. Use the thumb walk to thoroughly cover this area, moving up, down, and/or diagonally. Pay special attention to the large liver area on the right foot.

3. At the kidney and adrenal reflexes (also in the soft center of the foot) use the "rotation on a point" technique. (See page 68.)

4. Many people with low thyroid hormones feel tired and sluggish much of the time. We recommend working the reflex zone for the thyroid gland (around the base of the big toe) by rubbing and pressing. The finger walk technique may be helpful here.

5. If you have observed people who are depressed, you have probably noticed that their posture is often stooped, as if they are carrying the weight of the world on their shoulders. If you investigated, you would probably find their breathing quite shallow. Shallow breathing doesn't bring in enough oxygen to energize the body, so a kind of vicious cycle is created. To open up the lung and chest area, thumb walk the chest and lung reflex zones on the ball of the foot (between the diaphragm line and the base of the toes). You can also finger walk the chest and lymph gland reflexes on the top of the foot. And take some deep breaths!

6. If you have time, work the toes, thumb walking up the bottom of the toes and paying special attention to the pituitary reflex in the center of the big toe. Use the "hook and back up" technique for pinpoint accuracy there.

Don't forget that you can work the same reflex areas on your hands. Refer to the hand diagrams on pages 47 and 48.

SHIATSU

Stand with the feet shoulder width apart. Start with the arms hanging loose at your sides. With deep, slow inhalation, slowly lift your arms to the sides and over your head, then turn the palms to face the ceiling with the fingertips pointing together. Look at the space between the tips of the fingers. On the exhalation, lower your arms. Repeat 10–12 times.

If your balance is good, try raising your heels off the ground as you lift your arms.

Stretching the arms above you and standing on the toes helps to open the channels and circulate the *ch'i*.

ADDITIONAL SUGGESTIONS

DEEP BREATHING. End your session with 3–5 minutes of deep, rhythmical breathing. Most people take shallow breaths, mostly from the chest. Begin your inhalation from the solar plexus, filling your belly, then fill the lungs, feeling the chest rise.

ST. JOHN'S WORT (HYPERICUM PERFORATUM). This Western herb has received a great deal of attention lately as an effective way to combat depression, partly due to the books of the noted psychiatrist, Harold H. Bloomfield, M.D. It has almost no side effects, but can increase sun sensitivity in a very few people, so avoid prolonged sun exposure. Also, give it time to work. It often takes 4 to 6 weeks of regular use before results become significant. The standard dosage is 300 mg. three times/day. If you are being treated for depression, it would be best to consult with your doctor about using St. John's Wort or any other herbal medication.

HAVE A GOOD CRY. Crying may be just what you need to release the pent-up emotions causing your low mood.

HAVE A GOOD LAUGH. Watch a funny video, or whatever elevates your spirits. You may think, "What's the point?" but that's your depression talking; it can really help.

GET MORE EXERCISE. Stagnant energy is surely one of the major causes of depression. Get it moving. Take a brisk walk, do some aerobic exercise such as bicycling or jogging (if you are fit for it), go dancing (even in your living room), take a swim—anything to get your energy flowing.

Note: Clinical depression is a serious medical condition that requires the supervision of a medical doctor. Mild cases may sometimes be completely healed using these natural techniques, and more serious cases can certainly be helped. But if you find that the remedies suggested here have not begun to significantly lift your spirits after a couple of weeks, we strongly urge you to seek appropriate professional help.

Dermatitis

See "Skin Problems"

Diarrhea

Diarrhea—abnormally frequent and watery bowel movements—has many possible causes. In some cases, such as food poisoning, the diarrhea is your body's way of getting toxins out of the system. Poor digestion, or eating some inappropriate food (such as dairy products if you are lactose intolerant) can also result in diarrhea, as can a bacterial infection or some antibiotics. Unusual stress or anxiety may also lead to a bout of diarrhea.

In most cases, there is no need to take medications; the diarrhea will subside naturally within 24 to 48 hours. But here are a few precautions:

- If the diarrhea lasts longer than a couple of days, or if it occurs more than just occasionally, we recommend consulting a doctor. When diarrhea persists, absorption of nutrients is curtailed, dehydration becomes a serious concern, and resistance to infection is reduced.

- Diarrhea in infants and the elderly can be quite dangerous, so it would be best to seek a doctor's advice if it continues more than a few hours. Watch out for symptoms of dehydration—sunken eyes, dry lips, light-headedness, dizziness, drowsiness. Dehydration is a serious medical problem that needs prompt attention.

The following pressure point suggestions will help to restore balance to your system so that healing can take place more quickly.

ACUPRESSURE

The first two points below (St 36 and Sp 6) are included in "Ten Master Pressure Points" (beginning on page 49) where you will find illustrations of the exact point locations and suggestions on how to press them for maximum benefit.

1. (St 36, Three Mile Foot) This point on the stomach meridian is helpful to harmonize the gastro-intestinal tract.

2. (Sp 6, Three Yin Meeting) This is the crossing point of the three *yin* meridians of the leg, the Spleen, Liver, and Kidney. In combination with St 36 it is very helpful for restoring normal function to the gastro-intestinal tract. Both points help to nourish the *ch'i* and increase vitality. **Caution:** This point should be avoided by pregnant women.

3. (Cv 6, Sea of *Ch'i*) As the name implies, this point has a powerful effect on energizing the body's *ch'i*, the basic life energy. It is located one and a half finger widths directly below the navel (belly button), in the center of the body. Use moderate pressure for about a minute. **Caution:** Pregnant women should not use pressure on this or any other points located on the abdomen.

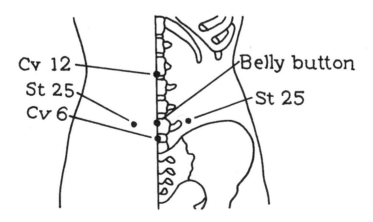

Fig. 86

4. (St 25, Heavens Pivot) This point on the stomach meridian is the most important one on the body for treating a wide range of intestinal disorders. You can use it for both constipation and diarrhea.

The point is located two thumb widths on either side of the belly button. Press on both sides at the same time, with medium to firm pressure for a minute. You can use your middle fingers or thumbs, whichever feels more comfortable and effective.

5. (Cv 12, Middle Stomach) Find a notch at the bottom of your breast bone. Cv 12 is midway between this notch and your belly button. Use firm pressure for about a minute here. You'll probably find pressing with your middle finger most workable.

If the diarrhea is from bad food or food poisoning, press St 44:

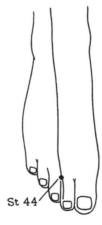

St 44

Fig. 87

6. (St 44, Inner Courtyard) St 44 is located on the top of the foot, in the web margin between the 2nd and 3rd toes. It is right in the center of the web. Use your thumb, and with firm pressure angle into the 'V.' Or, put your thumb underneath your foot, with the middle finger on the point. Apply pressure by squeezing the thumb and finger together.

REFLEXOLOGY

A good foot massage can help alleviate the stress or tension that is sometimes the cause of diarrhea. Beyond that, a number of specific reflex points on the foot are helpful for regulating intestinal functioning.

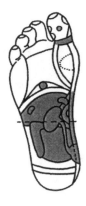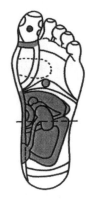

Fig. 88

1. Start by taking a few minutes to massage your feet, both by just rubbing them and kneading them, then by using the relaxation techniques described in the Reflexology Warm-Up in the box on page 69. Be sure to include the thumb press on the solar plexus point.

2. To help normalize the body's metabolism, work on your thyroid reflex, located around the base of the big toe. Rub and press this area; try the thumb or finger walk.

3. To help regulate hormonal balance and reduce stress, press on the reflex for the pituitary gland, located in the center of the big toe. Use the "hook and back up" technique for pinpoint accuracy. (See page 68.)

4. Next, put your attention on the stomach, small intestine, colon, and abdominal organs. The reflex points and zones you will want to work on are in the lower part of the foot, between the diaphragm line and the heel. Spend at least 5 minutes on this area on each foot.

Thumb walk up from the heel to the diaphragm line, then down, horizontally across, and diagonally, covering the entire area from all directions. In this way you will stimulate the stomach, kidneys, liver, gall bladder, adrenals, small intestines, and the various aspects of the colon (ascending, descending, transverse) related to digestion and peristaltic action.

5. The lower spine contains the nerves leading to the intestines, so we recommend spending some time working on the spine reflexes, located on the inside edge of both feet (zone 1). They extend from the heel nearly to the top of the big toe, and working the entire length will aid relaxation, but our concern now is primarily with the lower spine, up to about the waist line of the foot.

When you work the spinal reflexes, work slowly up and down the foot using the thumb walk technique. You will need a little extra strength on the thick skin of the heel area.

6. Finally, you might wish to go back and spend a little extra time working specifically on the colon reflexes.

SHIATSU

Here is a simple Shiatsu routine that will help stop your diarrhea and make you feel better.

1. Rub the palms of your hands together rapidly for 10–20 seconds, until they get nice and warm. Place one palm on the back of the other hand, and put your hands all the way down on the lower left side of your abdomen. Slide your hands up to just below the rib cage, and then across the top of the abdomen and down the right side. Slide across the bottom of your abdomen back to where you started. Press with a gentle pressure as you go. It should take 6–7 seconds to complete one full circle. Do this for 4–5 minutes.

You are moving in a counterclockwise direction, which is opposite the normal direction of the flow of the large intestine. This will help stop the diarrhea and will soothe the intestines and bowels. You'll feel the warmth and the soothing effect immediately!

2. Next, stimulate the Stomach meridian, which runs between the 2nd and 3rd toes, across the top of the foot and up the front of the ankle.

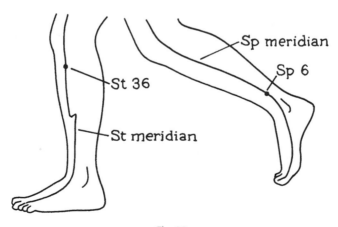

Fig. 89

From the ankle it continues up the front of the leg, about 1 finger breadth to the outside (little toe side) of the shin bone. So, pick one foot, and start at the second toe on the little toe side, using the press and release technique. (It's just what it sounds like: Press for 6–7 seconds, release, move a little way along the channel and press again.) Continue along the entire channel. Four finger widths below the lower edge of the kneecap is St 36. End with an extra minute of "press and release" on this key point. Then work on the other foot and leg in the same way.

ADDITIONAL SUGGESTIONS

DRINK A LOT. The most dangerous effect of simple diarrhea is dehydration. Drink plenty of water, mild fruit juice, herb tea, or clear broth. Avoid milk products, alcohol, and anything with caffeine.

TRY CAROB. Roasted carob powder has been used traditionally for diarrhea in Mediterranean cultures. Mix it with water the way you might make cocoa or coffee—but milk is not recommended when you have diarrhea.

BARLEY. A helpful dietary suggestion from Chinese medicine is pearl barley. This is an example of a food that is also used medicinally. You can eat it as a cooked grain (like oatmeal) or add it to soups. If you have chronic diarrhea, adding a little barley and roasted carob powder to your diet on a regular basis will help prevent recurrences.

MORE FOOD REMEDIES. Two other foods that may help are applesauce (better than buying a jar, just peel and cut up two or three fresh apples and cook until soft), or a little cooked rice with one or two spoonfuls of fresh yogurt.

Dizziness

Dizziness—that uncomfortable sense of lightheadedness, or the feeling that things are spinning—can have many origins, ranging from the serious to the merely uncomfortable. It may also be due to migraines, menopause, or motion sickness, and is one of the symptoms of the inner ear condition known as Ménière's disease. Look up the appropriate section in the book for help with most of these conditions.

Dizziness may also be symptomatic of a stroke or heart attack, especially if it comes on suddenly and is accompanied by chest pain, numbness, blurred vision, or an impairment in your speaking ability. Seek medical help *immediately!*

In Chinese medicine, dizziness has two main causes, each treated a little differently. You shouldn't have much difficulty deciding which category you fall into.

The first is a mild dizziness common to older people, postpartum mothers, and people who have a chronic illness or are in a delicate state of health. They often feel an underlying, constant tiredness; sometimes they also have mild headaches or poor appetite. This is a deficiency type of dizziness, and the goal of treatment is to boost overall vitality, strengthen the *ch'i*, and nourish the blood.

The second type is due to excess, usually an abundance of very strong emotions, such as anger or intense frustration. People who have these strong feelings but repress them and keep them bottled up inside, may also experience this type of dizziness. Treatment for this uses points that pacify the effects of excess emotion.

Points for deficiency dizziness:

The first two points below (Sp 6 and St 36) are included in "Ten Master Pressure Points" (beginning on page 49) where you will find illustrations of the exact point locations and suggestions on how to press them for maximum benefit.

1. (Sp 6, Three Yin Meeting) This is one of the most important of all Acupressure points. Located at the crossing point of the three *yin* meridians of the leg (Spleen, Liver, and Kidney), it nourishes the overall *yin* of the body by simultaneously nourishing the *yin* of these meridians. **Caution:** This point should be avoided by pregnant women.

2. (St 36, Three Mile Foot) This is the major point to tonify the *ch'i* and blood. In combination with Sp 6, it strongly revitalizes the entire body.

3. (Cv 12, Middle Stomach) Find a notch at the bottom of your breast bone. Cv 12 is midway between this notch and your belly button. Use firm pressure for about a minute here. You'll probably find pressing with your middle finger most workable, or the middle finger of both hands together. This

point strengthens the stomach and digestive system, what is called the "middle burner" in Chinese medicine. This is the primary source of our energy, and it must be functioning well if we hope to rebuild vitality and stamina.

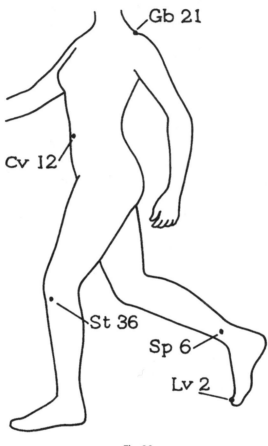

Fig. 90

Points for excess-type dizziness:

4. (Gb 20, Wind Pool) Place your thumbs on your earlobes, then slide them back toward the center of your neck. You should be approximately one thumb width above the hairline of the neck. Your thumbs will fall into a depression on either side of the vertebra of your neck, at the base of your skull. The depressions may be more evident if you slowly bend your head forward and then back again. Gb 20 is located in these depressions. It is easiest to use the thumbs to apply Acupressure on these points. Use

medium to firm pressure, and hold for a minute or more, remembering to breathe deeply and to build up and release pressure gradually.

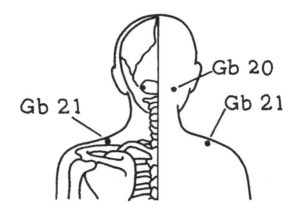

Fig. 91

5. (Gb 21, Shoulder Well) Place your right hand on your left shoulder. Midway between the neck and the outer edge of the shoulder, on the highest point of the shoulder, is Gb 21. Don't be surprised if this point is quite tender. Use your middle finger to press firmly on the point. Or, you can press both shoulders at the same time by curving the left hand over the left shoulder and right over the right.

Increase pressure gradually, then press quite firmly for up to 2 minutes and gradually release. Remember to take slow, deep breaths as you do this and the other techniques. This point helps to balance the excess of *ch'i* that can build up in the upper part of the body.

In Chinese medicine, anger is understood to make the *ch'i* rise up, which leads to an unhealthy excess of *ch'i* in the head. The quick uprushing of *ch'i* to the head creates this type of dizziness.

Caution: Don't use this point if you are pregnant.

6. (Lv 2, Moving Between) This point is located in the web margin between the big toe and second toe (see Fig. 90). Use medium pressure with your index fingers, pressing on both feet at the same time if that is comfortable, otherwise one at a time. This point is useful in balancing the excess *ch'i* created by strong emotions.

7. (Sp 6, Three Yin Meeting) See Point #1 on page 177. This point nourishes the overall *yin* of the body. A healthy state of *yin* helps keep the emotions more even.

REFLEXOLOGY

1. To help you settle into your Reflexology session, spend a few minutes massaging your feet and relaxing them with the techniques described in the Reflexology Warm-Up in the box on page 69. This is an important step that helps you relax, tones the energy of the whole body, and prepares your feet to be worked on; please don't skip it!

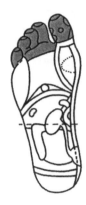 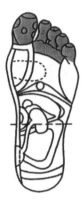

Fig. 92

2. Next, work on your toes, where reflex zones to the ear are located. (Disturbances in the inner ear are the source of many instances of dizziness.) On the bottom of your foot, work the fleshy part of all the toes, but especially the second and third. Use the thumb walk for maximum benefit, or at least give them a good rubbing with your thumb.

3. There is also a reflex zone for the inner ear on the top of your foot, in the groove between the second and third toe. (It doesn't go all the way up the groove, just an inch or an inch and a half.) Work this with your index finger, using the finger walk technique. Use substantial pressure, unless it is very tender.

4. Some dizziness is due to lack of blood flow to the brain. To help relax the neck and shoulder areas, press on the cervical spine reflex, along the outside edge of your big toe. Use the thumb walk and go over the area several times. (To directly enliven the brain, press on the brain reflexes at the tip of each toe by rolling the tip of your index finger from side to side.)

5. Finally, work the neck reflexes on both feet. To do this, walk the ridge at the top of the ball of the foot (at the base of the toes). You will need

to use the inside corner of either your thumb or index finger (usually you use the outside corner). Pull the flesh of the pad of the foot down and away from the ridge with your other hand, to increase access to the ridge. Walk in both directions.

Earache

Earaches, common to both adults and children, come in many guises: they can be dull, sharp, burning, constant, or on-and-off. They may come from an infection in the outer ear canal, or from deep in the inner ear. They may occur during a plane ride, when changes in cabin pressure cause unequal pressure on the two sides (inner and outer) of the eardrum.

Try these pressure point remedies. You can use most of them (the ones on your hands and head) even on a plane to relieve sudden pressure. Children can do them, or you can do them on your child. But if the discomfort doesn't subside in a couple of days, seek medical advice; complications from ear infections, though fairly rare, can be serious, including hearing loss and spread of the infection to the brain.

ACUPRESSURE

Note: Even though you probably have pain in only one ear, for best results please use these Acupressure points on *both* sides of the body.

1. (Li 4, Adjoining Valley) For an illustration of the exact location of this important point, and instructions on how to press it most effectively, please see page 49 for the beginning of "Ten Master Pressure Points."

2. (Tw 5, Outer Gate) Hold your left arm in front of you with the palm down facing the floor. Measure two thumb widths above the wrist. The point is right in the center between the two forearm bones. Press with your thumb or middle finger for about a minute. The Tw (triple warmer) channel runs up the back of the arm to the shoulder and neck, then moves around to the side of the neck and from there enters the ear. Stimulating points on this meridian's pathway—especially this and Tw 17 (see next page)—can be beneficial for any ear problems.

3. (Tw 17, Wind Screen) This point, also on the triple warmer meridian just before it enters the ear, is located in the natural depression right behind the earlobe. Apply pressure with your index or middle finger. Use mild to moderate pressure, as this point may be tender.

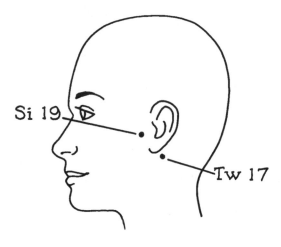

Fig. 93

4. (Si 19, Listening Palace) To locate this point, place your index fingers on the side of your face, next to where the ear is attached. Open and close your mouth a few times to feel the jaw bone moving under your fingers. Si 19 is in the depression that forms when the mouth opens. Stimulate the point with your mouth open. Use mild pressure, right in the center of the depression. For maximum effectiveness, try using your second, third, and fourth fingers together (little finger pointing up, thumb down). Two other valuable points are in this depression, just above and just below Si 19, and that way you will stimulate all three.

REFLEXOLOGY

Reflex points on the feet can facilitate the healing of earaches. Start by massaging your feet and relaxing them with the techniques described in the Reflexology Warm-Up on page 69. Don't skip this important step; it helps you relax, tones the energy of the whole body, and prepares your feet for the rest of the sequence.

The remainder of the Reflexology session will be dedicated primarily to reflex zones on and around your toes, related directly to the ear and to your neck, throat, shoulders, chest, and jaws—all closely connected to the health of the ear.

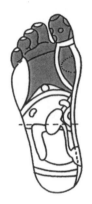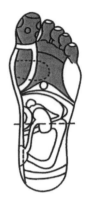

Fig. 94

1. Start by working the chest and lung area on the soles of your feet, to help clear any congestion and stimulate healthy breathing. Thumb walk the chest and lung reflex zones, located on the ball of the foot between the diaphragm line and the base of the toes. Then finger walk the chest and lymph gland reflexes on top of the foot.

2. Next, use your thumb or index finger to walk the ridge at the base of your toes, at the top of the ball of the foot. Use your other hand to pull down on the pad of the foot so you can get closer down to the bone of the ridge. You'll need to use the inside corner of your finger (usually you use the outside corner). Walk in both directions. This is a very important zone for helping to heal ear problems of all kinds, so spend several minutes here.

3. Work the fleshy pads of all your toes, especially the 2nd and 3rd, where the reflex zones to the ears are located. Use the thumb walk for maximum benefit, or at least massage the toes well between your thumb and index finger.

4. There is also a reflex zone for the ear on the top of your foot, in the groove between the second and third toe. (It doesn't go all the way up the groove, just an inch or an inch and a half.) Work this with your index finger, using the finger walk technique. Use substantial pressure, unless it is very tender.

5. To help relax the neck and shoulder areas and increase blood flow to the head, press on the cervical spine reflex, along the outside edge of your big toe. Use the thumb walk and go over the area several times. Use your thumb or index finger to walk the seventh cervical area in the groove at the base of the big toe (on the top and sides of the toe.) You may find it quite tender.

6. Finally, use your thumb or index finger to walk the top and sides of the big toe from the base to the bottom of the nail. Work in as many directions as you comfortably can, across the toe and up and down.

Remember that you can also work these areas on your hands.

SHIATSU

1. Find the space in your foot between the 4th and 5th toes. This is the territory of the Gall Bladder meridian. Start at the web margin and move up the channel using the press and release technique: press for 6–7 seconds, release, move a little way along the channel, and press again. Continue moving along in this manner until you are about halfwayup the foot and no longer feel a space between the toe bones. Repeat on the other foot.

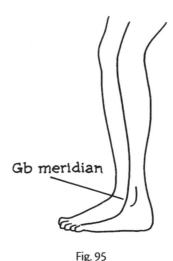

Gb meridian

Fig. 95

2. Use the press and release technique on Li 4, the point on your hand that we recommended as point #1 in the Acupressure section on page 181. When you squeeze your thumb against the other fingers, Li 4 is

located in the middle of the fleshy mound between the thumb and the index finger Because of the importance of this point in pain control, continue stimulating for 2 minutes. Be sure to do both hands.

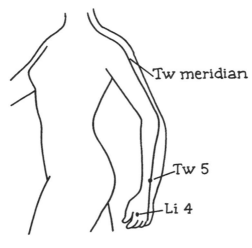

Fig. 96

3. This next sequence stimulates the Triple Warmer meridian, which has many points beneficial for the ear. Start at the tip of your 4th finger, on the little finger side. With your index finger, use a press and release technique for this exercise. Press once for 6–7 seconds, then release. Move half an inch or an inch along the channel, then press again.

From the tip of the 4th finger move slowly along the side of the finger to the web margin between the 4th and 5th fingers. Do two or three extra presses and releases on this point, with your thumb underneath the webbing for support. Then continue forward along the groove between the 4th and 5th fingers. About halfway between the knuckles and the wrist you will be over Tw 3. Give a little extra stimulation on this point.

As you approach the wrist, you will notice that there is no longer a groove beneath your fingers. Instead you are feeling the small bones of the wrist. When you feel that you're no longer in a groove, angle slightly inwards toward the center of the wrist. Continue up the center of the forearm until you get about halfway to the elbow.

Now go back and follow the same path on your other arm.

When you are done with both arms, press Tw 17 (in the natural depression right behind the earlobe—see Fig. 93) several times with the index or middle finger of both hands, using the press and release technique.

ADDITIONAL SUGGESTIONS

VITAMIN C   and the herb echinacea can boost the body's natural immune system to help combat any infection.

A DIET CHANGE.   If you have chronic earaches or ear infections, cut back on sweets, fats, and dairy products.

GARLIC.   Try eating one or two cloves of raw garlic each day. Garlic has natural antibiotic qualities that may be able to kill the germs that cause earaches. If the raw garlic upsets your digestive system, try taking your garlic in capsule form.

Eating Disorders

See also, Stress; Weight Control; Depression; Anxiety

In Chinese medicine, eating disorders of all types, from simple overeating to more extreme conditions like anorexia or bulimia, are seen primarily as an imbalance in the earth element within the body. The earth element is the nourishing, nurturing aspect of life. It promotes the feeling of being rooted or grounded, of having a sense of security or belonging. Treatment is focused on balancing this element and restoring emotional well-being. The meridians in the body associated with the earth element are the Spleen and Stomach meridians. For a simple Shiatsu routine to help balance these meridians, see page 187.

From a more Western point of view, most eating problems are associated with stress and psychological conditions such as depression, anxiety, grief, and low self-esteem. As someone said, "Eating disorders are usually more about emotions than about appetite." Our sections on "Depression" and "Anxiety" offer many helpful suggestions, involving pressure point therapy as well as dietary and exercise recommendations and more. Rather than repeat all the treatment recommendations offered in those sections, we would like to refer you directly to them.

Whether you feel your eating problems are a result of stress or are causing you stress (it's probably both), using the recommendations in the section on "Stress" will help you gain balance and control.

You will also find helpful suggestions in the section, "Weight Control."

Important: Eating disorders may seriously endanger your health or even be life threatening. To fully heal them you may require psychological or psychiatric counseling. If that is what you need, please don't put it off! These conditions can be treated, and your life can dramatically improve.

SHIATSU

As promised previously, here are simple methods to help balance the Spleen and Stomach meridians.

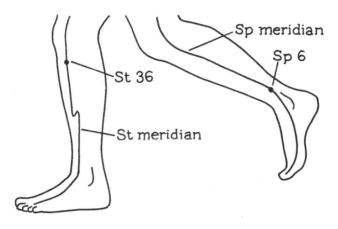

Fig. 97

   1. Begin with the Stomach meridian, which runs between the 2nd and 3rd toes, across the top of the foot and up the front of the ankle. From the ankle it continues up the front of the leg, about 1 finger breadth to the outside (little toe side) of the shin bone. Pick one foot, and start at the second toe on the little toe side, using the press and release technique: Press for 6–7 seconds, release, move about half an inch along the channel and press again. Continue along the entire channel. Four finger widths below the lower edge of the kneecap is a point known as St 36. End with an extra minute of press and release on this one key point. Then work on the other foot and leg in the same way.

   2. The Spleen meridian starts at the big toe. The first point is very close to the nail cuticle at the inside corner of the big toenail. From there, the meridian follows along the side of the big toe bone, at the inside of the foot, up the side of the ankle and the inside of the leg. Along the leg it follows just below the bone. Use the press and release technique from the big toe to just below the knee. (See Fig. K on page 43.)

When you are finished with one foot and leg, be sure to repeat the procedure on the other side.

This press and release exercise is just one small suggestion. Please be sure to see the other recommended chapters for much more that can help you.

Eczema

See "Skin Problems"

Energy Tune-Up

See also, "Daily Health 'Builder'"

Fatigue and feelings of low energy are so common today that tiredness could easily be called an epidemic. In this section we will offer you three different pressure point approaches to increase energy on a daily basis. If you use even one of them each day, you will feel the results! Please also check out the additional recommendations at the end of the section for more helpful hints.

ACUPRESSURE

The first two points below (Sp 6 and St 36) are fully described in the section, "Ten Master Pressure Points" (beginning on page 49) where you will find illustrations of the exact point locations and suggestions on how to press them for maximum benefit. (Also see Fig. 97.)

1. (Sp 6, Three Yin Meeting) This is one of the 12 most important Acupressure points on the body. The crossing point of three *yin* meridians (Spleen, Liver, and Kidney), it nourishes the overall *yin* of the body. Combined with St 36 it strengthens both *ch'i* and blood, and promotes vitality. **Caution:** Pregnant women should not press this point.

2. (St 36, Three Mile Foot) This is the best point to strengthen the *ch'i* and blood. Legends say that soldiers in ancient China relied on this point to sustain themselves when exhausted or weakened by lack of food. In combination with Sp 6, it strongly revitalizes the entire body.

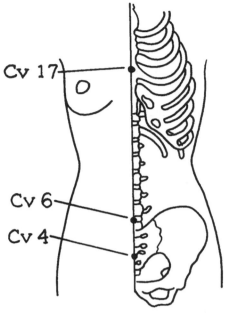

Fig. 98

3. (Cv 4, Gate of Original *Ch'i*) Located 4 finger widths directly below your navel (belly button), Cv 4 is also looked upon as one of the major points on the body. Its function is very similar to the combination of Sp 6 and St 36. The difference is that this point (as its name, Gate of Original *Ch'i*, implies) stimulates your constitutional *ch'i* or original *ch'i* while the former two points stimulate the *ch'i* that your body produces from the food you eat and the air you breathe.

Cv 4 is often used to promote strength in individuals with weak constitutions or who are run down from chronic illness. It is more for chronic, deep-seated fatigue, rather than ordinary day-to-day tiredness.

This point is the *dan tien* that various forms of martial arts, *tai chi*, and *ch'i gong* cultivate for power, centeredness and well-being. It taps the body's deepest energy reserves and therefore should be used wisely. In other words, if what you really need is more sleep and less caffeine or other stimulants, use this point sparingly. Instead of draining your savings account, it's better to live within your budget.

Use moderate pressure on Cv 4. A circular motion while pressing works well at this point. **Caution:** Pregnant women should not use pressure on this or any other abdominal points.

4. (Cv 6, Sea of *Ch'i*) This point is about one and a half finger widths directly below the navel. Place the middle finger of both hands there, and press inward with the fingertips of both hands to a depth of about an inch. Use moderate pressure and hold for a minute or two, breathing deeply.

This point has a powerful effect on energizing the *ch'i* and circulating it throughout the body. While involved with the *dan tien* energy, its focus is more on the distribution of that energy. You might try lying on your back to work this point, as well as Cv 4. Start by taking a few deep breaths to relax.

Caution: Again, pregnant women should not use pressure on any abdominal points.

5. (Cv 17, Chest Center) This point is also known as the Upper Sea of *Ch'i*. It strengthens and circulates *ch'i*, especially the *ch'i* of the chest which is derived from the air we breathe. It is located right in the center of the chest, on the breastbone. Traditionally it is said to be "even with the nipples" and men will easily locate it that way. For women, using this direction may be misleading, due to the wide variation in the shape of the female breast from individual to individual. Rather, locate the point by going about 3 finger widths up from the bottom of the breastbone. Be sure to measure from the bottom of the bone itself, *not* including the springy cartilage at the lower end of the bone.

Hold your index, middle, and ring finger together and press on this point for about 1 minute with your middle finger, with your eyes closed. If you are not sure you are locating it precisely, don't worry; simply press with all 3 fingers. Use medium pressure, or, if the spot is quite tender, use lighter pressure, then rub it lightly for a few seconds after you finish pressing. Remember to breathe slowly and deeply.

REFLEXOLOGY

This energy tune-up is adapted from Reflexologist Laura Norman, who lays it out in full in her book, *Feet First*. She says it produces "a different quality of energy to replace the nervous, fidgety energy that characterizes so much indoor activity," and promotes creativity and concentration. She recommends that you take half an hour or more for the complete session.

1. Start with a warm-up to relax your feet and settle down. Use the techniques described in our Reflexology Warm-Up on page 69. This is an important step that tones the energy of the whole body, and prepares your feet to be worked on; please don't skip it!

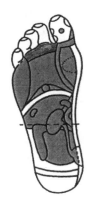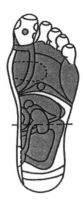

Fig. 99

2. Since much of our energy comes from the air we breathe, start to open up your breathing by thumb walking the chest and lung reflex zones on the ball of the foot (between the diaphragm line and the base of the toes). Spend some time "walking" across the diaphragm line. Then rotate or flex your foot (with your holding hand) to help work this key area. This will help send fresh oxygen to the cells.

3. Work the neck and shoulder reflexes on both feet. Walk the ridge at the top of the ball of the foot (at the base of the toes). Pull the flesh of the pad of the foot down and away from the ridge with your other hand, to increase access to the ridge. Walk in both directions. Then work the shoulder reflex area in Zone 5, reaching from the base of your little toe to the diaphragm line. This will help relax your neck and shoulder muscles, thus increasing blood flow, a key to increased energy.

4. Many people with low thyroid hormones feel tired and sluggish much of the time. To stimulate more balanced and healthy thyroid activity, work the reflex zone for the thyroid and parathyroid glands (around the base of the big toe) by rubbing and pressing.

5. To further relax the neck and shoulder areas and increase blood flow to the head, press on the cervical spine reflex, along the outside edge of your big toe. Use the thumb walk and go over the area several times. Use your thumb or index finger to walk the seventh cervical area in the groove at the base of the big toe (on top of the foot). You may find it quite tender.

6. To stimulate the endocrine glands to function more efficiently, work the pituitary gland in the center of the pad of the big toe. Massage with your thumb or use the "hook and back up" technique (on page 68) for pinpoint accuracy.

7. The liver has over 500 known functions, most having to do with manufacturing nutrients for the blood and cleansing it. When not functioning at its best, this vital organ can be a source of stagnant energy leading to fatigue and even depression. To stimulate the liver (as well as the small intestines, stomach, and other internal organs) work the entire area in the arch of your foot, from the pelvic line up to the diaphragm line. Use the thumb walk to thoroughly cover this area, moving up, down, and/or diagonally.

8. At the kidney and adrenal reflexes (also in the soft center of the foot) use the "rotation on a point" technique. (See page 68.) In Chinese medicine the kidneys are considered the seat of our energy reserves.

9. After this lengthy session, spend a minute or two gently rubbing your feet to relax, and use the thumb press on the solar plexus point.

SHIATSU

Use the press and release technique to stimulate your Spleen and Stomach meridians (see Fig. 97). The technique is just what it sounds like: Press for 6–7 seconds, release, move a fraction of an inch along the channel, press again.

1. The Spleen meridian starts at the big toe. The first point is very close to the nail cuticle at the inside corner of the big toenail. From there, the meridian follows along the side of the big toe bone, at the inside of the foot, up the side of the ankle and the inside of the leg. Along the leg it follows just below the bone. Use the press and release technique from the big toe to just below the knee. Give special attention to Sp 6, a very important point located about one palm width above the center of the ankle bone, just off the bone toward the back of the leg. Be sure to work on both legs.

2. Next, energize the Stomach meridian, which runs between the 2nd and 3rd toes, across the top of the foot and up the front of the ankle. From the ankle it continues up the front of the leg, about 1 finger breadth to the outside (little toe side) of the shin bone. Pick one foot and start at the second toe on the little toe side, using the press and release technique. Continue along the entire channel. Four finger widths below the lower

edge of the kneecap is St 36. End with an extra minute of press and release on this one key point. Then work on the other foot and leg in the same way.

3. Press and release on Cv 4 three times and then Cv 6 three times (see Fig. 98).

4. Next, rub the palms of your hands together rapidly for 10–20 seconds, until they get nice and warm. Place one palm on the back of the other hand, and put your hands flat on your abdomen. Make a circular movement in a clockwise direction. The movement should be slow and deliberate and the hand pressure firm. Let your attention follow your hand.

Repeat step 4 three times. Keep your breathing deep and rhythmical.

5. End with 2–3 minutes of the horse posture. In Chinese medicine, the Kidneys are considered the root of vitality, and one of the best exercises to cultivate Kidney *ch'i* is the horse stance. Because of its effectiveness, this posture is widely used in almost all martial art forms. When done properly it builds stamina, cultures *ch'i*, and promotes circulation. If you have not exercised for a while, you will find this posture quite strenuous at first. It may be difficult to hold for more than 20–30 seconds. Over time you can gradually build up to the point where you can hold the stance up to 5 minutes. Some martial arts practitioners can maintain this posture for 30–60 minutes or even more.

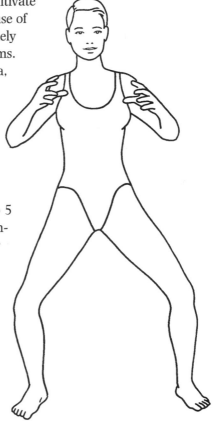

Stand with your feet about shoulder width apart. You'll find that your feet will naturally want to point slightly outward, but position them so they are pointing as straight ahead as you comfortably can. This may feel a little odd at first. Do the best you can if you can't get them completely straight.

Fig. 100

Hold your arms in front of you, elbows slightly lower than the hands. Hands should be about 8–12 inches apart and roughly parallel (palms facing each other), but with the index fingers slightly closer to each other than the little fingers. Pretend you are holding a dinner plate in your hands, which is parallel to the floor. Let your fingers naturally curl with the thumb slightly apart from the fingers. Also let your fingers space themselves naturally.

Keep your back straight, and bend the knees. The more you bend your knees, the more difficult the exercise becomes, so start with just a slight bend. Over time, as you build strength, you can increase the amount of bend. If you can eventually sink 6–8 inches into the bend that's enough.

Now for the important part: Relax! Don't strain when doing this exercise. Holding your muscles tight will constrict the flow of *ch'i* along the meridians. When you start to get tired, it's better to return to a normal pose for a few moments, rest and then step back into the horse stance again. This will be more effective than straining to hold the posture longer. See if you can feel the *ch'i* flowing, especially between your hands. It may feel like a soft breeze or a tingling in your hands.

ADDITIONAL SUGGESTIONS

Here are several suggestions from top health experts on how to increase your energy level.

GET ENOUGH EXERCISE.   Many people feel tired because they don't do enough. Exercise is critical for vitality; it pumps oxygen-rich blood to the cells, feeding your brain and body with fuel. However, over-exercise can be draining. Find the amount that works to energize you, and do it regularly. A brisk daily walk, and some Yoga stretching or *tai chi,* is all most people need. An excellent Yoga energy tune up is the Sun Salutation, a series of 12 postures that stretch the whole body. The Shoulder Stand tones the thyroid gland and promotes energy and balance.

EAT A HIGH-OCTANE BREAKFAST.   Proteins and complex carbohydrates early in the day will keep your energy supply stable and strong for many hours. Avoid those coffee and doughnut breakfasts; they'll give you a quick boost and drop you back down just as quickly.

GET ENOUGH SLEEP. Rest is the basis of effective activity. If you're serious about increasing your energy, there's no better place to start than with a good night's rest—every day!

TAKE A BREATHING BREAK. Several times a day, set aside a few minutes and take five long, deep breaths. Breathe slowly, through your nose. To best energize your blood with oxygen, fill your belly first, then your chest.

TAKE NAPS. A brief nap of five to ten minutes can take the edge off fatigue and recharge your batteries.

TAKE AN ACTION BREAK. If you spend most of your day sitting down, get up and take a brisk walk, ride a bicycle, climb some stairs, or whatever you need to get your blood and energy flowing.

USE ENERGIZING HERBS. Perhaps the best known Chinese vitalizing herb is ginseng, a wonderful herb with many healing and strengthening properties. However it is not appropriate for everyone. There are two main types of ginseng, Korean and American. The Korean variety has very warming properties and should definitely be avoided by anyone with hypertension or other conditions considered to be caused by excess heat. (This is best diagnosed by a qualified practitioner.) American ginseng has a cooling property and is safe for everyone as a general tonic. Ironically, the qualities of American ginseng are so revered in the Orient that the bulk of North American production is exported.

Eye Strain

Almost everyone experiences strained and tired eyes once in a while, and many of us—computer users, tv watchers, commuter drivers—endure strained eyes almost daily. This is particularly true for those of us over 40, which is when the eyes often start having trouble focusing.

Pressure point therapy is very effective for relieving tired eyes. Use these recommendations, and the Additional Suggestions at the end of this section, to regain rested, bright, comfortable eyes! You don't have to wait for your eyes to become tired and sore; use these points regularly for routine maintenance to keep your eyes healthy and your vision strong.

ACUPRESSURE

A number of the points that energize the eyes are located close to them; in working these points, the technique will be to use a series of short presses rather than the longer presses we usually recommend. For best results, use the recommended procedure.

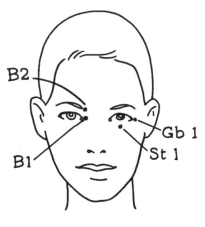

Fig. 101

1. (B 1, Eye Clarity) This point is located between the eyebrow and the eye, where the eye socket touches the nose. Use your thumbs. The side of each thumb will be against your nose, and the flat part will be underneath the bone that forms a ridge below the eyebrow. Press gently in towards the nose and upward. Gradually increase the pressure, hold with firm pressure for two seconds and release. Repeat ten times, and end with five seconds of steady pressure.

Caution: Use caution with points close to the eye. These points cannot be safely done with long fingernails.

2. (B 2 Collecting Bamboo) Directly above B 1 at the level of the eyebrows is B 2. Use the thumbs of both hands. Close your eyes and breathe deeply as you press. You may allow your head to lean forward into your fingers. Use either steady pressure or a circular motion. As with B 1 (above), gradually increase pressure, hold about two seconds, and release. Repeat ten times, and end with five seconds of steady pressure.

Then with your thumb underneath the eyebrow and your index finger above, pinch the eyebrow starting from the inside and working to the outside. Go back and repeat this pinching five or six times.

3. (Gb 1, Pupil Crevice) From the outside of the eyebrow let your fingers drop down even with, but outside the eye socket. Slowly move the skin over the skull and you will feel a pronounced depression. Press firmly with the middle fingers of each hand. Apply pressure slightly upward and outward. Again, gradually increase pressure, hold about 2 seconds, and release. Repeat 10 times, and end with 5 seconds of steady pressure.

4. (St 1, Contain Tears) Place your middle finger just below the eye socket, in line with the center of the pupils. Now gently roll up on the pads of your fingers until you feel the ridge of the bone of the eye socket. With gentle sideways movement you should feel a small notch in the bone. St 1 is located at this notch. Press straight in toward the bone.

Use gentle pressure on this point. (You won't be able to work on this point with long fingernails.) Press and release 5 times and end with 5–6 seconds steady pressure.

From this point, move your fingers along the ridge of this bone one half the distance from St 1 to the outer edge of the eye socket. Press and release on this point 5 times, and again end with 5–6 seconds of steady pressure.

5. (Ear lobe) A point in the very center of the earlobe is helpful for strengthening eye function. Remove any earrings and press and hold this point for 30 seconds. Hold between your thumb and index finger.

"BLIND WITH RAGE"

In traditional Chinese medicine, vision problems are intimately connected to the Liver meridian, which starts at the top of the big toe and runs up the entire body to the eyes. Treatment for various eye complaints frequently involves stimulating the Liver meridian points to benefit vision. An important point for this is Lv 3, which you will work on in a moment. Interestingly, this is also one of the most effective points for calming tension, or for helping people who are prone to anger. Perhaps the expression "blind with rage" refers to this intimate connection.

6. (Lv 3, Bigger Rushing) For an illustration of the exact location of this important point, and instructions on how to press it most effectively, please see page 49 for the beginning of "Ten Master Pressure Points." (See also Fig. 103.)

7. To close your Acupressure session, sit comfortably or lie down. Rub your hands together vigorously for about 15 to 30 seconds. Cup your palms and place them *lightly* over your eyes. (Don't press on the eyeballs.) Visualize and feel healing energy flowing from your palms and soothing your eyes. Continue for 1–3 minutes. You can do this any time, as a break from your work, or when you stop for a while during a long drive, to soothe your eyes.

REFLEXOLOGY

One of the main principles of Oriental medicine, and of the new paradigm emerging in Western medicine, is that all things are interconnected. Thus, even though we know precisely where the reflex zones are to treat the eyes, we also want to promote relaxation of the entire system, more energy and increased oxygen supply to the brain, and so on.

1. We recommend that you start your Reflexology session for tired, strained eyes by massaging your feet for a few minutes and relaxing them with the relaxation techniques described in the Reflexology Warm-Up on page 69. This is an important step that helps you relax, tones the energy of the whole body, and prepares your feet to be worked on.

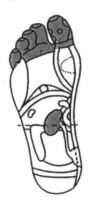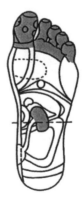

Fig. 102

2. Now turn to the eye reflex area, which is located on the bottom of both feet, on the ridge at the base of the smaller toes. This area is also connected to the neck, which is another reason to work on it; relaxation of the often tense neck area increases blood flow to the brain and eyes and is helpful for vision.

Work this area by "walking the ridge" at the top of the ball of the foot, using either your thumb or index finger, whichever feels easier. Pull the flesh of the pad of the foot gently down and away from the ridge with your other hand. "Walk" in both directions. Be sure to work both feet.

3. Next, work on all your toes. Use the finger walk or thumb walk to go up and down the toes, paying special attention to the big toe. It has all 5 of the body's reflex zones represented on it, so working on it has a wide-ranging effect. Dwight Byers, author of *Better Health with Foot Reflexology* and one of the leading Reflexology educators in the world, says that "because of the zone lines, working all the toes is very helpful for many eye problems."

Work especially on the fleshy pad of the toes on the bottom of your feet, but make sure to also do the tops and sides. To work on the brain reflex, place your index finger at the tip of the toe and roll your finger back and forth to press on the toe.

End by giving all the toes a good wiggling and some gentle twisting and pulling to further loosen them up.

4. Return to the area at the base of the big toe, where it is joined to the foot, and spend some time working all around in a circle, as if there were a ring around the toe.

5. Dwight Byers also recommends working the kidney reflex in the center of the foot, using the "rotation on a point" technique described on page 68. "The kidneys are in the third zone of the body," he says, "the same zone as the eyes. Through many years of Reflexology, I have found that working the kidney reflex is very helpful for some eye problems."

6. Finally, work the cervical spine reflex. This will help relax the neck and shoulder areas and increase blood flow and energy to the head. This reflex is along the outside edge of your big toe. Use the thumb walk and go over the area several times. Then use your thumb or index finger to walk the seventh cervical area in the groove at the base of the big toe (on top of the foot).

SHIATSU

1. Sit or stand comfortably. Vigorously rub the palms of your hands together for 30 seconds. Get them good and warm. Now, using the tips of your fingers, rub with moderate pressure all around the eye (not *on* the eye) for 1 minute.

2. Using more of the palms, make circular motions around the eye starting from your cheeks, in toward the nose, up over the eyes, then out across the forehead and temples. Just pretend you're washing your face, except you're not using water. Do this for 1 minute.

3. Close your eyes. Very gently place your 2nd, 3rd, and 4th fingers on your closed eyelids. Use no pressure. Without moving over the surface of the skin, move your eyelid over your eyeball in tiny circles. Remember: no pressure on the eyeball!

4. Look back at the Acupressure section, on page 196, and follow the instructions for B 1 and B 2. (See Fig. 101.) When you've finished, place 3 fingers on each eyebrow and slide to the outside, toward the temples. Use moderate pressure. When you get to the temples, make 3 circular strokes. Repeat 9 times. Do both sides simultaneously.

5. Finish your Shiatsu session by stimulating the Liver channel on your foot. Sit cross-legged on the floor, bed, or sofa, or cross one leg over the other while sitting in a chair. Put the tips of the fingers of your right hand in the space between the big toe and the second toe of your left foot. Position your little finger at the web margin between the toes. Apply pressure beginning with the little finger and rippling up toward the index finger. Use firm pressure. Keep applying a rippling wave of pressure for a full 1 minute. Then use your left hand for the right foot. (If you are pretty limber you can do both feet at the same time.)

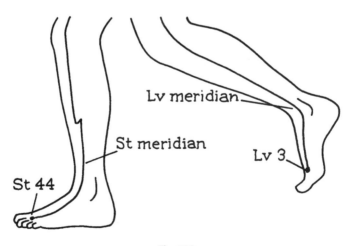

Fig. 103

ADDITIONAL SUGGESTIONS

SIP CHRYSANTHEMUM TEA. A great tasting tea that is widely acclaimed for its beneficial effect on the eyes is chrysanthemum flower tea. This is available in packets of presweetened, freeze dried granules at some health food stores and almost any Chinese grocery store. It has a soothing and cooling effect on the Liver meridian, which opens directly into the eye.

TRY BILBERRY EXTRACT. Another important herb for eye health is extract of bilberry. It is widely used as an antioxidant specific to the structures of the eye. British pilots during World War II were encouraged to eat bilberry preserves for its beneficial effect on night vision. Bilberry extract standardized to contain 25% of the main active ingredient (anthocyanidin) is available at natural food stores. Standard dose: 120 mg. three times a day.

TAKE A BLINK BREAK. Interrupt your work occasionally and blink your eyes a few times. Each blink lubricates and cleanses the surface of the eyes and gives them a mini massage.

REST YOUR EYES. The best way to relieve eyestrain may be the simplest and cheapest: rest. Whenever you can, just close your eyes for a minute or two. You can do this when you're on the phone, or sitting on a plane or train or if someone else is driving. Commercial breaks on tv shows are an ideal time to rest your eyes. You'll be surprised how much this can help relieve eyestrain and fatigue.

HELPFUL YOGA. The Yoga inverted poses (including Shoulder Stand and Plow, and the Forward Bend, all increase circulation in the upper body and are said to soothe and nourish the eyes. Headstand is *not* recommended unless you have been trained by a qualified Yoga teacher.

Fever

Fever may be a sign of infection, or, a more common view in Eastern schools of medicine, a sign that the body is working to eliminate accumulated toxins. In either case, it is not good for the brain and body to get too hot; pressure point therapies provide a simple means to help pacify or "drain" the heat from the system.

ACUPRESSURE

1. (St 44, Inner Courtyard) This point is located on the top of the foot, in the web margin between the 2nd and 3rd toes. (See Fig. 103.) It is right in the center of the web. Use your thumb, and with firm pressure angle into the 'V.' This is the most powerful point on the Stomach meridian to clear heat in the Stomach channel.

For illustrations of the exact location of the next two key points, and instructions on how to press them most effectively, please see page 49 for the beginning of "Ten Master Pressure Points."

2. (Li 4, Adjoining Valley) This point is beneficial for many cold symptoms, including headaches and congestion, and is also effective in clearing heat.
3. (Li 11, Pool at the Crook) Li 11 helps to clear heat from the body, and thus is good for fever.

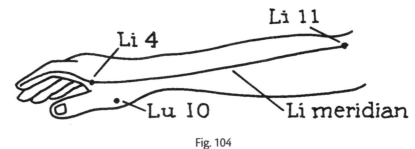

Fig. 104

4. (Lu 10, Fish Border) This point is on the meaty part of the hand leading up to the thumb, at the midpoint between the wrist and the first knuckle of the thumb. You'll find a little depression just below the bone. It clears heat from the lung meridian and is used for sore throat as well as fever. Use firm pressure and hold for about one minute.

REFLEXOLOGY

There are a number of reflex areas you can press to help reduce a fever and help your body heal the infection or eliminate the toxins causing it. However, we recommend that you start by massaging your feet and relaxing them with the techniques described in the Reflexology Warm-Up on page 69. This brief sequence of steps helps you relax, tones the energy of the whole body, and prepares your feet to be worked on; please don't skip it!

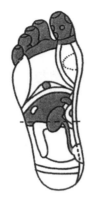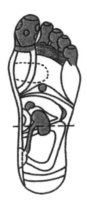

Fig. 105

1. To stimulate a more balanced and healthy thyroid activity (the thyroid regulates metabolism, which directly affects body temperature), work the reflex zone for the thyroid gland (around the base of the big toe) by rubbing and pressing. The finger or thumb walk technique is best here.

2. The toes hold reflex areas for the head: eyes, ears, sinuses, temples, forehead, pituitary, and brain. Spend quite some time working them carefully. On the bottom of your foot, work the fleshy part of all the toes. Use the thumb walk for maximum benefit, or at least give them a good rubbing with your thumb. Some simple massaging and wiggling of the toes will also help.

3. The pituitary gland located right in the center of the pad of the big toe is a major key to health. Known as the "master gland," it regulates the secretion of hormones, controls body temperature and metabolism, and governs energy level. To press on this point, massage with your thumb; it is best to use the "hook and back up" technique described on page 68.

4. Next, press the brain reflexes, located on the tips of the toes. The special way to work this area is to use the top of your index finger and roll it back and forth over the tip of each toe.

5. Finally, spend some time on key internal organs. The liver helps clear toxins from the blood; the adrenals fight inflammation; the spleen fights infection; the kidneys filter toxins from the blood and regulate fluid balance. All these are important. Rather than giving you specific points to press, we recommend that you carefully and thoroughly work the entire area on the bottom of your foot from the diaphragm line to the base of the heel. Thumb walk up, down, diagonally, horizontally. Spend several minutes here.

6. We suggest that you finish your session by repeating some of the relaxation presses from step #1, or just give your feet a gentle massaging. The thumb press on the solar plexus point is also very relaxing.

SHIATSU

This Shiatsu sequence stimulates the Large Intestine and Stomach channels to help clear heat from those meridians. Figure 104 shows the Large Intestine meridian; the Stomach meridian is in Figure 106.

1. The Large Intestine channel (see Fig 104) begins at the tip of the index finger and runs along the thumb side of the finger bone to the wrist, up the forearm to the elbow, and then continues on. Start at the tip of your left index finger (on the thumb side) and use the press and release technique. Press for 6 or 7 seconds; release; move a little way along the channel; and press again. Use firm pressure with your thumb.

When you come to the knuckles, press just under the bone on both sides of the knuckle, not on the knuckle itself. Follow the channel as it moves upward, close to the side of the finger bone in the hand up to Li 4 in the center of the web margin between the thumb and the index finger. Keep following it with the press and release technique.

From here the meridian follows a virtually straight line to the outer edge of the elbow crease. To be sure you are on the right line, position your arm in front of you with the palm facing your stomach about 4–5 inches away from your body. Imagine the line drawn on your arm in this position. Press and release along the entire length of your forearm to the elbow. Stop at the elbow crease. Be sure to do both arms.

2. To work the Stomach meridian start at the tip of your second toe, slightly on the little toe side, and move upward using the press and release technique to move along in small increments. The meridian runs over the

top of the foot between the 2nd and 3rd toes, and up the front of the ankle. From the ankle it continues along the front of the leg about 1 finger breadth to the little toe side of the shin bone. Stop just below the knee. Use firm pressure.

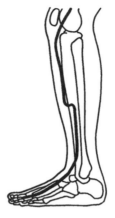

Fig. 106

ADDITIONAL SUGGESTIONS

1. Drink a lot. You tend to perspire a lot when you have a fever (perspiration helps cool the body), so you need to drink to replenish the liquid loss. Although you may think cold drinks would be helpful, they are not; stick to room temperature water or juices, or drink hot herb teas. Grape juice is a good cooling drink; add a little cumin and fennel (about ½ teaspoon each) to increase the cooling effect.

2. Rest. It's best not to exercise or travel when you have a fever. Rest as much as you can until the fever breaks.

3. The herb goldenseal is widely used as an herbal antibiotic and can help reduce fevers. It's available at any health food store and in many regular drug stores.

4. For high fever, place cool compresses on the forehead. Keep changing them each time the compress warms up to body temperature. You can increase the cooling effect by also putting a compress over the navel area.

5. Fast. The old saying "Feed a cold and starve a fever" holds a lot of truth. Fasting for a day or two will help eliminate the accumulated toxins that are most likely causing the fever. But be sure to have enough to drink.

6. Watch for danger signs. Mild fever is not dangerous, but here are 5 instances when you should seek medical help:

1. Any fever in a baby under 4 months old.
2. Fever above 104 degrees F. in an adult.
3. Fever above 101 degrees F. in a person over 60.
4. Fever that lasts more than 3 days.
5. Any fever in a person who has chronic illness such as heart disease, diabetes, or respiratory disease.

Hay Fever

See "Allergies"

Headaches

Headaches may well be the most common health complaint. Although some headaches are due to problems in the head itself, such as sinus congestion, generally headaches are a symptom of a health problem elsewhere in the body. Indigestion, constipation, poor posture, muscle tension, fatigue, and stress are common causes. Allergies, including hay fever and food reactions, are also at the root of many headaches.

Eyestrain is another common cause of headaches. Too much studying or sitting in front of a computer screen without a break, or an out-of-date eyeglass prescription can strain your eyes and result in quite a strong headache.

The most common origin is muscle tension. Due to a wide variety of causes, the muscles in our neck, shoulders, and head tighten up and constrict the blood vessels, partially preventing the flow of blood to the brain. The reasons we tighten up can be physical, mental, or emotional, and include such factors as stress, slumping and other forms of poor posture, anger, anxiety, and worry.

From an Eastern point of view, this muscle tension has the deeper effect of blocking the flow of energy (*Ch'i* or *Prana*) to the head. When neither oxygen nor Life Energy is flowing adequately, the body cries out in pain.

According to the theory behind all the finger pressure therapies, energy channels from all over the body, including the internal organs, are connected to the head. That's why headaches can result from such a wide variety of problems.

When a headache strikes, our culture offers an array of pain killers, including aspirin, acetaminophen (Tylenol®) and ibuprofen (Advil®) to mask the pain. Although these are often called "remedies," they do little or nothing to eliminate the root cause of the problem. A pill may make the headache disappear for a while, but it won't cure constipation, remove the cause of our anxiety, or help us sit up straight so sufficient oxygen can flow to nourish our brain cells.

Pressure point therapy allows us to relieve the pain not by avoiding it, but by helping to relax the tensed muscles and release the blocks in the energy channels.

A headache, like any pain, is a signal from the body that something is wrong that needs attention. Be sure to see a doctor if your headache persists or is severe.

ACUPRESSURE

The first two points (Li 4 and Gb 20) are described in the section, "Ten Master Pressure Points" (beginning on page 49) where you will find illustrations of the precise point locations as well as suggestions on how to press them for maximum benefit.

1. (Li 4, Adjoining Valley) This is one of the most effective of all pressure points for relieving pain. **Caution:** pregnant women should not press this point; it can stimulate premature uterine contractions.

2. (Gb 20, Wind Pool) When you've located this point, press for 2 minutes, remembering to build up and release pressure gradually. After you finish the steady pressing, find all the tender spots within about an inch of this point, and rub them with small circular motions.

3. (Extra Point Tai Yang) This point is located about 1 thumb width outside the outer edge of the eye socket. You'll find a natural depression, halfway between the eyebrow and the outer edge of the eye socket.

The point is in this depression. Press with the middle finger while making slow circles. After going clockwise for 30 seconds reverse and go the other way.

4. (Gb 13, Mind Root) This point is just inside the hairline, directly above the outer edge of the eye socket. (If your hair is receding, locate the point where your hair used to be. It should be approximately 4 finger widths above your eyebrows.) This point calms the mind and relieves headaches. Use the middle finger and apply steady pressure for 1 to 2 minutes.

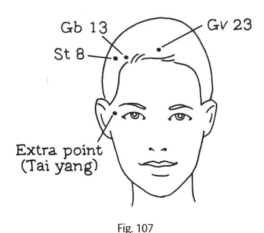

Fig. 107

5. (St 8, Skull Support) This point is at the same level as Gb 13 (above) but one more inch toward the outside of the head. It is also very effective for headaches. Press with the middle fingers with steady, firm pressure. Hold for 1 to 2 minutes.

Most headaches are related to stress. *For stress headaches or migraine headaches,* be sure to add:

6. (Gb 41, Falling Tears) This point is on the top of the foot in the channel between the little toe and the 4th toe, a little less than halfway between the ankle bone and the web margin between the toes. (It's closer to the toes.) This point is effective in restoring the smooth flow of *ch'i* which can be interrupted by stress, worry, and anxiety. It relieves headaches by removing obstructions and restoring balance. Once you locate the point, press firmly for about a minute with your index or middle finger.

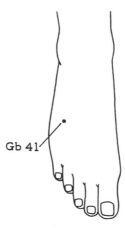

Fig. 108

7. (Tw 5, Outer Gate) Hold your left arm in front of you with the palm down facing the floor. Measure two thumb widths above the wrist. The point is right in the center between the two forearm bones. (See Fig. 109.) Press with your thumb or middle finger for about a minute; then switch arms. Tw 5 has a synergistic effect when paired with Gb 41. The two points are excellent for relieving migraines, or any headaches felt primarily on the sides of the head.

For frontal headaches add:

8. (Gv 23, Upper Star) This point is one thumb width inside the hairline of the forehead, directly above the nose (Fig. 107). It is also good for sinus and nasal congestion. Use firm pressure with your index or middle finger for about a minute.

For headaches associated with the common cold add:

9. (Lu 7, Broken Sequence) Hold one hand out in front of you with the palm facing down. Start from the V shape formed by your thumb and index finger. Use the index finger of the other hand to trace along the top of the thumb to the wrist. Your finger will fall into a natural depression where the base of your thumb joins the wrist. Keep going another inch and a half and you will be on Lu 7. This point is the command point for the head and is frequently used to treat colds in Chinese medicine. It is also healing to the lungs. Maintain firm pressure (you can use your thumb or index finger) for about a minute, then switch hands.

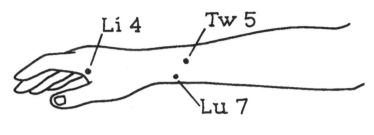

Fig. 109

REFLEXOLOGY

The hands and feet contain many pressure points that can be massaged to help alleviate headaches. Since you can always press your hands no matter where you are, let's start with a few key points there.

1. According to Mildred Carter, author of *Body Reflexology*, our thumbs represent the head. She suggests pressing on the pad of the thumb (using your opposite thumb), then squeezing the sides of the thumb by pressing alongside the nail. Move to the area just below the thumbnail and press along the width of the finger. Finally, look for tender spots as you press firmly all around the thumb. When you find a tender spot, massage it with a rotating pressure for several minutes. See pages 47 and 48.

2. If your headache is related to your sinuses, press the tips of your fingers. If you suspect eyestrain, the bottom of each finger (just above where it joins the hand) is a key area to massage. Also, press into the notch between the index and middle finger, using a rotating motion with your opposite index finger. Be sure to do both hands.

3. Mrs. Carter also suggests applying pressure across the center of the hand. This is where the stomach, colon and other aspects of the digestive and elimination system are located. Use the "thumb walk" to move along both palms, searching for tender spots and working them for up to several minutes when you find them.

4. Pressure points on your feet are located in similar places to points on the hand. When you work on your feet, begin with the Reflexology Warm-Up on page 69, a sequence of steps that help you relax as well as toning the energy of the whole body and preparing your feet to be worked on.

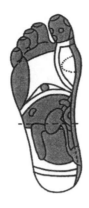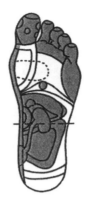

Fig. 110

5.   Then apply pressure to various points on the big toe, starting at the top and working toward the base. Circle the whole toe in search of spots that are tender, and use your thumb to work out the soreness. Move on to the other toes. These may be easier to work using the "finger walk," applying pressure with your fingers. Again, work from the top of the toe to the base. If your sinuses are congested, you will probably find a great deal of soreness in the toes. Be sure to work on both feet.

6.   To help relieve tension and congestion in the neck, work your way across the ridge at the base of the smaller toes. Support your foot and pull the pad of the foot downward with one hand while you "walk" with your thumb or index finger across the ridge from the little toe to the big toe, applying firm pressure. Spend more time on tender spots.

7.   Thumb walk the shoulder area (on the sole of the foot, below the little toe), to further eliminate tensions.

8.   Pressing the solar plexus point that you pressed during the Reflexology Warm-Up is very relaxing; try repeating it several times to help eliminate your headache.

9.   Dwight Byers, author of *Better Health with Foot Reflexology*, recommends working the spine reflexes for headache relief. These reflexes are located on the inside edge of both feet (zone 1), extending from the heel nearly to the top of the big toe, opposite the root of the toenail.

When you work the spinal reflexes, work slowly up the foot using the thumb walk technique. You will have to use a little extra strength in the heel area, as the skin is thicker there.

Thumb walk all the way down the spinal reflex area, and then take some time to walk across small areas horizontally, moving up the foot from the heel to the big toe.

10. Since indigestion and constipation are often at the root of a headache, take some time to work the entire soft part of the sole, from the heel line up to the diaphragm line. This area includes the reflexes for the stomach as well as the large and small intestines and the colon.

SHIATSU

Try this simple, 10-step Shiatsu sequence for headache relief. At each position, start lightly, gradually increase pressure, hold for about 5–7 seconds, then gradually release.

1. Use your index fingers to press the inside corner of each eye socket, at the bridge of the nose.

2. With thumb and index finger, pinch the bridge of your nose.

3. With your thumbs, press several points under your eyebrows, at the top of the eye socket. Start at the inside, next to your nose, and move outwards. Remember to start with light pressure, build up slowly, hold a few seconds, then gradually release the pressure. These points may be very sensitive; don't press too hard.

4. Pinch along your eyebrows, using thumb and index finger.

5. With your fingers spread, work along parallel lines from the middle of your forehead to the back of your neck. Press with 4 fingers; move about half an inch and press again, and continue onto the ropy muscles of the neck.

6. Lightly rub circles on your temples with your fingertips. Don't press.

7. With your thumbs, find the indentations on the back of the skull, just behind your ears. Press and hold for 15 seconds. Breathe deeply.

8. With your thumbs still locked in the same position, move your head slowly forward and back 3 times. Release gradually.

9. Squeeze the back of your neck for 5 seconds. Release. Repeat.

10. Close your eyes and sit quietly for 1 to 2 minutes to let the energy settle in a new pattern.

ADDITIONAL SUGGESTIONS

DRINK ENOUGH WATER.   Water helps with elimination (some headaches are caused by a build-up of toxins or impurities in the body), and provides a vital source of oxygen for your brain.

GET OUTSIDE.   When you have a headache, a walk in the fresh air can often be enough to relieve it. Many people fall prey to headaches from stuffy air.

EXERCISE.   Getting adequate exercise every day is an effective preventive measure. Exercise increases the flow of oxygen to the brain and also helps the system eliminate metabolic wastes. Yoga postures also improve circulation and elimination. An excellent daily all-round Yoga exercise is the Sun Salutation, a series of 12 postures that tones the entire body.

WATCH YOUR DIET.   A crucial factor in preventing constipation (a very common cause of headaches) is getting sufficient fiber in your diet by eating plenty of fruit, vegetables, and whole grains. Avoid red meat, white sugar, and white flour. Other foods that have been known to trigger headaches include red wine, chocolate, heavy cream, coffee, cheese, and bacon. Try to notice if your headaches occur after eating any of these foods.

KEEP THE LID ON STRESS.   Since the majority of headaches are caused by muscle tension, you need to relax. Tense muscles in the face, skull, neck, shoulders, and upper back can easily lead to headaches. Everyone has his or her own favorite ways to relax: a hot bath, a massage, listening to soothing music, doing Yoga postures, sitting in meditation, going swimming or getting some other type of exercise—whatever works for you, do it!

CORRECT POOR POSTURE.   If you slump when you stand or sit, you may be putting strain on your muscles and reducing oxygen flow to your brain. Stay straight but relaxed, with your shoulders dropped (not up around your ears!) and slightly back, and your pelvis tucked.

REDUCE EYESTRAIN.   Many headaches are the result of tired or strained eyes, due to driving, sitting in front of a computer screen, and numerous other causes. To relax your eyes, vigorously rub your palms together for a full 30 seconds until they become quite warm, then close your eyes and place your palms lightly over the eyes. Don't press on the eyeballs. Keep your hands there for 1 minute. (If you feel that eyestrain is causing the headache, see "Eyestrain" for more suggestions.)

Hearing Problems

Chinese medicine divides hearing problems into two main types. The *deficiency* type, associated with improperly functioning kidney *ch'i*, typically takes the form of a gradual loss of hearing as we age, due to waning vitality of energy in the Kidney meridian. To treat this, the kidney *ch'i* must be strengthened or "tonified."

The less frequent *excess* type of hearing problems, generally due to an abundance of stagnated *ch'i* in the Liver or Gallbladder meridians, may take the form of an abrupt loss of hearing over a few days. Treatment for this involves "draining" the energy to restore balance.

Tinnitus is another common hearing complaint. This is the subjective experience of hearing a shrill or high pitched sound (associated with stagnant or excess *ch'i*) or a lowpitched sound (associated with a lack of Kidney *ch'i*) in one or both ears.

The best treatment results with Acupressure are found for the excess type. That's because it is easier to drain an excess than to build up a deficiency. Deficiency disorders tend to be long-standing, chronic conditions, and they respond rather slowly to treatment. Results can definitely be achieved if you persevere—but don't look for them overnight.

ACUPRESSURE

Use the first three points for both types of condition:

1. (Tw 3, Middle Islet) On the back of your hand, between the little finger and 4th finger, find the depression about halfway between the knuckles and the wrist. Use your thumb and apply moderate pressure for about a minute. This point has a reputation for achieving very good results for ear disorders.

2. (Tw 17, Wind Screen) This point, also on the Triple Warmer meridian just before it enters the ear, is located in the natural depression right behind the earlobe. Apply pressure with your index or middle finger. Use mild to moderate pressure, as this point may be tender.

3. (Si 19, Listening Palace) Place your index fingers on your face where the ear is attached. Open and close your mouth a few times to feel the jaw bone moving under your fingers. Si 19 is in the depression that forms when the mouth opens. Stimulate this point with your mouth open. Use mild pressure with your index or middle fingers. Be sure you are pressing right in the center of the depression.

Two other points in this depression (about ½ inch above and ½ inch below) will also be stimulated. Si 19 has a beneficial effect on the ears and is also a crossing point of the Gallbladder and Triple Warmer meridians.

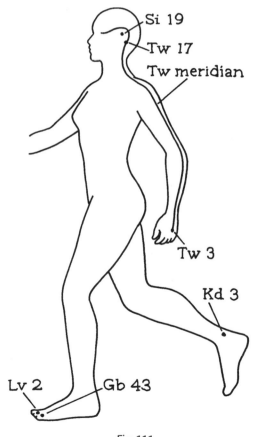

Fig. 111

For deficiency type hearing problems, add the following two points (Kd 3 and B 23) to the previous routine. For complete descriptions and location illustrations for these points, as well as instructions on how to press them most effectively, please see page 49 for the beginning of "Ten Master Pressure Points."

4. (Kd 3, Supreme Stream) The Kidney energy in Chinese medicine is considered the root of the *yin* and *yang* of the entire body, and Kd 3 is considered the source point for the Kidney meridian. Thus it not only exerts a powerful influence on the entire meridian, but gives support and nourishment to all the other energy systems of the body. Since the hearing loss we are considering is from deficient Kidney energy, pressing this point will be very helpful.

5. (B 23, Associated point of Kidney) This point in combination with Kd 3 greatly strengthens the Kidney *ch'i.*

For excess type hearing problems, press the following two points in addition to points 1 through 3 above:

6. (Gb 43, Clamped Stream) Gb 43 is located in the web margin between the 4th and 5th toe. It tends to be very tender. Use your index finger and apply mild to moderate pressure for a minute. The "excess" pattern for hearing problems typically has a Gallbladder meridian involvement; Gb 43 is the best point to drain excess from this meridian.

7. (Lv 2, Moving Between) This point is located in the web margin between the big toe and second toe. Use medium pressure with your index fingers, pressing on both feet at the same time if that is comfortable, otherwise one at a time. Just as Gb 43 is the best point to drain excess from the Gallbladder meridian, Lv 2 is the best point for draining excess energy from the Liver meridian.

REFLEXOLOGY

Your Reflexology session for hearing problems will focus mainly on reflex areas for the upper part of your body—shoulder and neck points for relaxation, spine points to stimulate the nervous system, as well as head, brain and specific ear points. We will also work the kidney reflex (which is in the same zone as the ears), since, as we have just seen, in Oriental medicine ear problems are frequently associated with weak Kidney energy.

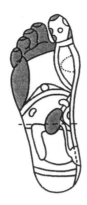 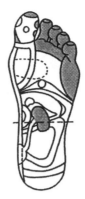

Fig. 112

1. Before moving to specific reflex points, however, we suggest that you begin by massaging your feet and relaxing them with the techniques described in the Reflexology Warm-Up box on page 69. This is an important step that helps you relax, tones the energy of the whole body, and prepares your feet to be worked on.

2. The reflex zones for your shoulders are located on the bottom of your foot in zone 5, under your little toe, and continuing out along the outside edge of your foot. It extends from the base of your little toe down to the diaphragm line. To relax your shoulders (and improve circulation to your head), work both horizontally and vertically along this zone. You'll probably find it easiest to use the thumb walk up the foot, the finger walk across, but do what works best.

3. To further relax the neck and shoulder areas and increase blood flow to the head, press on the cervical spine reflex, located on the opposite end of your foot, along the outside edge of your big toe. Use the thumb walk and go over the area several times. Use your thumb or index finger to walk the seventh cervical area in the groove at the base of the big toe (on top of the foot). It may be quite tender.

4. Circulation in the neck and temples can be stimulated by pressing along the inside side of your big toe, between the bottom of the nail and the base of the toe. You may find a lot of tenderness there. Don't press too hard on the joint.

5. You can also work on your neck as well as the inner ear area by "walking the ridge" at the top of the ball of the foot (at the base of the toes).

Use your thumb or index finger. Pull the fleshy pad of your foot down and away from the ridge with your other hand. Walk in both directions.

6. Ear reflexes are located on the bottom of your feet, on the fleshy part of the four smaller toes. Use the thumb walk for maximum benefit, or at least give them a good rubbing with your thumb.

There's also a reflex zone for the inner ear on the top of your foot, in the groove between the second and third toe. (It doesn't go all the way up the groove, just an inch or an inch and a half.) Work this with your index finger, using the finger walk technique. Use substantial pressure, unless it is very sensitive.

7. Now work the reflex zones for the brain, the central switchboard for all the senses. You'll find this key reflex on the very tip of all your toes. Work on it by pressing down with your index finger and rolling it back and forth across the top of each toe.

8. Finally, press the kidney reflexes located in the soft center of the foot. Try the "rotation on a point" technique described on page 68, or at least work the area well with the thumb walk.

After working on all these reflex areas, take a few minutes just to relax, massaging your feet and using the relaxation techniques, ending with the thumb press on the solar plexus point for half a minute.

SHIATSU

A Shiatsu routine helpful for any kind of ear or hearing difficulty is to stimulate along the Triple Warmer meridian. This channel runs up the arm to the shoulder and neck, circles around, enters the ear, re-emerges from the ear onto the face, and ends at the outer edge of the eyebrow. (See Fig. 111.)

Start at the tip of your 4th finger, on the little finger side. With the index finger of the other hand, use a press and release technique for this exercise. Press once for 6–7 seconds, then release. Use firm pressure. Move half an inch or so along the channel, then press again.

From the tip of the 4th finger move slowly along the side of the finger to the web margin between the 4th and 5th fingers. Do two or three extra presses and releases on this point, with your thumb underneath the webbing for support. Then continue forward along the groove between the 4th and 5th fingers. About halfway between the knuckles and the wrist you will be over Tw 3. Give a little extra stimulation on this point.

As you approach the wrist, you will notice that there is no longer a groove beneath your fingers. Instead, you'll be feeling the small bones of the wrist. When you feel that you're no longer in a groove, angle slightly inwards toward the center of the wrist. Then continue up the center of the forearm until you get about halfway toward the elbow.

At this point, switch to a new technique to stimulate the channel. The meridian continues over the back of the elbow and up the triceps to the shoulder, neck and ears. Cup your hand, and slap your arm. Start behind the elbow, and continue up over the shoulder to where the shoulder meets the neck. Don't slap your neck or ears.

Now go back and start with the other arm.

When you have completed this entire routine on both arms, press Tw 17 (in the natural depression right behind the earlobe) several times with the index or middle finger of both hands, using the press and release technique. End by pressing Tw 23, which is the last point on the channel. It is located at the outer edge of the eyebrow. Feel for a natural depression. Press and release. (See Fig. 66 on page 134.)

ADDITIONAL SUGGESTIONS

HERBAL FORMULA.   As we have mentioned, in Chinese medicine the ears are said to be governed by the Kidneys, and hearing loss is often associated with a weakening of the Kidney *ch'i*. One of the most famous Kidney tonics in Chinese medicine is Six Rhemania Formula (Liu Wei di Huang Wan), a tonic for the *yin* aspect of the Kidney. Many health food stores are starting to carry Chinese herbal preparations.

TRY MAGNESIUM.   If your hearing loss is due to excess noise exposure, magnesium supplements may help.

KEEP FIT.   Some research suggests that people who are more generally fit suffer less from hearing impairment than people who are more sedentary and less fit. This may be because adequate exercise maintains good circulation to the brain and the inner ears, which depend on good blood flow for proper functioning.

YOGA STRETCHING.   For good circulation, Yoga postures are always very helpful. Be sure to include the Shoulder Stand in your daily routine, as it tones the whole body and improves circulation throughout.

Heart Disease

See "Heart Tune-Up"

Heart Tune-Up

The heart, that most vital of our vital organs, works non-stop 24 hours a day pumping blood throughout the body. That life-giving blood brings nourishment, oxygen, hormones, and antibodies to every cell. When the heart stops, life stops.

Your heart pumps about 4,000 times an hour. It beats 100,000 times every day, moving about 2,000 gallons of blood through an estimated 70,000 miles of blood vessels. In the course of a year it beats almost 40 million times!

To keep this vital organ healthy is absolutely essential for a long, healthy life. Yet the typical American lifestyle, which combines too little exercise and too much stress with a very unhealthy diet, has led to an unprecedented amount of heart disease. The U.S. has the highest death rate from heart disease in the world. Over 60 million of us suffer from some form of it, and more of us will die from heart disease than from any other cause. Although much publicity surrounds breast cancer, heart disease takes the life of far more women every year. Keeping the heart healthy is thus not only helpful for a better quality of life, it is truly a matter of life and death.

Conventional medicine treats heart disease with powerful drugs to reduce cholesterol and high blood pressure, along with high-tech options such as angioplasty and bypass surgery. In addition to being dangerous and/or involving uncomfortable side effects, these methods are terribly costly; the medical cost for cardiovascular disease is approximately $60 billion every year.

In Chinese medicine, the heart is considered the ruler of all the other organs. But its importance goes far beyond the obvious requirement for blood circulation. The heart is also intimately connected with the inner being of the person, the *shen* (consciousness or spirit). Thus it is not just a physical organ; it is also deeply involved in our mental, emotional, and spiritual well-being.

This connection is a two-way street. High stress levels, discordant feelings and emotions, and lack of peace can have a deleterious effect on the heart, as harmonious feelings and a peaceful mind support its health. The bottom line is that a healthy heart requires more than just regular aerobic exercise! You need to work on maintaining overall balance in your life as well.

Fortunately, research shows that the risk of heart attacks and stroke can be greatly decreased through natural means. Here are some ways to keep your heart functioning at its best.

ACUPRESSURE

1.   (Ht 7, Mind Door) This point is on the palm side of your hand, on the wrist crease, directly below your little finger. Find the bony knob on the outside of your left wrist (the little finger side). The point is next to that, in a small indentation. Press for 30 seconds with your thumb; release gradually; switch hands. This point, considered the "source point" of the Heart meridian, is very nourishing to all aspects of the heart. As the heart influences our mental, emotional, and spiritual well-being, this point not only nourishes the physical aspect of the organ, but helps calm the mind and soothe the emotions.

2.   (Pc 6, Inner Gate) You will find this point on the palm side of your wrist, two thumb widths above the wrist crease in the center of the arm. Pc 6 regulates *ch'i* as well as blood in the chest. It is important for regulating anything to do with the heart; another name for it is "Heart Protector." Pressing this point helps strengthen the heart; it's also helpful to relieve pain or discomfort of the chest.

You can stimulate this point with your thumb, or by curling one hand around the opposite wrist and using the middle finger. Use moderate to firm pressure. Remember to build up gradually, hold about a minute, and gradually release. Be sure to do both hands.

The combination of Li 4 and Lv 3 (coming up next) is a famous combination known as "the four gates." It is unparalleled in its ability to circulate *ch'i* through the entire meridian network. This is healthy physically and also emotionally: by breaking up stuck energy it helps balance and harmonize us emotionally, which has a direct benefit on maintaining a healthy heart.

These two points are fully described in the section, "Ten Master Pressure Points" (beginning on page 49) where you will also find illustrations of the precise point locations and suggestions on how to press them for maximum benefit.

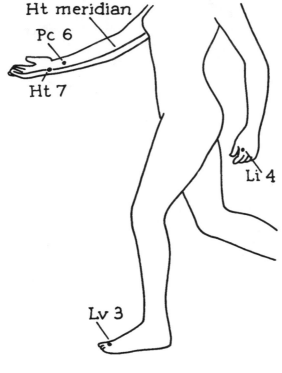

Fig. 113

3. (Li 4, Adjoining Valley)

4. (Lv 3, (Bigger Rushing) The source point of the Liver meridian, Lv 3 helps stimulate the Liver energy do its main job—keeping all the *ch'i* in the body flowing smoothly. When the Liver energy goes out of balance, it can cause stagnation and imbalance everywhere else. Of all the many points on the body, this is the most effective for regulating the smooth flow of *ch'i*.

REFLEXOLOGY

Here is an effective heart tune-up that you can do in just 10 minutes.

1. Begin with the Reflexology Warm-Up on page 69. This is an important step that helps you relax, tones the energy of the whole body, and prepares your feet to be worked on.

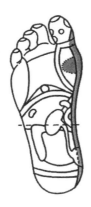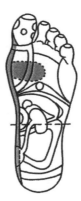

Fig. 114

2. Following the warm-up, begin specific treatment on your heart by working the heart reflex zones. Authorities are not all agreed on the precise location of the reflex zone for the heart, but all place it on the sole of the left foot, between the diaphragm line and the base of the toes. Some locate it more on the inside of the foot, toward the big toe; others place it a little more toward the little toe. For safety, work the entire area, thumb walking up, down, and across, giving even pressure as you work.

   Also work zones 1 and 2 (below the big toe and first toe) of the right foot, using the thumb walk.

3. Then, on the top of your foot, work the chest area, which runs from the base of the toes up about 2 inches toward your ankle. Use the finger walk in the grooves between the toes.

   Also work the corresponding areas on the palm of your left and right hands.

4. It is also helpful to work the spine reflex, especially the upper and mid-spine, on both your hands and feet. These reflexes are located on the inside edge of both feet (zone 1). Work slowly up and down the foot using the thumb walk technique.

SHIATSU

Here is a 5-step heart strengthening tune-up from the Shiatsu tradition.

1. Use 3 fingers (index, middle, and ring finger) of both hands to press between your ribs. Spread your fingers and place them so that they fit

between the ribs. Start close to the breastbone, at the top of the rib cage, below the collar bone, and move outward. Then move down to the next set of ribs. Apply pressure for 5 to 7 seconds at each place. (See Fig. 60) Women: don't press directly on the breasts; press only above, around, and below the breasts where you can work directly over the ribs.

2. Apply 3-finger pressure in the groove where your left arm meets your chest. Start at the top, beneath the collarbone, and move down an inch or so at a time, pressing about 10 seconds at each location.

3. Press the points along the Heart meridian (see Fig. 113) on the inside lower part of your right arm, from the armpit down to your wrist. Hold each point for about 10 seconds. You may find these points easily, as they may be tender. Don't worry if you don't locate them precisely; you will be moving along the meridian and stimulating it in a positive way even if you are not on the exact spot.

4. Hold the little finger of your left hand between your right thumb and index finger. Press between the joints and at the tip of the finger for 10 seconds each time. Repeat with the same points on your left ring finger.

5. Place your right palm just below your rib cage, in the center (below the breastbone). Place your left palm on top of the right, and press firmly with both hands for 10 seconds. Repeat. (This is the solar plexus area.)

ADDITIONAL SUGGESTIONS

The recommendations in the section, "11 Simple, Universal Guidelines for Good Health" on page 77, provide excellent tips for heart health. Of particular importance:

LOW FAT DIET.   To lower your risk of heart disease, reduce the amount of fat in your diet. Programs such as the Pritikin diet and Dean Ornish's "Program for Reversing Heart Disease" have been successful in slowing or even reversing heart disease in patients whose diet contained only 10 percent of calories from fat. Cut down (or eliminate) red meat, butter, cheese, ice cream, and other foods high in saturated fat; reduce your intake of fried foods. Eat several portions of fresh fruit, vegetables, and whole grains every day.

REDUCE STRESS.   Stress and tension not only put pressure on the circulatory system, reducing blood flow to the heart, they also create wear and tear on the body and generate free radicals, major villains in heart disease. To keep stress in check, spend at least 15 to 20 minutes (twice a day is best) practicing Progressive Relaxation, Transcendental Meditation, the Relaxation Response, visualization, or whatever helps you deeply relax.

EXERCISE.   Regular exercise is essential for maintaining a healthy heart. Research suggests that vigorous aerobic exercise is not necessary for heart health; a 30- minute daily walk is quite sufficient. If you are a heart patient or are over 40 and have not been exercising regularly, consult a doctor before beginning any exercise program.

QUIT SMOKING.   Smoking puts an enormous amount of damaging stress on the cardiovascular system, weakens the heart and lungs, and almost certainly shortens the life span. Experts agree that if you are a smoker, quitting is the best thing you can do for your heart and your health.

YOGA.   Yoga stretching can improve circulation to the heart. Unless you have a heart condition, do several cycles of the Sun Salutation every day (slowly), as well as the Cobra and Locust poses (which will help stretch the coronary arteries and increase blood supply to the heart). A gentle Spinal Twist will also be effective.

Hemorrhoids

Hemorrhoids are swollen veins (like varicose veins) in the rectum or anus which may bleed and become painful. Though many people are too embarrassed to admit they have hemorrhoids, they are extremely common, striking about eight out of every ten of us over the course of a lifetime. Men and women are equally susceptible, despite the fact that many women suffer from hemorrhoids when they are pregnant, as the swollen uterus restricts blood flow in the rectal area. Straining during delivery exacerbates the problem.

Aside from pregnancy, there are two major causes of hemorrhoids. First is a diet lacking in sufficient fiber. Fiber (found in whole grains, vegetables, and fruit) makes the stool softer and bulkier. Processed food such as refined flour and sugar, so common in the Western diet, tends to produce hard, dry stools which can both cause and irritate hemorrhoids. The second main cause is straining while moving the bowels—usually due to the first problem!

In this section we will suggest some effective pressure point remedies, as well as a few other simple suggestions to help prevent and relieve hemorrhoids.

ACUPRESSURE

1. (B 57, Support the Mountain) One of the main points used in Oriental medicine to relieve hemorrhoids, B 57 is located in the center of the "V" formed by the lower border of the calf muscles. (It's approximately halfway between the ankle bone and a point directly behind your knee). A good way to work on this point is to put both thumbs together and press with strong pressure. Hold for about a minute. Remember to start lightly, build up, hold, and gradually release.

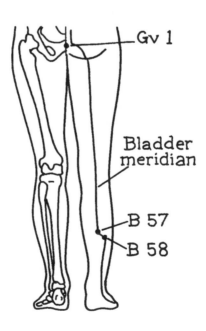

Fig. 115

2. (B 58, Soaring Upwards) About one thumb width below and to the outside of B 57 (in #1). Use the same technique and pressure. This point reinforces the effect of B 57. Stimulating these points on the Bladder meridian is effective for hemorrhoid relief because a branch of the meridian circles the anus.

3. (Gv 1, Long Strong) This point is located between the tip of the tail bone (coccyx) and the anus. You may find it easier to press on it if you first lie down on your side, then press with the middle finger with moderate pressure. It is used both for its local effect and to stimulate the entire Gv meridian, which also winds around the anus.

4. (Sp 10, Sea of Blood) As Sp 10 is the main point in Oriental medicine to break up blood stagnation, it is helpful in treating hemorrhoids. For an illustration of the exact location of this point, and instructions on how to press most effectively, see page 49 for the beginning of "Ten Master Pressure Points."

REFLEXOLOGY

Effective reflexology self-treatment for hemorrhoids involves a number of areas on your feet.

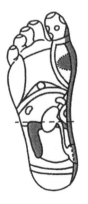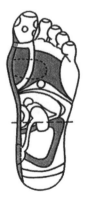

Fig. 116

But before you treat specific reflex areas, begin with the Reflexology Warm-Up on page 69. This important step helps you relax, tones the energy of the whole body, and prepares your feet to be worked on; please don't skip it!

1. Since hemorrhoids are related to the circulatory system (they are essentially varicose veins in the rectum), we suggest working the heart reflex. Use your thumb to walk up and down on your left foot between the diaphragm line and the base of the toes. Some Reflexologists believe there is an additional area for the heart on the ball of the right foot; spend some time pressing there.

2. Next, work on your lower spine. The spine reflexes are located on the inside edge of both feet (zone 1), extending from the heel nearly to the top of the big toe, opposite the root of the toenail. If you have time, first briefly work the entire spine, going once up and once down using the thumb walk. Otherwise, concentrate on the coccyx and the sacral and lumbar areas, which run from your heel (about an inch up from the back of your foot) to the midpoint or center line of the foot.

3. Now work on the reflex areas for the colon. As you can see from Fig. M on page 45, there are several reflex areas involved here, on both feet, between the heel and midline of the foot. Work these reflexes thoroughly and carefully using the thumb walk technique.

4. Finally, there is an area specific to the rectum. It is sometimes referred to as the "chronic area." It runs up along the Achilles tendon on the back of the foot, from the heel up the ankle to the bottom of the leg. You can work it both on the inside and outside of your foot. This area is likely to be very sensitive, so don't press too hard. You can use either the thumb walk or finger walk.

SHIATSU

1. To stretch and open the Bladder meridian, we suggest the heel and calf stretch. Here's how to do it:

Place your left foot slightly in front of you, at a 45-degree-angle from the right foot. Your feet should be about shoulder width apart.

Now angle your right foot so that the toes are pointed to the left. Now, shift most of your weight to the left (forward) foot. Keep your right (rear) heel on the ground and feel the stretch in the heel and calf as you shift your center of gravity toward your left foot.

Hold the stretch for 30–60 seconds. Try to relax into the stretch. The relaxation is an ongoing process as the muscles loosen up. Switch to the other side. After doing both sides, go back and repeat both legs twice more for a total of three on each side.

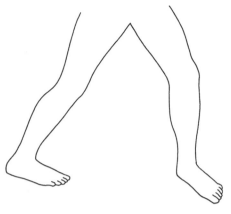

Fig. 117

2. To further work on the Bladder meridian, use the press and release process along the entire channel. (See Fig. 115.) Start at the little toe and press along the side of the bone. Press for 6–7 seconds, release, move up ½ inch to an inch, and repeat.

At the "knuckle" where the little toe joins the foot, press slightly below the bone on both sides of the joint. Keep moving along the bone, just slightly below it. Move up to the ankle bone and press just below it. Next, move to a point at the level of the ankle bone, midway between the ankle bone and the Achilles tendon at the back of the ankle. Move up the leg between the Achilles tendon and the leg bone.

When you get to the calf muscle, change the procedure. From here, the meridian will move to the center of the back of the leg and runs up the back of the leg to the buttocks. Instead of pressing and releasing, to stimulate the channel between the calves and the buttocks we'll use loose fist slapping. Make a loose fist, and, starting at the calves, rhythmically strike the back of the legs all the way up to the buttocks and onto the low back as far up as you can reach. Start over again at the calves and repeat the process twice more.

Make sure to do both legs. Work on both simultaneously if you can do it comfortably.

ADDITIONAL SUGGESTIONS

EAT MORE FIBER.   As we mentioned, fiber in your food (vegetables, fruits, whole grains such as brown rice, oatmeal, whole wheat bread) makes stools much bulkier and softer. Cut down on refined sugar and refined flour, meat, coffee, and alcohol which have the opposite effect.

DRINK MORE WATER.   You need at least 6 glasses of water a day to keep the stools soft and avoid irritation that may lead to bleeding and pain.

TAKE A SITZ BATH.   When hemorrhoids are painful, sit in your bath-tub with your knees raised, in a few inches of warm water. The warm water soothes the pain, and simultaneously increases blood flow, which in turn can start shrinking the swollen veins.

TRY WITCH HAZEL.   This very inexpensive, simple astringent avail-able in any drug store can slow or stop bleeding and shrink the swelling of external hemorrhoids. Moisten a cotton ball and apply for a few minutes.

DON'T PUSH IT.   Try not to strain on the toilet when you move your bowels. Straining makes the blood vessels in the rectum swell up and become susceptible to being scraped and irritated.

WASH INSTEAD OF WIPING.   Instead of using toilet paper after emp-tying the bowels, wash yourself with warm water and pat dry. Toilet paper, especially if it is rough, can easily irritate.

TRY YOGA.   Several Yoga stretches are traditionally said to help relieve hemorrhoids. These include the Fish, Bow, and Shoulder Stand.

Herpes

Herpes simplex is a viral infection, transmitted by contact with a person who has it, that can cause painful blisters and sores on the body. Type I generally affects the lips and the area around the mouth; Type II affects the genitals. Once a person is infected with the virus, it will remain in the system permanently (there is no known cure), and there is a 90% chance of recurrences, especially when under stress, which depresses immune function and allows the virus to emerge from its dormant state. The Western treatment with anti-viral medications effectively relieves symptoms, and can prevent or at least increase the time between recurrences. Oriental medicine classifies herpes as a condition of damp heat in the Liver and Gallbladder meridians. (The Liver meridian encircles the genitalia).

ACUPRESSURE

For thorough descriptions and location illustrations for the first two points (Li 11 and Sp 10), as well as instructions on how to press them for maximum benefit, please see page 49 for the beginning of "Ten Master Pressure Points."

1. (Li 11, Pool at the Crook) Li 11 is one of the best points for clearing damp heat, and is widely used in many skin conditions.
2. (Sp 10, Sea of Blood) Sp 10 helps to remove excess heat in the blood which may be contributing to skin disorders. It also helps promote better circulation.

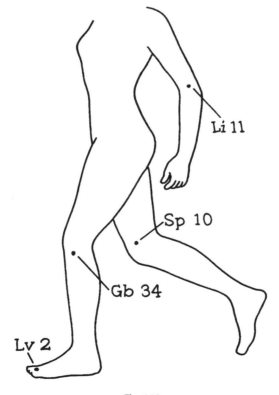

Fig. 118

3. (Gb 34, Yang Hill Spring) At the lower border of the kneecap, slide your finger off the shinbone toward the outside (little toe side). Two bones come together here. Press in the soft tissue area between them, using your thumb or your index and middle fingers together (3rd on top of 2nd). Gb 34 clears damp heat from the Liver and Gallbladder.

4. (Lv 2, Moving Between) This point is located in the web margin between the big toe and second toe. Use medium pressure with your index fingers, pressing on both feet at the same time if that is comfortable, or one at a time.

REFLEXOLOGY

Reflexology cannot cure herpes, or heal an outbreak of the virus. However, there is a clear correlation between stress and recurrences in people who already have the herpes virus. So we recommend a Reflexology relaxation session for stress reduction. For this, turn to page 69 and follow the step-by-step instructions in the section, "How to Use Reflexology for Prevention and Healing." We believe you will find this very soothing, calming, and relaxing. Alternatively, use the sequence in the section, "Stress."

SHIATSU

We will work on releasing heat and stimulating the free flow of energy in the Gallbladder and Liver meridians.

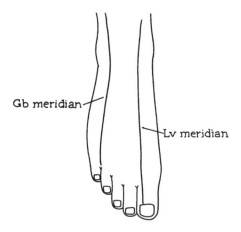

Fig. 119

1. Start in the middle of the top of your foot, in line with the space between your big toe and 2nd toe. Using the press and release technique (press for 6–7 seconds with your thumb, release, move a fraction of an inch along the meridian, and press again), start working toward the toes. As you get closer to the toes, be sure to be in the channel between the big toe and 2nd toe. Work down to the web margin between them. From here go along the top of the big toe and stop at the nail. Do both feet.

2. Now find the space in your foot between the 4th and 5th toes. Start at the web margin and stimulate the channel with the press and release technique. Press for 6–7 seconds, release, move a little way along the channel and press again. Continue this about halfway up the foot, to where you no longer feel a space between the toe bones.

ADDITIONAL SUGGESTIONS

BOOST YOUR LYSINE COUNT.   The amino acid arginine is a key part of the reproduction cycle of the herpes virus, so try to avoid arginine-containing foods such as nuts and—we're sorry to say—chocolate. Fortunately, another amino acid, lysine, helps to block the reproductive process. Legumes (peas, beans, lentils) and many vegetables are high in lysine. Consider a supplement to increase your lysine intake to 1000 mg. per day.

VITAMIN C.   Keep your vitamin C intake high. Vitamin C is contained in most fresh fruits, many vegetables, and in rose hips tea. Consider supplementing your vitamin C intake if you don't already take a multi-vitamin.

HERBS.   A Chinese herbal remedy that specifically clears Liver/Gallbladder damp heat is *Long dan xie gan tang.* It is very cooling but, over time, can adversely affect the Spleen/Stomach function. Don't take it for more than 3 weeks without professional supervision.

RELAX.   The connection between stress and herpes outbreaks is well established. Prolonged stress encourages repeated attacks by depressing your natural immune function. So find a good way to relax and deal with the daily stress of life. Try meditation, Progressive Relaxation, visualization, deep breathing, Yoga stretching, listening to soothing music—whatever works for you. See the "Additional Suggestions" in the Anxiety chapter for a simple meditation practice.

ST. JOHNS' WORT.   Try placing a few drops of the tincture directly on the affected area to help heal lesions.

Hiccups

Hiccups are uncontrollable, rhythmic contractions in the lungs, diaphragm, and throat. No one knows for sure what causes them, and Western medicine is pretty much at a loss for certain ways to stop them. Luckily, hiccups usually stop by themselves in a few minutes, but if they don't, the following pressure point strategies may help. The more you can relax, the more effective pressing these points will be, so sit comfortably, close your eyes, and breathe deeply while working with these points.

ACUPRESSURE

1. (B 2, Collecting Bamboo) This point is located where the bridge of your nose runs into the ridge of the eyebrows. (See page 196.) It's directly above the inner corner of your eye sockets. You'll feel a small indentation there. Use the thumbs of both hands to press up and into this point for 2 to 3 minutes with steady, moderate pressure. You may allow your head to lean forward into your fingers. Close your eyes and breathe deeply as you press. Or try this: Take a deep breath, and hold it. When you have to, exhale slowly. Then take a few normal breaths and again take a deep breath and hold. Do this until you have stimulated B 2 for 2 to 3 minutes.

2. (Pc 6, Inner Gate) You will locate this point on the palm side of your wrist, two thumb widths above the wrist crease in the center of the arm. This point regulates *ch'i* as well as blood in the chest. As it regulates the chest, it also helps restore normal function to the diaphragm. Use medium pressure; build up gradually, hold about a minute, and gradually release. Be sure to do both hands.

3. (Cv 17, Chest Center) This point is also known as the Upper Sea of *Ch'i*. It not only strengthens and circulates *ch'i*, but also helps "descend" rebellious *ch'i* and can help minimize hiccups. The point is located right in the center of the chest, on the breastbone. Traditionally it is said to be "even with the nipples" and men will easily locate it that way. For women, using this direction may be misleading, due to the wide variation in the shape of the female breast from individual to individual. Instead, locate the point by going about 3 finger widths up from the bottom of the breastbone. Be sure to measure from the bottom of the bone itself, *not* including the springy cartilage at the lower end of the bone.

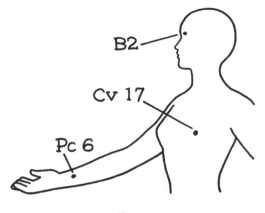

Fig. 120

Hold your index, middle, and ring finger together and press on this point for about 1 minute with your middle finger, with your eyes closed. If you are not sure you are locating it precisely, don't worry; simply press with all 3 fingers. Use medium pressure, or, if the spot is quite tender, use lighter pressure, then rub it lightly for a few seconds after you finish pressing. Remember to breathe slowly and deeply.

REFLEXOLOGY

The Reflexology strategy for relieving hiccups centers around relaxing the diaphragm, the chest area, and the neck and shoulders. This relaxation and releasing helps stop the hiccuping. Be sure to work all areas on both feet.

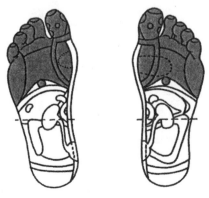

Fig. 121

1. Begin by massaging your feet to promote relaxation of the feet and the entire body. Follow the steps in the Reflexology Warm-Up on page 69. This sequence not only helps you relax, it also tones the energy of the whole body, and prepares your feet to be worked on.

2. The main reflex area for the chest is located on the top of your foot. Start in zone 1, in the webbing at the base of the big toe, and work upward a total of about 2 inches, toward your leg. Press in the troughs between the toes. Continue working each zone, ending in zone 5 near the outside edge of your foot. Work with your index finger, using the finger walk.

3. To open up the lung area, thumb walk the chest and lung reflex areas on the ball of the foot (between the diaphragm line and the base of the toes). Remember to take some deep breaths.

4. Next work on your toes, where reflex zones to various parts of the head are located. On the bottom of your foot, work the fleshy part of all the toes, but especially the second and third toe. Use the thumb walk for maximum benefit, or at least give them a good rubbing with your thumb.

5. To help relax your shoulders, press on the shoulder reflex area. This is on the bottom of your foot, below your little toe, stretching from the base of the toe down to the diaphragm line. Use the thumb walk.

6. The shoulders and neck are also associated with the ridge that runs along the base of all the toes. To work this area, "walk the ridge" with your thumb or index finger. Pull the pad of the foot down and away from the ridge with your other hand, and walk in both directions.

7. To finish the session, briefly work the entire area from the diaphragm line up to the base of the toes. Thumb walk up and down each zone. You can also rub the foot and, holding the toes in one hand and the heel in the other, bend the toes and twist the foot a little to loosen it up and relax it. These extra relaxation steps should help if the hiccups are still there. Close by pressing on the solar plexus point for about 30 seconds.

ADDITIONAL SUGGESTIONS

Virtually all the additional suggestions for relieving hiccups are of the home-grown variety, strategies people have tried that worked. Here are a few. Give them a try.

HOLD YOUR BREATH.   Take a deep breath, and for as long as you can, hold it, then gradually exhale. Some people recommend that you also swallow when you feel the urge to hiccup. Repeat several times.

BROWN BAG IT.   Hold a paper bag up to your mouth. Breathe in and out without taking the bag away. Make sure the bag fits tightly around your mouth. Don't do this for more than a minute or so, or you might faint.

WATER.   Drink a glass of water non-stop.

PULL ON YOUR TONGUE.   Don't pull too forcefully; just give a gentle yank.

COMPRESS YOUR CHEST.   Curl up with your knees up to your chest, or sit in a chair and bend forward.

EAT SOME SUGAR.   Try a spoonful of plain sugar, swallowed dry.

High Blood Pressure (Hypertension)

Blood pressure is the force exerted by the blood against the walls of the arteries. High blood pressure increases your risk of cardiovascular diseases such as heart attack and stroke. About 55 to 60 million Americans suffer from this condition. Although Western medicine cautiously continues to say that the causes of high blood pressure are "unknown," a very close association has been demonstrated between this condition and several key lifestyle factors, including a high fat, high cholesterol diet; insufficient exercise; smoking; being overweight; and stress.

In addition to pressure point self-treatments, we'll include some lifestyle recommendations that can help you control your blood pressure. If you're currently taking antihypertensive drugs, please don't quit or cut down on the medications without your doctor's knowledge and advice.

ACUPRESSURE

Four of the following six points (Gb 20, Li 11, St 36, and Lv 3) are fully described in the section, "Ten Master Pressure Points" (beginning on page 49) where you will also find illustrations of the precise point locations and suggestions on how to press them for maximum benefit.

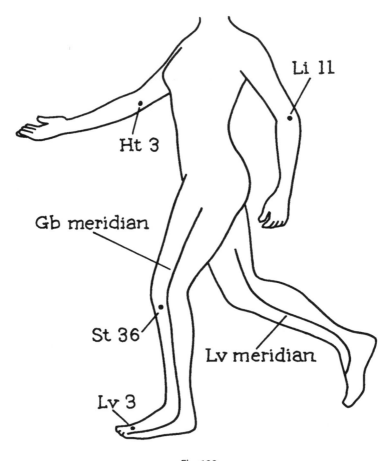

Fig. 122

1. (Gb 20, Wind Pool, see pages 53–54.)

2. Press Li 11 and Ht 3 simultaneously. To find Li 11, hold your arm in front of your chest, as if you were holding a cup in your hand. The point is at the outside end of the crease on your arm at the elbow joint.

3. To find Ht 3 (Lesser Sea), hold your palms facing up. From Li 11 (in Fig. 122) slide your fingers across the elbow crease until you feel the bony projection of the outside of your funny bone. Just above this bony projection is a natural depression; Ht 3 is in this depression. Place your thumb on Ht 3 and your middle finger on Li 11 and apply strong pressure for about a minute.

4. (St 36, Three Mile Foot) This is the most effective point to rejuvenate the *ch'i* and blood. The combination of Li 11 and St 36 is used extensively to treat hypertension.

5. (Lv 3, Bigger Rushing) In traditional Oriental medicine, hypertension is said to be intimately connected with blockages in the Liver meridian. Lv 3, as the source point of the Liver meridian, exerts a powerful, beneficial influence on all aspects of the body associated with the meridian, helping to normalize their functioning.

6. (Kd 1, Bubbling Spring) Kd 1 is on the sole of the foot between the second and third toe bone, two thirds of the distance from the heel to the base of the second toe. It's just below the ball of the foot. Press firmly for about a minute.

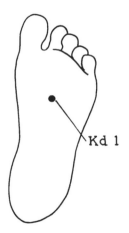

Fig. 123

REFLEXOLOGY

Your Reflexology session for hypertension will focus on relaxation, reducing your feelings of stress and pressure, and improving the functioning of your heart and circulatory system.

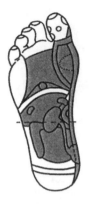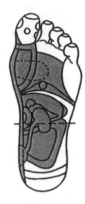

Fig. 124

1. Before you treat specific reflex areas, start with the Reflexology Warm-Up on page 69 to help you relax, tone the energy of the whole body, and prepare your feet to be worked on. Please don't skip this important step!

2. Now start directly on the heart and chest area. This stretches from the diaphragm line to the base of the toes on both feet. Use the thumb walk to work this area thoroughly. Concentrate on the heart reflex on your left foot, to help strengthen and regulate your heart. Reflexologist Laura Norman, author of *Feet First*, teaches that there is an additional area for the heart on the ball of the right foot; work that area also.

3. While on the bottom of your foot, thumb walk over the diaphragm line running just below the ball of the foot. This will help deepen and open your breathing and bring more oxygen and *ch'i* or *prana* to each cell.

4. Now work on the reflex areas for your chest located on *top* of both feet, in the troughs between the toes. Start in zone 1, at the base of the big toe, and work up toward your leg, about 2 inches up from the webbing. Continue working each zone, ending in zone 5 near the outside edge of your foot. Press with your index finger, using the finger walk. This area may be quite tender, so don't press too hard.

5. Around the base of your big toe (on the bottom of your foot) is the reflex area for the thyroid and parathyroid glands, which regulate pulse rate and help with calcium absorption. (Studies show that

insufficient calcium may raise blood pressure levels.) To stimulate more balanced and healthy thyroid activity, work the reflex zone for the thyroid gland by rubbing and pressing. The finger or thumb walk technique is best here.

6. Working the spine reflexes nourishes the nervous system that feeds the entire body. These reflexes are located on the inside edge of both feet (zone 1), extending from the heel nearly to the top of the big toe, opposite the root of the toenail. When you work the spinal reflexes, work slowly up the foot using the thumb walk technique. You will need a little extra strength on the thick skin of the heel area. Thumb walk all the way down, and take some time to walk across small areas horizontally, moving up the foot from the heel to the big toe.

7. Finally, work on the soft center of your foot, from the diaphragm line down to the midline. This will stimulate the liver, kidneys, adrenals, and other organs vital for circulation and the regulation of water levels in the body. Use the thumb walk to thoroughly cover this area, moving up, down, and/or diagonally. Pay special attention to the large liver area on the right foot.

SHIATSU

1. Find the space on the top of your foot, between the 4th and 5th toes. This is in the territory of the Gall Bladder meridian. (See Fig. 119 on page 232.) Start at the web margin and stimulate the channel with the press and release technique. Press for 6–7 seconds at the first point, release, move about ½ inch along the channel and press again. Continue like this about halfway up the foot to where you no longer feel a space between the toe bones.

2. Then stimulate the Liver meridian (also on Fig. 119). Start in the center of the top of your big toe. Using the press and release technique, progress along the toe to the web margin between the big toe and second toe, then move up the channel between the big toe and second toe. From the ankle, the channel proceeds up the inside part of the leg, along the bone. Use only mild to moderate pressure along the bone. About halfway up the leg the meridian comes off the bone but continues up the middle of the inside of the leg. Stop around the knee. Be sure to work on both feet.

ADDITIONAL SUGGESTIONS

MINIMIZE STRESS. Hypertension is often associated with excessive stress, so take time every day for meditation, deep breathing, quiet listening to soothing music, Yoga stretching, and other activities that help you decompress from the day. Research funded by the National Institutes of Health has shown Transcendental Meditation (TM) to be as effective as anti-hypertensive medication, with no side effects and for a lower long-term cost. See the section, "Stress," for pressure points and other helpful stress-reducing suggestions for your daily routine.

LEAN YOUR CUISINE. A diet high in fat and cholesterol clogs the arteries, leading to atherosclerosis (hard fatty deposits on artery walls). The more clogged the arteries, the higher your blood pressure becomes, and the harder your heart has to work to pump the blood. So cut down on meat (especially beef and pork), dairy (except for non-fat milk), heavy desserts, and all fried foods. A vegetarian (or almost vegetarian) diet rich in fiber is by far the healthiest for your heart and your blood pressure.

QUIT SMOKING. Experts say that if you are a smoker, the best thing you can do for your health is to quit smoking.

CUT DOWN ON SALT. Sodium (especially in the form of table salt) increases the amount of fluid in your vascular system; the more liquid flowing through your arteries, the higher your blood pressure. Learn to eat without adding salt either when you cook or at the table.

EXERCISE REGULARLY. Get your body moving for half an hour three to four times a week. A vigorous daily walk is easiest and best. Yoga, tai chi, or other exercises that increase flexibility and improve circulation are wonderful for cardiovascular health. But please be sure to consult with your doctor before beginning any exercise program. Helpful Yoga postures include the Shoulder Stand, Cobra, and, for deep relaxation, the Yogic rest pose (Savasana) in which you lie flat on your back, arms at your sides, eyes closed, and follow your breathing.

MAINTAIN A HEALTHY WEIGHT. Being overweight is clearly associated with high blood pressure and risk of heart attack and stroke.

Hot Flashes
See "Menopause Problems"

Immune System Tone-Up

Your immune system is a vast, complex network that involves virtually every aspect of your mind and body. From your skin (the first defense against bacteria and viruses), to your stomach lining (which secretes a highly concentrated form of hydrochloric acid that kills microbes on contact), to your lymph glands (which produce and store literally trillions of white blood cells), to your thoughts (which can either increase or decrease immunity depending on their nature), this system protects you by finding, identifying, and destroying foreign microbes including pollen, dust, and environmental chemicals as well as viruses and bacteria.

The following pressure point recommendations will help you keep this marvelous, sensitive, living mechanism functioning at its best.

ACUPRESSURE

The first two points (Sp 6 and St 36) are described in the section, "Ten Master Pressure Points" (beginning on page 49) where you will also find illustrations of precise point locations and suggestions on how to press for maximum benefit.

1. (Sp 6, Three Yin Meeting) This important Acupressure point is the junction of three *yin* meridians. In combination with St 36 (below), it nourishes both *ch'i* and blood and brings vitality. **Caution:** This point should be avoided by pregnant women.
2. (St 36, Three Mile Foot) This is the major point to strengthen the *ch'i* and blood. Legend has it that soldiers in China relied on this point to sustain themselves when exhausted or weakened by lack of food. In combination with Sp 6, it strongly revitalizes the entire body and boosts the immune function. Pressing on this point can increase white blood cell count.

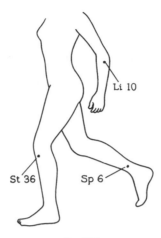

Fig. 125

3. (Li 10, Arm Three Mile) Hold your left arm in front of you, close to your stomach, with the arm flexed and thumb side of the hand pointed toward the ceiling. From the elbow crease, on the top of your forearm, move two thumb widths toward the hand. Find the most sensitive point in this area. If there are several sensitive points near here, stimulate them all. Use your thumb and apply strong pressure. Hold for 1 to 2 minutes. This point may be considered the St 36 of the arm; it has many of the same very beneficial effects.

REFLEXOLOGY

Try this immune-boosting Reflexology workout regularly (perhaps two or three times a week), if you feel you may be overtired, or if you're susceptible to getting sick.

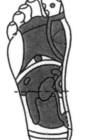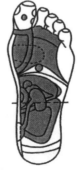

Fig. 126

1. Begin by massaging your feet and relaxing them with the Reflexology Warm-Up on page 69. This important step helps you relax, tones the energy of the whole body, and prepares your feet to be worked on; please don't skip it!

2. Thumb walk reflex areas for the heart and chest on the bottom of your feet, between the diaphragm line and the base of the toes. Pay special attention to the heart area on the sole of the left foot. Because authorities differ just a little on the location of the heart reflex, to be sure you stimulate it work the entire area, thumb walking up, down, and across.

3. To stimulate immune activity, work on the reflex area for the thymus. On the foot, the gland is located in a narrow strip along the reflex for the spine, in zone 1, on the inside (big toe side) of the foot from the base of the big toe to the ball of the foot. Work both feet with the thumb walk.

4. Next, stimulate the lymph glands, key participants in the immune system, by working the reflex area for the lymph system. You'll find this in the channel between your big toe and second toe, on the top of your foot. Use the finger walk to work on this area for a minute or so.

5. Continue working on the lymph system by stimulating the reflex area for the neck. Work the neck reflexes on both feet by "walking the ridge" at the top of the ball of the foot (at the base of your toes). Pull the flesh of the pad of the foot down and away from the ridge with your other hand. Walk in both directions.

6. Also massage all around the base of your big toe, top, bottom, and sides to energize the neck, thyroid, parathyroid, and tonsils.

7. An important area to press is the reflex for the pituitary gland, located in the center of the pad of the big toe. Known as the "master gland," it regulates the secretion of hormones, controls body temperature and metabolism, governs energy level, and has hundreds of other functions, many directly related to immune function. Massage with your thumb or use the "hook and back up" technique described on page 68 for pinpoint accuracy.

8. Next, work on your internal organs (especially the spleen, liver, and adrenals) by working the area in the arch of your foot, from about the midline of the foot up to the diaphragm line. Use the thumb walk to thoroughly cover this area, moving up, down, and/or diagonally. Pay special attention to the large liver area on the right foot.

9. Now work the area from the heel (pelvic line) up to the waist or mid-line. Here you will primarily be stimulating the intestines and facilitating the elimination of wastes and toxins. Note that the kidneys are partially above and partially below the midline; we suggest taking some time to work directly on that area.

10. Finally, bring this session to a close by soothing your entire foot with a minute or two of relaxation exercises and by pressing on the solar plexus point, as in step #1.

SHIATSU

Stand with your feet about shoulder width apart. Make a loose fist with both hands. Lean forward and beat lightly on the inside of your legs with moderate force. Start at your ankles and come up the leg to the inside of the thighs. Cross over at the hips and go back down the outside of the legs back to the ankles. Repeat 3 times.

Now do the same with your arms, except you'll have to do one arm at a time. Start on the "back-of-the-hand" side of your arm and work up to the shoulder, then down the palm side of the arm. Then slap lightly on your abdomen for a few moments (pregnant women should skip this part). In the same way, stimulate the lower part of your back. Work slowly up the back as far as you can reach. This exercise enlivens the flow of *ch'i* in the meridians.

Now we are ready for deep breathing. You are still standing with your feet shoulder width apart. Start with your arms hanging loosely at your sides. Imagine you are holding a large ball, the size of a basketball, in your palms. With a single deep, slow inhalation, slowly lift the imaginary ball in front of you until you are holding it with arms stretched above your head.

Now, imagine letting go of the ball. It becomes very light and rises above your head, out of sight.

Now exhale, slowly lowering your arms back to the starting position. Continue this for a full 3–5 minutes.

Throughout the exercise, imagine your hands becoming energized and tingling. With each breath, feel that the air you breathe is alive and vibrant with energy and vitality, and that this new vitality is starting to circulate throughout your body.

ADDITIONAL SUGGESTIONS

The essential ingredients needed to maintain a healthy immune system working at peak performance levels include regular exercise, sufficient sleep, stress management, good nutrition, and, believe it or not, staying happy. We discuss these and other key points in our 11 Simple, Universal Guidelines for Good Health on page 77. Here are some highlights:

LIFT YOUR SPIRITS. Recent research has strikingly demonstrated that our thoughts and emotions have a powerful influence on the effectiveness of our immune system. In fact, an entire new branch of science, known as psycho-neuroimmunology, has sprung up to study this relationship more fully. In a nutshell, the studies have shown that depression, anger, unhappiness, and other negative thoughts and emotions can decrease the effectiveness of the immune system, while love, joy, a sense of peacefulness, and other harmonious thoughts and feelings can boost the body's defense system.

So if you feel you are being unduly gripped by negative emotions, take action! Walk outside in nature, listen to music, do something for fun. One study found that people who watched a comedy video increased their production of white blood cells by about 40% while decreasing a stress hormone about 45%.

EXERCISE. One excellent way to raise your energy and happiness levels and to boost immune system function is to get some exercise. Take a walk in the park; do some extra deep breathing as described in the Shiatsu section above. Both the exercise and the deep breathing help get the *ch'i* flowing harmoniously again and can be powerful tools for regaining emotional equilibrium. Yoga postures are also very beneficial. The Sun Salutation (a cycle of 12 postures) tones the whole body. The Shoulder Stand is also excellent; its Sanskrit name is "Sarvanga Asana," meaning a pose beneficial for the whole body.

MEDITATE. To reduce stress and negative feelings and gain emotional and physiological balance, practice some form of meditation or relaxation, such as Progressive Relaxation, Transcendental Meditation (TM), the Relaxation Response, guided imagery, mindfulness or insight meditation, or whatever you have found that helps you relax. See "Anxiety" for a simple meditation practice.

SLEEP ENOUGH.   A huge number of Americans are sleep-deprived. Sleep is vital to revive your body's infection-fighting cells. As difficult as it is in this hectic world, do your best to get as much sleep as you need.

EAT RIGHT.   Eat fresh fruit and vegetables, whole grains, and leafy greens, all rich in Life Energy as well as the vitamins and minerals your immune system needs to fight off invaders. Stay away from fast food and junk food such as soda, candy, heavy meats, fatty dairy products, etc. If you don't take the time to eat properly, be sure to take some vitamin and mineral supplements, but this is no substitute for proper eating. Be sure your supplement includes Vitamin A, Beta-carotene, Vitamin B6, Vitamin C, Vitamin E, and a little magnesium.

Impotence
See "Sexual Problems"

Incontinence

Urinary incontinence—inability to completely control urination—is a problem that affects some 10 to 20 million Americans. This embarrassing condition is not a disease, but it might as well be, as it keeps people home, afraid to go to the theater or on social visits, or to take trips if there isn't immediate access to a toilet.

Incontinence is more common among women, primarily because their urethra is shorter, a basic fact rarely mentioned in discussions about incontinence. It is also more frequent among the elderly, but it can become a problem in middle age, when it usually manifests in a milder form, or may be triggered by an external cause, such as sneezing, coughing, laughing, bending, or jumping. It may be experienced as a limited ability to hold the urine, or a need to urinate frequently. Quite a few women also have an incontinence problem after giving birth.

According to Chinese medicine, incontinence is primarily due to a deficiency in Kidney and/or Spleen energy. The Kidneys govern the opening and closing of the lower bodily "gates" or orifices, so weakened Kidney energy can lead to urinary (or bowel) incontinence. Spleen energy regulates the body's muscle tone; decreased muscle tone is frequently a significant part of incontinence. Most often the condition is due to a combination of the two deficiencies.

Incontinence can almost always be brought under control. Katherine Jeter, Ed.D., who founded the organization called Help for Incontinent People, said that "nearly everybody can be made better or cured." So take heart! The following pressure point recommendations, combined with the "Additional Suggestions" at the end of the section, can help you solve this problem.

Childhood incontinence—bed wetting—is discussed separately at the end of this section.

ACUPRESSURE

For descriptions and illustrations for two of the following points (Sp 6 and St 36), as well as instructions on how to press them most effectively, please see page 49 for the beginning of "Ten Master Pressure Points."

1. (Sp 6, Three Yin Meeting) Pressing Sp 6 nourishes the Spleen *ch'i* and helps to remove any stagnation of *ch'i* in the lower part of the body. **Caution:** This point should be avoided by pregnant women.

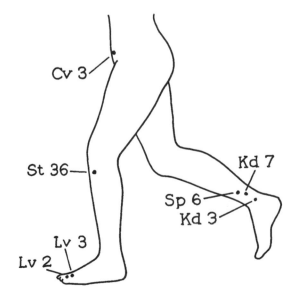

Fig. 127

2. (Kd 7, Returning Current) This is a key point on the Kidney meridian. The easiest way to locate it is to first locate Kd 3. On the inside of the ankle (big toe side), Kd 3 is halfway between the ankle bone and the Achilles tendon at the back of the ankle. Place your thumb on the prominence of the ankle bone and let it slide down toward the Achilles tendon. Kd 3 is in the depression, halfway between the bone and the back edge of the ankle. From Kd 3 go up two thumb widths toward the knee. This is Kd 7. Use firm pressure with your thumb for about a minute.

3. (St 36, Three Mile Foot) This is the most effective point for strengthening the *ch'i* and blood. In combination with Sp 6 it strongly revitalizes the entire body. Both points may be stimulated either with the heel of your opposite foot, or with your fingers.

4. (Cv 3, Central Pole) First locate Cv 4, which is four finger widths directly below the navel. Cv 3 is one thumb width below Cv 4. Its influence is specific to bladder dysfunction. Use moderate pressure with your thumb or middle finger. You can add a small circular motion with steady pressure. You may want to empty your bladder before pressing on this point. **Caution:** Pregnant women should not use pressure on this or any other abdominal points.

5. (B 28, Associated point of Urinary Bladder) B 28 is approximately 1-½ inches on either side of the spine, in the mid-sacral area of the back. The best way to stimulate these points is to lie on your back on the floor, with a tennis ball beneath you. Slowly roll up and down on the ball, first on one side of the spine, then on the other. (Or, put two tennis balls in a sock; this will enable you to work both sides at once.) Many valuable points alongside the spine on both sides will be stimulated with this technique; spend several minutes working them. Like Cv 3, B 28 is specific to urinary bladder function.

REFLEXOLOGY

To help reduce and eliminate problems of incontinence, your Reflexology session will center around reflex points for the urinary system: the kidneys, ureters, and bladder. We'll also work on the lower spine, to soothe and nourish the nerves which feed the urinary system.

1. First, massage your feet and relax them, using the techniques in the Reflexology Warm-Up on page 69. This is an important step that helps you relax, tones the energy of the whole body, and prepares your feet to be worked on; please don't skip it!

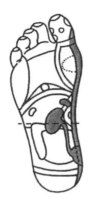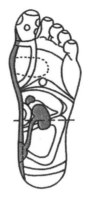

Fig. 128

2. The reflexes for the spine are located on the inside edge of both feet (zone 1), extending from the heel nearly to the top of the big toe, opposite the root of the toenail.

For incontinence, focus mainly on the lower spine area, from the heel up to about the waist line or midline of the foot. Work slowly up the foot using the thumb walk technique. Then thumb walk all the way down, and take some time to walk across small areas horizontally, moving up the foot from the heel to the big toe.

3. Next, work the kidneys and adrenals. These reflex areas are in the center of the foot, above and below the waist line and on the inside of the large tendon running up the foot. Use the thumb walk and, for best results, the "rotation on a point" technique. (See page 68.)

4. Finally, massage the bladder and ureters. Their reflex zone is located mostly in zone 1 (beneath the big toe). The ureters stretch down from the kidneys to the bladder, located where the heel begins. If you can, stretch your foot slightly backwards to extend the tendon while working on the ureters. Work up from the bladder, then cross the big tendon and work up or across the kidney reflex. Use the thumb walk technique.

SHIATSU

You will find the horse posture helpful in controlling incontinence. As mentioned previously, weakened Kidney energy is almost always involved in incontinence. In Chinese medicine, the kidneys are considered the root of vitality, and one of the best exercises to cultivate Kidney *ch'i* is the horse pose. When done properly it builds stamina, cultures *ch'i*, and promotes circulation. Please turn to page 193 (Fig. 100), where you will find an illustration and detailed instructions for the horse pose.

Unless you feel comfortable with this pose right away, start with about 30 seconds and build up to 3–5 minutes. In addition to strengthening the Kidney *ch'i* and helping with your bladder control, you should find your energy level improving as well.

BED WETTING IN CHILDREN

When children repeatedly wet their bed, there is almost always an underlying emotional factor. In many cases the underlying emotion is fear. In most Oriental systems of medicine, fear is associated with the kidneys. Excess fear impairs kidney function and lessens control over urination.

Another emotional factor is plain old stress (yes, even children can get quite stressed out). The stress causes emotional upset, which can easily turn into excess heat in the Liver meridian, as stress usually hits the Liver meridian first. An excess of Liver heat can also adversely affect urinary control.

The points selected below are designed to be effective regardless of the specific cause.

ACUPRESSURE (FOR CHILDREN'S BED WETTING)

You can make Acupressure a fun experience for your child. Use it as a chance for some extra quality bonding time. Don't create extra anxiety or pressure by promising that this will stop the bed wetting; if you want, just say that gradually, over time, this will help.

When you use pressure on your own body, you can press to the point of some discomfort. But children are very responsive to Acupressure and don't need as much stimulation as adults, so adjust the pressure to stop before the point of discomfort. In addition, use less time on each point. Half a minute is enough.

Ask your child to participate by putting attention on the spot you are pressing. Even briefly will be helpful. Get creative in drawing your child into the process. For example, you can say the points are like "on" switches that help make them strong and healthy when you push them.

If you think it's appropriate, tell the child that two extra ingredients help make it work better—the love you put into the point while you are pressing, and her/his imagining a bright, healthy, and happy feeling coming in as you press.

In finding the points on a child's body, use the width of the *child's* thumb or palm in measuring distances, not your own hand. Figure 127 (on pg. 249) shows the pressure points you will need.

1. (Lv 2 and Lv 3, Moving Between and Bigger Rushing) Lv 2 is located in the web margin of skin between the big toe and second toe. Start pressing here. If your thumb is too big to fit in this space use your index or middle finger. Since these points can be quite sensitive, start gently. Use a press and release technique: press for 6–7 seconds, and release. Repeat three or four times right at the web margin. Then gradually move up in the space between the big toe and second toe. Use the press and release technique every half inch or so along this space between the toe bones, until you've gone about one third of the way up the foot. You'll stimulate both Lv 2 and Lv 3, and the beginning of the Liver meridian. This will not only release excess heat if there is any, but will also relieve stress and have a calming effect on the mind.

Remember, light pressure here is usually enough.

2. (Sp 6, Three Yin Meeting) This point is located on the inside portion of the leg above the ankle bone. From the center of the ankle bone slide up four fingers' width. Remember to use your child's palm as the measure. The point is just off the bone (toward the back of the leg). When you find it, gradually increase pressure until you are pressing quite firmly, but be sure not to cause pain. Hold about half a minute and gradually release.

Sp 6 is used here as much for its calming effect on the mind as for its beneficial effect on urinary dysfunction. You can use your thumbs to stimulate this point on your child. Use moderate pressure.

3. (Kd 7, Returning Current) The easiest way to locate Kd 7 is to first locate Kd 3. On the inside of the ankle (big toe side), Kd 3 is located halfway between the ankle bone and the Achilles tendon on the back side of the ankle. Place your thumb on the prominence of the ankle bone, and let it slide down toward the Achilles tendon on the back edge of the ankle. Kd 3 is in the depression, approximately halfway between the bone and the back edge of the ankle.

From Kd 3 go up two (child-size) thumb widths, toward the knee. This is Kd 7. Use your thumb to apply moderate pressure for about half a minute. This is the "tonification point" on the Kidney meridian, and is directly helpful for urinary incontinence.

4. (Ht 7, Mind Door) You will find this point on the palm side of the hand, on the wrist crease, directly below the little finger. (See Figure 113, page 222.) Find the bony knob on the outside of the left wrist (the little finger side). The point is next to that, in a small indentation. Press for about 30 seconds with your thumb, and release gradually. You can do both hands at once, or do one first and then switch hands. This point is used primarily for the calming effect it has on the mind and emotions.

5. (B 28, Associated point of Urinary Bladder) B 28, which is specific to urinary bladder function, is located approximately 1-½ half inches on either side of an adult's spine, in the mid sacral area of the back. The distance is proportionately less on a child's body. There are many valuable points throughout the sacral area, so begin by giving a gentle massage to the whole area. Then press along both sides of the spine starting at the sacral region and working up the low back to just below the midpoint of the back.

ADDITIONAL SUGGESTIONS

REGULATE YOUR DRINKING.   Six to eight 8-ounce glasses of fluid a day is about right. Don't drink much at night, especially the last 2–3 hours before you go to bed.

MINIMIZE YOUR CONSUMPTION OF ALCOHOLIC BEVERAGES.   Cut down on caffeine (tea, coffee, sodas), and grapefruit juice. These are diuretics which increase urine production and may increase the urgency of your need to "go."

TRY CRANBERRY JUICE.   It is justly famous for its beneficial effects on the bladder and urinary system.

QUIT SMOKING.   Nicotine adversely affects the bladder and urethra; also, smoker's cough may trigger sudden urine loss.

DO KEGEL EXERCISES.   Many women have already learned these exercises, which can be helpful in childbirth and are frequently recommended to improve sexual pleasure and the ability to experience orgasm. Step one is to tighten the sphincter (the ring of muscles) around the anus. These are the muscles you would use to hold back a bowel movement. Tighten them without tensing the muscles of your legs, belly, or buttocks.

Next, when you're urinating, practice stopping the flow about 5 times each time you go. These are the front pelvic muscles.

Now, combine these two sets of muscles. Work from back to front— tighten the anal sphincter muscles, then tighten the front muscles. Do this *slowly*, to a count of 4 or 5, and hold for a second or two before gradually releasing. Repeat 4 more times. This is one "set." Do at least 3 sets of 5 every day, gradually increasing the number of repetitions in each set until you're doing about 100 repetitions a day.

Individuals with an incontinence problem may find it difficult to do even 1 set of 5—the muscles may be very weak. But with practice, they will gain strength.

A HELPFUL YOGA POSTURE.   The Forward Bend is said to help with bladder and incontinence problems.

Indigestion

Indigestion has many causes and takes many forms. Tainted food, overeating, wrong food combinations, consuming specific foods that don't agree with us, may give rise to heartburn, stomach cramps, even vomiting and diarrhea. Several of these problems we consider in separate sections. (See "Constipation," "Diarrhea," "Nausea and Vomiting.") Food poisoning— when food contaminated with toxic bacteria causes cramps, nausea, vomiting, diarrhea, and sometimes dizziness—generally passes by itself in 24 to 48 hours; about all you can do is drink clear liquids to prevent dehydration, and take it easy. (For children, the elderly, or someone already sick, or if there is high fever or the condition persists more than a day or two, call the doctor.)

Most stomach upsets are due to simple overeating, wrong food choices or combinations, and acid reflux (gastroesophageal reflux), the back-up of digestive acids from the stomach into the esophagus that causes the feeling we know as heartburn. The following pressure point strategies and suggestions will help you prevent and heal your tummy aches.

ACUPRESSURE

This sequence of Acupressure points is a simple but highly effective combination to settle the stomach. In addition to providing symptom relief, these points will have a long-term strengthening influence on the digestive system.

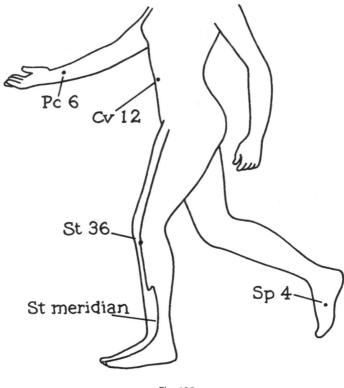

Fig. 129

1. (Pc 6, Inner Gate) You will find this point on the palm side of your wrist, two thumb widths above the wrist crease and in the center of the arm. Pc 6 has a wide-ranging influence on the body. It can be used to alleviate chest discomfort and angina, it calms the mind, helps regulate menstruation and has a profoundly harmonizing effect on the stomach. Use medium pressure; build up gradually, hold about a minute, and gradually release. Be sure to do both hands.

2. (Cv 12, Middle Stomach) Find a notch at the bottom of your breast bone. Cv 12 is midway between this notch and your belly button. This point has a powerful effect on the stomach and is a part of almost every point combination involving the digestive system. Use firm pressure for about a minute here. You'll probably find pressing with your middle finger most workable.

3. (St 36, Three Mile Foot) For an illustration of the exact location of this important point, and instructions on how to press it most effectively, see page 49 for the beginning of "Ten Master Pressure Points." It has a beneficial effect on digestion as well as a strengthening effect on the *ch'i* and blood.

4. (Sp 4, Grandfather Grandson) Start at the joint where the big toe connects to the foot. Slide along the underside of this bone. From the center of the joint, go approximately two thumb widths toward the ankle. Sp 4 is not on the side of this bone, but just below it. This point helps harmonize the *ch'i* of the stomach. For future reference, it is also very helpful for any type of menstrual disorder.

REFLEXOLOGY

To help you remedy your indigestion—and to strengthen the digestive system to prevent future problems—we suggest working on your stomach, intestines, liver, gallbladder, pancreas, and several other reflexes. Working the colon reflexes will help relieve constipation or soothe diarrhea, as well as eliminate toxins, which may be partially to blame for your upset stomach.

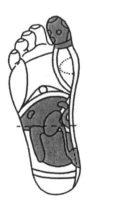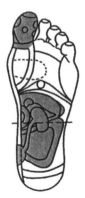

Fig. 130

1. To start your session, settle in and relax by massaging your feet and using the techniques in the Reflexology Warm-Up on page 69. This is an important step that helps you relax, tones the energy of the whole body, and prepares your feet to be worked on.

2. Since digestion begins in the mouth, with the salivary glands, we recommend working all around your big toe, from the base all the way up to the tip. (Don't press on the nail on the top of the toe, however.) Use the thumb walk technique. Work up and down the big toe, and where you can, work around the circumference as well.

3. To stimulate both the liver and stomach, work the entire area from the midline of your foot up to the diaphragm line. Use the thumb walk to thoroughly cover this area, moving up, down, and/or diagonally. Note that the liver reflex is on the bottom of your right foot, the stomach reflex on the left. The adrenal glands are also in this area, as are the duodenum and pancreas, key elements in the digestive process.

Study the master foot maps on pages 45 and 46 to gain a greater understanding of their location. If you were a professional Reflexologist, you would carefully work each reflex area individually (the stomach, pancreas, etc.). If you have time and patience, that would be best. But you'll derive great benefit just by thoroughly covering the entire area.

4. Moving down the foot, spend some time working specifically on the colon reflexes. Note that the reflexes for various aspects of the colon are divided between the two feet, with the ascending colon in zone 1 of the right foot, the descending colon reflex area in zone 1 of the left foot, etc. Again, work these reflexes individually if you can; at least be sure to cover the general area thoroughly.

5. Conclude your session with some extra relaxation by repeating step 1 for at least a couple of minutes.

SHIATSU

1. Rub the palms of your hands together rapidly for 10–20 seconds until they get nice and warm. Now with one palm on top of the back of the other hand, place your hands on the lower right side of your abdomen. Slide your hands up to just below the rib cage and then across the top of the abdomen and down the left side. Slide across the bottom of your abdomen back to where you started. Press with a gentle pressure as you go. It should take 6–7 seconds to complete one full circle. Do this for 4–5 minutes. This will help soothe and settle the stomach.

2. Next, directly stimulate the Stomach meridian, which runs between the 2nd and 3rd toes, across the top of the foot and up the front of the ankle.

(See Fig. J or Fig. 129.) From the ankle it continues up the front of the leg, about one finger breadth to the outside (little toe side) of the shin bone.

Pick one foot, and start at the second toe on the little toe side, using the press and release technique. (Press for 6–7 seconds, release, move a little way along the channel and press again.) Continue along the entire channel. Four finger widths below the lower edge of the kneecap is St 36; end with an extra minute of press and release on this key point. Then work on the other foot and leg in the same way.

ADDITIONAL SUGGESTIONS

EAT SMALLER MEALS.   One of the main causes of indigestion is eating too much food at one time. The stomach simply can't handle it, and it lets you know. Also, an overfull belly tends to force acids back up into the esophagus. There's only one way to prevent this problem, and you know what it is! Ayurveda, the ancient Indian system of natural medicine, says a meal should consist of the amount of food you could hold in two cupped hands.

SLOW DOWN.   Eating too fast is one of the most common causes of upset stomachs. Take some time to sit quietly and eat your meals.

TAKE AN ANTACID.   Over-the-counter remedies are effective for most people, and, if not used too often, are relatively harmless.

FOODS TO AVOID.   For many people, eating spicy food, pickles, hot peppers, and citrus fruits are a virtual guarantee of heartburn or stomach upset, so avoid these food culprits. Other foods to avoid or minimize include anything with caffeine; alcohol; mints; milk; fatty meats; and all greasy, fried foods.

TWO NATURAL HEARTBURN REMEDIES.   For a soothing herbal cure for heartburn and acid stomach, try 2 tablespoons of pure aloe vera gel. Add a pinch of baking soda to increase effectiveness.

Another simple heartburn remedy is a cup of room temperature water, to which you add about 10 drops of lime juice and ½ teaspoon of sugar (preferably a natural, unrefined type). Just before you're ready to drink it, add about ¼ teaspoon of baking soda. The drink will fizz up; drink it down quickly while it's bubbling.

FIRE UP YOUR DIGESTION.   If you're prone to chronic stomach aches, it may be because your digestion is weak. To promote better digestion, use some ginger. Just before eating, chop or grate a little fresh ginger root, add a few drops of lime juice and a pinch of salt, and eat the mixture. Alternatively, make some ginger tea (either with slices of fresh ginger root or dry, powdered ginger) and drink it 2 or 3 times a day. You can add a little honey if you like.

YOGA.   Helpful Yoga poses include the Fish, Cobra, and Locust, all of which stretch and massage the abdominal area. Also try the Knee-chest pose, which is simply lying on your back, bringing the knees to the chest, and wrapping your arms around your knees.

Insomnia

In Chinese medicine, *yang* is an active, outward energy, while yin is more restful and inward. During the day, when we are engaged in activity, the *ch'i* flows predominantly in the *yang* meridians, then enters the *yin* meridians more during the night. This transition from a *yang-* dominated cycle to a *yin-* dominated cycle should proceed smoothly, with our energy flowing naturally from one to the other. If the flow is interrupted, the *ch'i* cannot enter the *yin* meridians and remains stuck in the *yang* channels at night as well. The result is insomnia, and about a third of us regularly suffer from some type of it —can't fall asleep; can't stay asleep; toss and turn; wake up early and can't get back to sleep.

From a Chinese medicine perspective, sleep is essential to nourish the overall *yin* of the body and maintain a healthy balance of *yang* and *yin*. We understand the importance of sleep from scientific studies as well as personal experience. Lack of sleep makes us more irritable and less efficient, not to mention the toll on our quality of life and enjoyment.

Yet the demands of modern life require prolonged work and ceaseless activity, with too little time for rest, recreation, and pursuits that nourish and replenish us. It seems there's never enough time to accomplish everything we need or want to do. So, instead of going to bed when we're tired, we often remain active until late at night, finishing some work we brought home or busy with household chores, phone calls, finances. Instead of a natural winding down before bed, many of us remain in a *yang* mode, active and focused.

Although insomnia may have many causes, Chinese medicine sees this type of stress as primary, and the pressure point strategies we recommend below are designed largely to help you unwind. (Please see the "Stress" and "Anxiety" chapters for more suggestions.) Use these techniques before going to bed at night. They can also be used during the day, to help create better *yin/yang* balance. We don't, however, recommend using pressure points if you wake up during the night.

Regarding prescription sleep medications: while these may be appropriate in some cases for short term use (less than one week, and only with the advice of your physician), they should never be considered a long-term solution.

ACUPRESSURE

For all types of insomnia:

1. (Ht 7, Mind Door) You will find this point on the palm side of your hand, on the wrist crease, directly below the little finger. Find the bony knob on the outside of your left wrist (the little finger side). The point is next to that, in a small indentation. Press for 30 seconds or a minute with your thumb; release gradually; switch hands. This point has a calming effect on the mind and emotions, nourishes the function of the heart and also promotes sleep.

2. (Gv 24, Mind Courtyard) This point is also just inside the hairline of the forehead (or what used to be your hairline!) directly above the nose. (See Fig. A on page 36.) Pressing here has a powerful calming effect on the mind. Use medium to firm pressure with your middle finger and hold for about a minute. Remember to always increase and decrease pressure gradually, not suddenly.

The next two points (Sp 6 and Lv 3) are fully described in the section, "Ten Master Pressure Points" (beginning on page 49) where you will also find illustrations of the precise point locations and suggestions on how to press them for maximum benefit.

3. (Sp 6, Three Yin Meeting) The crossing point of three *yin* meridians of the leg (Spleen, Liver, and Kidney), this is an excellent point to nourish *yin* energy, which helps settle the mind. The combination of the *yin* nourishing and calming effect of this point makes it important for relieving insomnia. **Caution:** Pregnant women should not press this point.

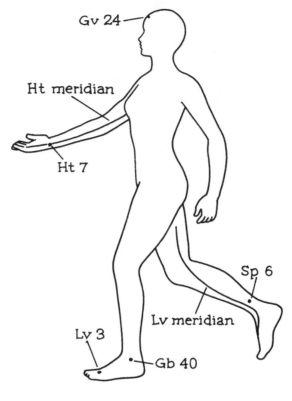

Fig. 131

4. (Lv 3, Bigger Rushing) This point helps neutralize all types of stress, and has a calming, relaxing effect on the mind.

If you wake up early and can't fall back asleep, there may be a deficiency in the Gallbladder meridian. If this pattern applies to you, add the following:

5. (Gb 40, Hills Ruins) Locate the ankle bone on the outside (little toe side) of your foot. Gb 40 is slightly below the high point of this bone and about one thumb width in front (towards the toes), in a natural depression between the tendons of the foot. This is the source point of the Gallbladder meridian. Source points strongly tonify all aspects of their meridian.

REFLEXOLOGY

It's always good to start your Reflexology session by massaging your feet and relaxing them with the techniques in the Reflexology Warm-Up on page 69. This is especially helpful for treating insomnia, which generally is due to anxiety or hyper-activity.

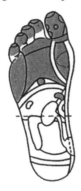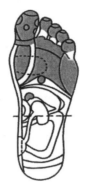

Fig. 132

　　1. Thumb walk the chest and lung reflex zones on the ball of the foot (between the diaphragm line and the base of the toes).
　　You can also finger walk the chest and lymph gland reflexes on the top of the foot in the solid part of the foot between the diaphragm line and the shoulder line. Work up from the webbing toward your leg, in the troughs between the toes. Start in zone 1—at the base of the big toe, and go up about 2 inches. Continue working each zone, ending in zone 5 near the outside edge of your foot. Work this area (which may be quite tender) with your index finger, using the finger walk.
　　And remember to take some slow, deep breaths!

　　2. A good neck and shoulder massage is one of the best ways to help relax. You can simulate that effect by working on the shoulder reflexes on your foot. These are located on the bottom of your foot in zone 5, under your little toe, and continuing out along the outside edge of your foot. It extends from the base of your little toe down to the diaphragm line. Work both horizontally and vertically along this zone using the thumb walk.

　　3. To work the neck reflexes on both feet, thumb or finger walk along the ridge at the top of the ball of the foot (at the base of the toes). Pull the pad of the foot down and away from the ridge with your other hand, to increase access to the bony ridge. Walk in both directions.

4. Another area for the neck (and also for the important thyroid gland, which regulates metabolism and how slow or speedy we are) is located in a narrow band around the base of the big toe. To stimulate more balanced and healthy thyroid activity, work the reflex zone for the thyroid gland by rubbing and pressing. The finger or thumb walk technique is best here, but you can also simply use a massaging kind of action.

5. Next, work on your toes, particularly the upper part of the toe (nearest the tip) where there are reflex areas for the brain, pituitary gland, and hypothalamus. Use the thumb walk to go up the fleshy part of the bottom of each toe. For maximum benefit, Laura Norman, author of *Feet First*, recommends walking all five zones of each big toe, and "making three passes down each of the smaller toes: once down the center of the toe and once on each side. Take about ten to fifteen tiny bites in each pass."

6. The reflex for the pituitary gland is located in the center of the pad of the big toe. Known as the "master gland," it regulates all the endocrine glands and governs our energy level. To press on this point, it is best to use the "hook and back up" technique described on page 68.

7. While in the area of your toes, stimulate the brain by placing the tip of your index finger on the tip of each toe, and rolling your finger back and forth to press on the toe. You can also use your thumbnail to roll across the tops of the toes.

8. The last major area to work on is the reflex for the adrenal glands. These important glands are central players in the "fight or flight" response to stress, when the body gears up for action by secreting more adrenaline, thereby increasing heart rate, breathing rate, oxygen consumption, and muscle efficiency, and undergoes numerous other changes. Perhaps the main cause of insomnia is this stress reaction, which plagues most of us in our high-speed, high-pressure lifestyle.

To help settle down, work on the adrenal glands, which are located about midway between the waist line and diaphragm line of both feet, at about zone 1, ½ below the big toe and second toe, right next to the large tendon running up the foot. It is likely to be quite tender, so be careful. Tilt the foot back to get better access to the area. Perhaps the best way to work on this very small area, recommended by Dwight Byers in his book, *Better Health with Foot Reflexology*, is simply to hold your thumb still on the area and rotate or flex your foot around the point.

If you have time, thumb walk across the entire area from the waist line to the diaphragm line; you will influence the liver, stomach, kidneys, gallbladder, and pancreas.

9. End your session by spending a few minutes just relaxing your feet, rubbing and massaging them slowly and gently. You could also use the relaxation techniques suggested in step 1 above. Finish with the thumb press on the solar plexus point for about half a minute.

SHIATSU

1. Cup your hands around your neck with the fingers on the back of your neck, on both sides of the spinal vertebrae. Start at the top, in the natural depression where the neck meets the skull. Using the press and release technique, slowly work down both sides to the upper shoulders. Press quite firmly, hold for 6–7 seconds, release, move your fingers a short distance (½ inch or so), press again.

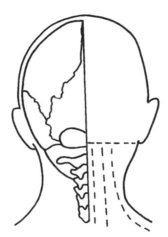

Fig. 133

Begin again at the upper portion of the neck, but this time start with your hands about an inch and a half outward, toward the sides of the neck. Work down along this line to the top of the shoulder.

Start a third time at the upper portion of the neck, with the tips of your fingers about 3 inches away from the vertebrae. Press along this line to the top of the shoulder.

Go back to the natural depressions in the neck where you started, but this time instead of working down toward the shoulders, follow along the base of the skull toward the earlobes. Spend extra time wherever you find a particularly sore spot.

2. Place the middle 3 fingers of each hand at eyebrow level, with the 4th fingers of each hand next to each other at the space between the eyebrows. With moderate pressure, slowly slide your fingers to the outside toward the temples. When you get to the temples make 3 circular strokes. Repeat 3 times.

Use the same sliding motion of the fingers, but this time start at the center of the forehead. Slide toward the temples and make three circular strokes. Repeat 3 times.

Now place your fingers at the center of the top of your forehead. Slowly slide toward the temples and again finish with circular strokes.

3. Now stimulate the Liver channel on your foot. (See Fig. 119 on page 232.) Sit cross-legged on the floor or put one foot on the opposite knee while sitting in a chair. Put the tips of the fingers of your right hand in the space between the big toe and the second toe of your left foot. Position your little finger at the web margin between the toes. With your fingers in place, apply pressure beginning with the little finger and rippling up toward the index finger. Use firm pressure. Keep applying a rippling wave of pressure for a full minute. Then use your left hand for the right foot. You can do both feet at the same time.

4. If you have time, add some stimulation along the Heart meridian. (See Fig. L, page 43.) Start by grabbing the tip of the little finger of your left hand between the thumb and first finger of your right hand. Position your hands so that the right thumb is on the inside and the first finger along the outside. (The meridian runs along the inside of the little finger, so be sure you are stimulating the sides and not the top and bottom of the finger.)

Press and release from the fingertip to the web margin between the 4th and 5th fingers. From the web margin, the meridian runs along the palm side of the hand between the 4th and 5th finger bones. Press into this groove with your thumb, until you reach the wrist crease. On the arm side right at the wrist crease, in line with the little finger, use a circular pressing motion with your thumb. Now switch to the other hand.

ADDITIONAL SUGGESTIONS

1. Try eating lighter at night. Chances are good that you will sleep better. Favor carbohydrates (pasta, hot cereal, potatoes) rather than protein (meat, fish, chicken).

2. Take time out for meditation, quiet listening to soothing music, or some sort of relaxing activity like a walk in the park. Try to get out in nature during your walk. For helpful suggestions on how to meditate, see the Additional Suggestions under "Anxiety."

3. Moderate or eliminate your use of stimulants such as caffeine.

4. The herb kava kava has been found effective for both anxiety and insomnia. This is widely available at health food stores and increasingly at your local pharmacy. The active ingredient is kavalactones. For insomnia the standard dose is 200 milligrams of kavalactones an hour before bed.

5. Valerian root is also widely used for insomnia. This is usually available as capsules of the dried root, in powdered form. Take up to one gram of the powder 30–45 minutes before bed. (Some people find the odor of valerian root disagreeable, but the herb is effective.)
    Both kava kava and valerian root are considered safe and can be used for temporary relief without the side effects of stronger medications. But remember: the long-term solution is in rebalancing the energy in the body.

6. Calcium and magnesium supplements may be helpful. Try taking 500 milligrams a day of each with either of the above herbs, or just by themselves.

7. A helpful Yoga posture is the Yogic rest pose (Savasana). Lie flat on your back, legs slightly apart, arms about 6 inches from your sides. This is very relaxing, even more so if you gently pay attention to your breathing.

Joint Pain

See "Arthritis" and "Pain"

Knee Pain
See "Arthritis" and "Pain"

Memory and Mental Clarity

In this age of computers, information, and increasingly rapid change, with new skills to learn and new technology to master almost every day, we all need sharp minds able to concentrate and sort through massive amounts of information, and strong, reliable memories. The following finger pressure recommendations and additional suggestions will be helpful for everyone, from students who are trying to optimize their mental performance, to people who notice that their memory may not be what it used to be.

In traditional Chinese medicine, brain function is very much associated with the healthy functioning of the *ch'i* in the Kidney meridian. The points below enliven the Kidney *ch'i* and in turn improve memory and brain/mind function.

ACUPRESSURE

Here are two points universally beneficial for improving mind/brain functioning. Afterwards we will include others specifically helpful for memory.

1. (St 36, Three Mile Foot) For an illustration of the exact location of this important point, and instructions on how to press it most effectively, please see page 49 for the beginning of "Ten Master Pressure Points." St 36 is the most powerful point for revitalizing the *ch'i* and blood of the entire body. It also helps to clear excess dampness. In Oriental medicine, "mental dampness" equates with cloudy thinking. Another colorful term often used for this condition is "brain fog."

2. (Gv 20, Hundred Meetings) All the *yang* channels of the body meet here. It is located on the midline of the top of the head, midway between the tips of the ears. Use all four fingers of both hands to stimulate this point and the area immediately surrounding it. (See Fig. C on page 37.)

To increase mental clarity and ability to concentrate, add:

3. (Sp 3, Supreme White) You will find it easiest to work this point if you sit cross-legged, or can comfortably put one foot on the opposite knee while sitting in a chair. You can also put your foot up on a stool. Place your thumb on the outside edge of your right big toe, and slide it up until it goes over the big joint at the base of the big toe, where the toe is connected to the foot. On the heel side of the joint, find the bone that connects to the joint. Sp 3 is just off the lower border of the bone. This point is frequently tender, so you may not be able to use firm pressure. Most people find it easiest to use the thumb for this point.

Sp 3 has a strong ability to clear congestion, even stronger when used in conjunction with St 40. It benefits mental alertness by clearing the mind of excess "mental dampness"—cloudy thinking.

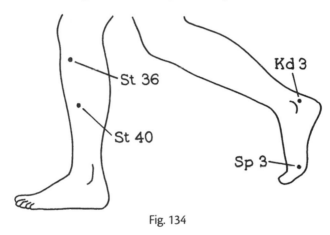

Fig. 134

For thorough descriptions and location illustrations for the following three points (St 40, Kd 3, and B 23), as well as instructions on how to press them most effectively, please see page 49 for the beginning of "Ten Master Pressure Points."

4. (St 40, Abundant Splendor) St 40 is very useful for reducing mucus and congestion which cloud the mind.

For improved memory, add

5. (Kd 3, Supreme Stream) Kidney energy, in Chinese medicine, is considered the root of the *yin* and *yang* of the entire body. Kd 3, as the "source point" for the Kidney meridian, exerts a powerful influence on the meridian and the entire body.

6. B23 and B 20 (Associated points of Kidney and Spleen) These points in combination with Kd 3 greatly strengthen the Kidney *ch'i*.

REFLEXOLOGY

Our Reflexology session will include both relaxation procedures (since tension reduces circulation to the brain and nervous system), and a specific focus on reflex areas for the brain, spine, and key endocrine glands.

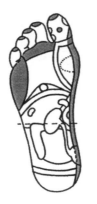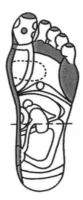

Fig. 135

But before you start on reflex areas to improve memory and increase mental acuteness, please be sure to begin with the Reflexology Warm-Up in the box on page 69. This is an important step that relaxes you and prepares your feet to be worked on; please don't skip it!

1. To further eliminate tension, work on the reflexes for the neck and shoulders. The neck reflexes are located on the "ridge" at the top of the ball of the foot (at the base of the toes). Work this area using your thumb, while pulling the pad of the foot down and away from the ridge with your other hand. Walk in both directions.

2. The reflex zones for your shoulders are located on the bottom of your foot in zone 5, that is, under your little toe, continuing out along the outside edge of your foot. They extend from the base of your little toe down to the diaphragm line, a total of only about 1 to 1-½ inches. To relax your shoulders (and thereby improve circulation to your head), work both horizontally and vertically along this zone using the thumb walk.

3. Learning, concentration, memory, information processing. . . these are functions of the gray matter between your ears! To stimulate the brain reflexes (located on the very tip of each toe), place the tip of your index finger on the tip of the toe, and roll your finger back and forth to press on the toe. You can also use your thumbnail to roll across the toe-tops.

4. The other major aspect of the nervous system is the spine, located on the inside edge of both feet (zone 1), extending from the heel nearly to the top of the big toe, opposite the root of the toenail. Work slowly up the foot using the thumb walk technique. (You will need a little extra strength on the thick skin of the heel area.) Also thumb walk all the way down, and work across small areas horizontally, moving up the foot from the heel to the big toe.

5. To stimulate the endocrine glands to function more efficiently, work the pituitary gland in the center of the pad of the big toe. Massage with your thumb or use the "hook and back up" technique for pinpoint accuracy.

SHIATSU

Here is a simple 3-step Shiatsu routine to increase circulation to the head and brain.

1. With your middle three fingers, press along the midline of your head from the hairline to just beyond the top of your head. Use a press and release technique: press with moderate to firm pressure for 6–7 seconds, release, move about ½ inch back, and press again. Repeat twice.

2. Again using 3-finger pressure, use both your hands to work along 6 rows of points on the top of your head. This time start from the crown of the head and work forward, toward the hairline. Start just outside the midline and work outward, moving out about ½ inch each time. Repeat twice.

3. Place your right palm on the front of your head (just above the forehead), put your left hand on top of the right, and press for 6–7 seconds. Move the two palms to the crown of the head, and repeat the pressure. Then press at the back of the head (at about the level of your forehead, not down at the neck). Finally, press both sides of the head, above the ears and slightly forward.

ADDITIONAL SUGGESTIONS

TAKE A HOLISTIC APPROACH. A strong mind—clear thinking, retentive memory, insight, foresight, etc.—can only be developed and sustained in the context of a healthy body and a healthy lifestyle. A nourishing diet, appropriate exercise, adequate rest, reducing stress, quitting smoking, etc. are extremely important for the short- and long-term optimum functioning of your body and mind.

Stress and tension (for example in your shoulders and neck) can restrict blood flow to your brain; insufficient sleep reduces alertness and ability to concentrate, as do even a couple of beers; caffeine is likely to produce insomnia, hence sleep deprivation; cigarettes impair memory and constrict arteries, reducing blood flow to the brain. Please read The 11 Simple, Universal Guidelines for Good Health on page 77 and put them into practice.

HERBAL BRAIN BUILDERS. Two herbs, ginkgo biloba and gotu kola, increase circulation in the brain and are good memory tonics. They have long been available in most natural food stores and are now in many regular pharmacies.

USE MNEMONICS. If you have a real memory problem (and you've ruled out, with your physician, the possibility of Alzheimer's or other organic conditions), pick up a book offering tips to help you remember. Many of these devices work quite well, such as the use of imagery, rhymes, or associations linked to a person's name, etc.

BE A YOGI. The inverted Yoga poses (Shoulder Stand, Headstand, Plow) help bring more blood to the brain. The Sun Salutation also increases circulation and energy flow throughout the body.

USE IT OR LOSE IT. Research clearly shows that the mind can remain alert, clear, and creative into our late years, if we keep using the mind actively. Read, think, and learn; do crossword puzzles; listen to beautiful music. Regardless of your age, do creative and mentally stimulating projects, whether large or small. One of the authors' mothers recently completed, at age 91, a 700-page book translation that is being published by a leading university press.

Menopause

Menopause—cessation of the monthly menstrual period—signals the end of a woman's fertile, childbearing years. For most women in our youth-oriented society, this is experienced as a loss, a sign of aging and decline. But there is another side to the coin: freedom from painful periods, PMS, the fear of pregnancy, the hassle of birth control. Liberated from her childbearing and childrearing responsibilities, she is ready for a new phase of life, a chance to use her creative energies and accumulated wisdom in new ways. Indeed many cultures, including the original Native Americans, consider menopause a special and even sacred event in a woman's life, a transition to a new status as a respected elder.

Menopause generally occurs during a woman's mid-40's to early 50's, though it can happen earlier or later to some individuals. Six months or more without menstruation is considered the "official" start of menopause, but experts caution that if you don't want to become pregnant, continue to use some form of birth control until a year has passed.

The term menopause is commonly used to indicate an ongoing process, the physical and emotional changes leading to the actual cessation of menstruation. Experiences and "symptoms" vary widely. Some women have quite a comfortable time; others endure a full range of symptoms: night sweats, hot flashes, vaginal dryness, mood swings, depression, irritability, fatigue. At least 80% of American women experience some of these menopausal symptoms, which are caused primarily by hormonal changes.

Hormones are chemicals that the body produces and secretes from endocrine glands such as the ovaries, adrenals, and pituitary. These chemicals are the body's way of controlling, regulating, and balancing its many functions. In menopause, production of two hormones in particular—estrogen and progesterone—slows down. Both these hormones originate in the egg-containing follicles of the ovaries. By the age of menopause, the majority of the follicles have been exhausted, resulting in greatly reduced hormone levels. The symptoms of menopause are caused both by this reduced level of hormones and by fluctuating imbalances between them.

According to Chinese medicine, menopause is a result of *yin* deficiency. *Yin* deficiency is like running your car engine without oil for lubrication, or without water in the radiator. The dryness or lack of internal cooling ability caused by insufficient *yin* results in heat symptoms—known as *yin* deficiency heat in Oriental diagnosis—such as hot flashes and irritability. The primary way to treat this is to stimulate points which nourish the *yin* and thereby restore a better *yin/yang* balance in the body.

ACUPRESSURE

1. (Lu 7, Broken Sequence) This point (especially paired with Kd 6, on the next page) has a special function: it opens the Cv (Conception Vessel) channel, which is also known as the Sea of *Yin.*

Hold one hand out in front of you, palm down. Start from the V shape formed by your thumb and index finger. Use the index finger of the other hand to trace along the top of the thumb to the wrist. Your finger will fall into a natural depression where the base of your thumb joins the wrist. Keep going another inch and a half and you will be on Lu 7. Press with your thumb or index finger for about a minute, then switch hands. There's not much tissue between the skin and the bone here so mild to moderate pressure is enough.

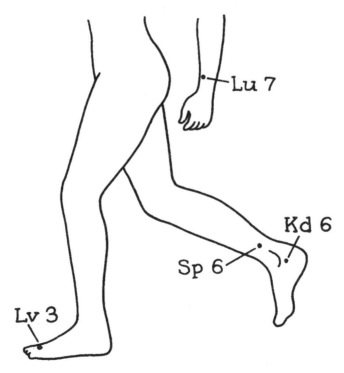

Fig. 136

2. (Kd 6, Shining Sea) From the ankle bone on the inside of your foot (the big toe side), slide straight down (toward the sole of the foot) one thumb width. Kd 6 is located here. Use your thumb to apply moderate to firm pressure. This is the primary point on the Kidney channel to strengthen the Kidney *yin*; it has a moistening, nourishing, and cooling influence and helps carry the Kidney *yin* energy upward. Stagnation of Kidney *yin* is frequently involved in menopause symptoms. Stimulating this point after Lu 7 helps open the Sea of *Yin*.

3. (Sp 6, Three Yin Meeting) For an illustration of the exact location of this important point, and instructions on how to press it most effectively, please see page 49 for the beginning of "Ten Master Pressure Points." The meeting point of three *yin* meridians (Spleen, Liver, and Kidney) Sp 6 nourishes the *yin* of the entire body. It is recommended here for its healing effect on the uterus as well.

4. (Lv 3, Bigger Rushing) This point is also described in "Ten Master Pressure Points" beginning on page 49. It helps balance the emotional component of menopause as well as nourishing the yin aspect of the Liver meridian energy.

REFLEXOLOGY

Menopause involves much more than hormones and hot flashes! The following Reflexology routine will not only help regulate body temperature and hormone production, it will also promote relaxation and stress reduction to help you maintain physical and emotional balance, and foster the circulation of blood and energy to the entire reproductive system. We suggest you spend from 15 minutes to half an hour, 2 or 3 times a week.

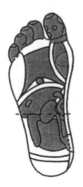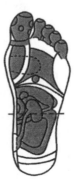

Fig. 137

1. Before you begin to treat specific reflex areas, turn to the Reflexology Warm-Up on page 69 and go through the recommended sequence. This is an important step that helps you relax, tones the energy of the whole body, and prepares your feet to be worked on.

2. To help relax, dissolve stress, and facilitate deep, regular breathing, work on the chest/lung areas on both the bottom and top of your foot. First, thumb walk the chest and lung reflex zones on the ball of the foot (between the diaphragm line and the base of the toes). Then finger walk the related reflexes on the top of the foot, in the solid part of the foot between the diaphragm line and the shoulder line. Use your index finger to work up from the webbing toward your leg, in the troughs between the toes. This area may be quite tender, so don't press too hard. And take some deep breaths!

3. To stimulate more balanced and healthy activity of the thyroid and parathyroid glands, work all around the base of your big toe (at the webbing, where it joins the foot).

4. Next, on the bottom of your foot, work the fleshy part of all the toes, especially the big toe. Use the thumb walk for maximum benefit. Work down the toe from the tip to the base, making three passes—both sides, and the center. Be especially thorough with the big toe. If you can, take five separate trips down that toe with your thumb, covering each of the five zones. Reflex zones for the hypothalamus (which regulates body temperature), pineal gland, pituitary gland, and brain are all located in the toes.

5. The pituitary gland is in the center of the pad of the big toe. This "master gland" governs energy level and is vital for healthy, balanced functioning of the entire hormone system. Massage with your thumb or use the "hook and back up" technique for pinpoint accuracy.

6. Continuing in the area of your toes, work on the brain reflex (located at the very tip of each toe) by placing the tip of your index finger on the tip of the toe, and rolling your finger back and forth to press on the toe. You can also use your thumbnail to roll across the tops of the toes. It hardly needs saying that the brain is the control center for all mind/body activity and holds the key to physical and emotional balance.

7. Thoroughly work the large area on the bottom of your foot between the diaphragm and the heel. This area contains reflexes for the liver, stomach, small intestines, kidneys, adrenals, and other internal organs. To help detoxify the blood, regulate fluid retention, control body heat, and stimulate production of new blood, work this entire area. Use the thumb walk to cover this area, moving up, down, and diagonally.

8. Now we will focus on removing blocks in energy circulation to the female organs, starting with the uterus. To locate it, make an imaginary line between the high point of your ankle bone on the inside (big toe side) of your foot, and the very back and bottom of your heel. The uterus reflex is at the midpoint of that line. (See Fig. 37 on page 74)

This point is likely to be very sensitive. Feel around for a tender spot with your index finger, and when you've found it (it may be in a slight indentation), work it gently with a circular motion. You can use your index finger, middle finger, or thumb.

9. The reflex for the ovaries is located in the same position on the *outside* (little toe side) of your foot. Again, when you find the spot (midway between the high point of the ankle bone and the back of the heel) work it with a slight circular motion. If these spots hurt a lot, ease off on the pressure; even stop for a few seconds, and then try again. But don't press too hard and hurt yourself. The ovaries regulate estrogen level, so don't skip this step.

10. Another "female" area to work is the reflex for the fallopian tubes. This is located in a band around the top of your foot, where the foot joins the ankle. It doesn't run in a circle around the ankle, but at an angle: Just as the actual fallopian tubes connect the ovaries to the uterus, the fallopian tube reflex connects these two reflex points. This also tends to be tender, so work it gently. Try using the finger walk with your index finger. If it's not too sensitive, use the thumb walk.

11. On the inside of each foot, along the Achilles tendon, is a long narrow zone that can help with chronic problems related to the uterus. Hold your foot at the toes with the opposite hand (right foot with left hand and vice versa), tilt the foot away from you a little, and work the area using the thumb walk. Start about six inches above the ankle bone and work down to the heel.

12. Take a few minutes to relax. If you like, repeat step 1: Rub your feet and use the relaxation techniques described on page 64. Finish with the thumb press on the solar plexus point for 15 to 30 seconds.

SHIATSU

Since deficiency of Kidney *yin* is the most important component of the *yin* deficiency behind most menopausal symptoms, we'll focus here on stimulating the Kidney meridian.

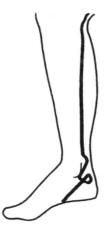

Fig. 138

Start on the sole of your foot, just below the ball of the foot, in the soft fleshy area. Work this area firmly with both thumbs, spending one or two minutes in the area of Kd 1. (See Fig. 5 on page 15) Use short, firm presses of 6–7 seconds each, repeating several times.

Then use the press and release technique to work in a line down the center of the sole of the foot to just in front of the heel. Press for 6–7 seconds, release, move half an inch to an inch along the channel, and press again.

Next, still pressing and releasing, work up to the area directly below the ankle bone on the big toe side of the foot. From here, move toward the Achilles tendon, paying special attention to any sore spots. Slowly move up in the space between the ankle bone and the Achilles tendon, and continue in a straight line up the leg, stopping once you get near the vicinity of the knee. Do both legs. Take at least 3 minutes on each leg.

ADDITIONAL SUGGESTIONS

TUNE UP YOUR DIET.   In many Asian cultures menopause symptoms are less frequent and severe. For example, only 15% of Japanese women report menopausal symptoms. One explanation may be the differences between Western and Oriental diets. The Japanese diet (typical of Asian diets in general) contains more fish and much less red meat, very little dairy, and liberal amounts of fresh produce, whole grains and soy products. Recent research has clearly demonstrated the beneficial effects of soy products such as tofu, miso, and tempeh. You may also find substituting soy milk for cow's milk helpful. Limit alcohol, sugar, salt, meat, fatty dairy products, and saturated oils such as coconut and palm.

GO HERBAL. The classic Chinese herbal formula for menopausal symptoms is *Zhi Bai di Huang Wan*. This is the most famous of all *yin* tonics, modified with additional heat-clearing herbs. You can find this highly effective formula in most Chinatowns, as well as some pharmacies specializing in natural medicines. Any practicing Acupuncturist should have it or be able to obtain it.

A Western herb that is helpful is black cohosh (Cimicifuga racemosa), especially for hot flashes or night sweats. It is considered safe and is commercially available in health food stores as Remifemin.

TRY VITAMIN E.   A supplement of 400-800 IU per day of Vitamin E may help.

CAREFULLY CONSIDER HRT.   A major, and very difficult decision menopausal women face is whether hormone replacement therapy (HRT) is appropriate for them. At first glance, it may seem obvious: HRT reduces hot flashes, prolongs youthful appearance, supple joints, and sexual fluids (to prevent vaginal dryness), and appears to protect from heart attack and osteoporosis. But: risk of breast cancer and uterine cancer significantly increase, as well as chances of gallbladder disease, asthma, and other unwelcome conditions.

So invest some time educating yourself on the issue, and discover what methods exist, both conventional and alternative. Conventional HRT offers many approaches, ranging from estrogen replacement alone to varying combinations of estrogen and progesterone. Herbs such as wild yam, and the Ayurvedic herbs shatavari and vidari, are food precursors of these two hormones, without side effects. Find a doctor who can discuss the advantages and disadvantages with you as well as the pros and cons of other options. *The Estrogen Decision Self-Help Book* by Susan M. Lark, M.D. is one of several books available on the topic.

EXERCISE TO AVOID OSTEOPOROSIS.   The risk of osteoporosis increases significantly in the menopausal and post-menopausal period. Regular weight-bearing exercise helps maintain bone density. (This does not necessarily mean weight *lifting*; it simply means walking, jogging, or any exercise other than swimming that puts weight on your bones. Weight lifting is also okay.)

YOGA IS EXCELLENT. For overall toning and to promote hormone production and balance, Yoga postures are outstanding. We recommend the Sun Salutation (up to 12 cycles a day, if you are fit for it), and a series of postures, some of which will strengthen the lower abdominal area, such as the Locust, Cobra, Bow, and Forward Bend. The Shoulder Stand is good for all organs. (Its name in Sanskrit is Sarvanga Asana, "a pose beneficial for the whole body.") Leg lifts are also helpful.

GET YOUR CALCIUM. For further osteoporosis prevention, be sure to get a minimum of 1200 mg of calcium per day. Consider a calcium supplement.

CUT DOWN ON COFFEE. According to one study (in the *American Journal of Epidemiology,* October 1990) 2–3 cups of coffee a day—*whether regular or decaffeinated*—increases the risk of osteoporosis-related fractures by nearly 70 percent. One suggestion: cut down on coffee and substitute green tea. In Chinese medicine, both coffee and black tea are considered to have a heating quality. Green tea is more cooling and has other recently documented beneficial effects.

MEDITATE. The unstable hormones flowing through your body at this time lead easily to shifting feelings and increased sensitivity to stress. Anger, depression, and sudden tears are common. To help maintain emotional equilibrium, spend some time every day in quiet meditation. If you've learned a technique that you like, practice it! If you haven't, turn to the Additional Suggestions in the "Anxiety" section for a simple meditation technique.

Menstrual Difficulties

See also, "PMS"

Almost all women experience unusual or abnormal periods at various times in their lives. Irregularity, longer or shorter periods, unusually heavy or light bleeding, spotting at midcycle, even missing a period—all this is common, once in a while. But if any of these factors occurs for three or more months, it needs looking into.

As Letha Hadady writes in her book, *Asian Health Secrets*, "The menstrual cycle is a good indication of general health. When the flow is adequate, on time, and without discomfort, blood production and circulation are in order. Stressful lifestyle, poor eating habits, and emotional upset encourage blood deficiency and stagnant *ch'i*, leading to irregularity and pain."

In this section we will suggest pressure points for alleviating pain and balancing the flow of *ch'i*, as well as some dietary and stress management suggestions to help keep your body healthy and your emotions balanced and harmonious. The section is organized into three parts:

1. Menstrual cramps and related pain (dysmenorrhea)
2. Lack of menstruation (amenorrhea)
3. Uterine bleeding (menorrhagia/metrorrhagia)

For suggestions on how to prevent and relieve PMS (premenstrual syndrome), please turn to that section.

By far the most common menstrual complaint is dysmenorrhea—pain, cramping, and general discomfort either in the lower abdominal area and/or the low back and sacral area. Fortunately Chinese medicine excels in bringing relief to this problem. Amenorrhea (no period) and uterine bleeding are less common but no less important; they too can be treated successfully with pressure point therapy combined with suggestions from both Oriental and Western medicine.

PAINFUL MENSTRUATION (DYSMENORRHEA)

According to Chinese medicine, the primary cause of menstrual pain is "blood stagnation," with "*ch'i* stagnation" a secondary factor. The pressure points you will be pressing are chosen with an emphasis on clearing these blockages, but are effective no matter what the origin of your discomfort.

Acupressure points can be extra-sensitive during your period, so be ready to reduce the amount of pressure you normally use if you feel it necessary.

Of the following 5 Acupressure points, start with 3 of them—Lv 3, Sp 4, and Sp 6—about 7 days before your period is due. Stimulate these points every day until your flow starts. Once it begins, add Sp 8 and St 29 and continue all the points until the end of your period.

You can also use some or all of these points if you experience pain or discomfort once your period starts.

After your period is over, use the "Daily Health Builder" (see that section starting on page 161) every day until 7 days before you expect your menses to start again, and follow the diet and stress management suggestions at the end of this section.

Expect good results from this program! If you use these points for 3-4 complete cycles of your menstrual period you will be amazed at the results.

Acupressure (for Painful Menstruation)

Three of the following points (Lv 3, Sp 6, and Sp 10) are described in the section, "Ten Master Pressure Points" (beginning on page 49) where you will find illustrations of the precise point locations and suggestions on how to press for maximum benefit.

1. (Lv 3, Bigger Rushing) Press for about 1 minute. This point can be very sensitive and often is especially so during menstruation. If you have trouble bending down and/or reaching your feet, try rubbing the area on your left foot with your right heel, and vice versa.

2. (Sp 4, Grandfather Grandson) Start at the joint where the big toe connects to the foot. Slide along the underside of this bone. From the center of the joint, go approximately two thumb widths toward the head. Sp 4 is not on the side of this bone, but just below it. This point has a very beneficial effect on any type of menstrual discomfort or imbalance; it is probably the single most important point for any type of menstrual pain. Use your thumbs to apply moderate pressure.

3. (Sp 6, Three Yin Meeting) At the crossing point of three yin meridians (Spleen, Liver, and Kidney), Sp 6 can nourish the overall yin of the body. It is thus an extremely important point for any gynecological complaints. It helps to stop pain and improves blood circulation in the uterus.

4. (Sp 8, Earth Pivot) Finding Sp 8 may be a little tricky the first time, but once you've located it, you'll be able to return easily whenever you need it. It's very helpful for stopping menstrual pain, so it's worth the effort.

Bend your leg at the knee. On the inside (big toe side) of your leg, slide your finger up along the lower border of the shin bone (tibia) until you are a few inches below the knee. Your fingers will fall into a natural depression. Sp 9 is in this depression, just below a rounded prominence in the top of the bone. Sp 8 is four fingers down the shin bone from Sp 9, toward the ankle. Press firmly for 1 minute.

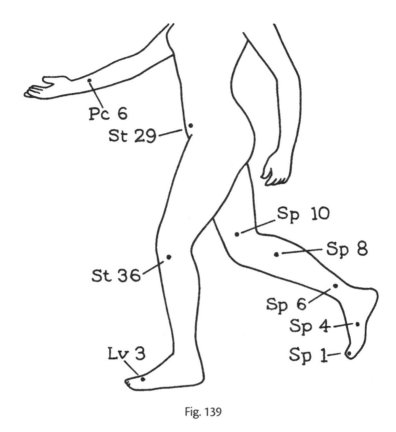

Fig. 139

5. (St 29, Returning) This point gets its name because of its power-ful ability to return the menstrual cycle to normal. Place the tips of your fingers on the pubic area above the genitals, and gently press until you feel the pubic bone under your fingers. St 29 is located one thumb width above this bone, and two thumb widths to either side of the midline of the abdomen. It is excellent for soothing menstrual pain. Press with your mid-dle or index fingers for about a minute.

If you have a lot of clots and the color of the blood is very dark, add Sp 10:

6. (Sp 10, Sea of Blood) About 2 thumb widths above the top edge of the knee you will feel a bulge in your thigh muscles. It's on the top of your leg, toward the inside. Press firmly for a minute with your thumb or the knuckle of your middle finger. This point effectively relieves blood stagnation.

Reflexology

The menstrual cycle is a very complex phenomenon, involving your body's entire hormone system, the brain and nervous system, and all the female organs. Thus our suggested Reflexology session is an unusually long one, with quite a number of reflex areas for you to massage and press. Professional Reflexologists have a great deal of success helping women regain menstrual regularity and alleviating cramps and other symptoms, such as tender breasts and intense emotional swings. You can achieve good results on your own, if you are patient and thorough.

Begin your self-treatments about a week before you expect your flow to begin, and continue throughout the week or so of your period. Spend at least 15 minutes, up to half an hour if you have time.

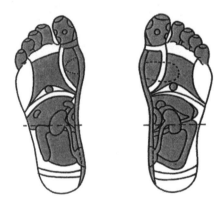

Fig. 140

1. Get started by simply massaging your feet and relaxing them with the techniques described in the Reflexology Warm-Up on page 69. Don't skip this important step, designed to help you relax, tone the energy of the whole body, and prepare your feet to be worked on.

2. To help relax, dissolve stress, relieve tenderness in your breasts, and facilitate deep, regular breathing, work on the chest/lung/breast areas on both the bottom and top of your foot. First, thumb walk the chest and lung reflex zones on the ball of the foot (between the diaphragm line and the base of the toes). Then finger walk the related reflexes on the top of your foot, in the solid part of the foot between the diaphragm line and the shoulder line. Work up from the webbing toward

your leg, pressing in the troughs between the toes. Start in zone 1, at the base of the big toe, and go up about 2 inches. Continue working each zone, ending in zone 5 near the outside edge of your foot. Work this area with your index finger, using the finger walk. This area may be quite tender, so don't press too hard.

3. While you are in this area, work all around the base of your big toe (at the webbing, where it joins the foot). This will stimulate more balanced and healthy activity of the thyroid and parathyroid glands. The thumb walk technique is best here, though some general rubbing and massaging will also be beneficial.

4. Next, work all your toes, especially the big toe. On the bottom of your foot, work the fleshy part of all the toes. Use the thumb walk for maximum benefit. Work down the toe from the tip to the base, making three passes—both sides, and the center. Be especially thorough with the big toe. If you can, make five separate trips down that toe with your thumb, covering each of the five zones. Reflex zones for the hypothalamus, pineal gland, pituitary gland, and brain are all located in the toes.

5. The pituitary gland reflex is in the center of the pad of the big toe. This "master gland" governs hormone secretion and energy level, and is extremely important for healthy, balanced endocrine function. Massage with your thumb or use the "hook and back up" technique for pinpoint accuracy.

6. Continuing in the area of your toes, work on the brain reflex (at the very tip of each toe) by placing the tip of your index finger on the tip of the toe, and rolling your finger back and forth to press on the toe. You can also use your thumbnail to roll across the tops of the toes.

7. Next, work on the spine reflexes. These are located on the inside edge of both feet (zone 1), extending from the heel nearly to the top of the big toe, opposite the root of the toenail.

When you work these reflexes, work slowly up the foot using the thumb walk technique. (You will need a little extra strength on the thick skin of the heel area.) Then thumb walk all the way *down* the spinal reflex area. Take some time to walk across small areas horizontally, moving up the foot from the heel to the big toe. Pay special attention to the lower spine (located around the heel and arch of the foot), to help increase blood flow and energy flow to the pelvic region. Aching back muscles may also be soothed by attention to the spine reflexes.

8. Thoroughly work the large area between the diaphragm and the heel. This area contains reflexes for the liver, stomach, small intestines, kidneys, adrenals, and other internal organs. To help detoxify the blood, regulate fluid retention, and stimulate production of new blood, use the thumb walk to cover this entire area, moving up, down, and/or diagonally.

9. You might wish to spend a little time working on the colon reflexes, to make sure elimination is regular and efficient. Note that the reflexes for various aspects of the colon are divided between the two feet (the ascending colon reflex is located on the right foot, the descending colon reflex on the left foot, etc.) Don't worry about the precise locations, but do cover the area thoroughly.

10. Now we finally arrive at the female organs. To locate the reflex for the uterus, make an imaginary line between the high point of your ankle bone on the inside (big toe side) of your foot, and the very back and bottom of your heel. The uterus reflex is at the midpoint of that line. (See Fig. 37 on page 74.)

This point is likely to be very sensitive. Feel around for a tender spot with your index finger, and when you've found it (it may be in a slight indentation), work it gently with a circular motion. Use your index finger, middle finger, or thumb. Another way to work this area is to hold one finger (probably your thumb) of one hand on the spot, while rotating your foot with the other hand.

11. The reflex for your ovaries is located in the same position on the *outside* (little toe side) of your foot. Again, when you find the spot (midway between the high point of the ankle bone and the back of the heel) work it with a slight circular motion. If these spots hurt a lot, ease off on the pressure; even stop for a few seconds, and then try again. But don't press too hard and hurt yourself.

12. The reflex for the fallopian tubes is located in a band around the top of your foot, where the foot joins the ankle. It doesn't run in a circle around the ankle, but at an angle: Just as the fallopian tubes connect the ovaries to the uterus, the fallopian tube reflex connects these two reflex points. This also tends to be tender, so work it gently. Try using the finger walk with your index fingers. If it's not too sensitive, use the thumb walk.

13. On the inside of each foot, in the area of the Achilles tendon, is a long narrow zone that can help with chronic problems related to the uterus. Hold your foot at the toes with the opposite hand (right foot with

left hand), tilt the foot away from you a little, and work the area using the thumb walk. Start about six inches above the ankle bone and work down to the heel.

14. After this long workout on your feet, take a few minutes just to relax! As in step 1, rub your feet and use the techniques described on page 69. Finish with the thumb press on the solar plexus point for 15 to 30 seconds.

Shiatsu

Two channels intimately connected with menstrual pain are the Liver and Spleen. The following Shiatsu routine enlivens both. Use the press and release technique—press for 6–7 seconds, release, move half an inch to an inch along the channel, and press again.

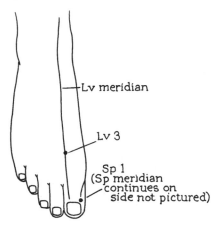

Fig. 141

1. To stimulate the Liver meridian, start in the center of the top of your big toe. Move along the toe to the web margin between the big toe and second toe, then up the channel between the big toe and second toe. From the ankle, the channel proceeds up the inside part of the leg, along the bone. (See Fig. 142.) Use only mild to moderate pressure along the bone. About halfway up the leg the meridian comes off the bone and continues up the middle of the inside of the leg. Above the knee, the pathway travels slightly higher than the middle of the inside portion of your thigh. Stop at the groin. On the thigh above the knee, you can use strong pressure.

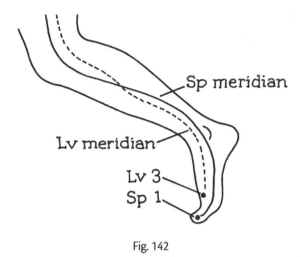

Fig. 142

2. The Spleen meridian also starts at the big toe. The first point is very close to the nail cuticle at the inside corner of the big toenail. From there, the meridian follows along the side of the big toe bone, at the inside of the foot, up the side of the ankle and the inside of the leg. Along the leg it follows just below the bone. Use the press and release technique from the big toe to just below the knee. Give special attention to Sp 6, located about one palm width (not including the thumb) above the center of the ankle bone, just off the bone toward the back of the leg. Be sure to work on both legs.

Additional Suggestions (For Painful Menstruation)

TRY HERBS. Chinese herbal prescriptions are tailored to the individual, based on an evaluation by a qualified practitioner. If your problem is severe, consider a consultation with an expert herbalist, as Chinese herbal formulas work very well for this problem. Typically, herbs are not used alone but are combined with up to a dozen other ingredients to build a formula that is specific both for the condition and the particular individual.

If you don't have a practitioner in your area, try taking Dang Gui (sometimes spelled Tang Kuei or Dong Quai) which is the Chinese name for *Angelicae sinesis*. It is sold in many health food stores, and even used alone it can be very effective. Start taking it 7 days before your period. If you have less pain and it seems to be helping, continue using it throughout the month. Otherwise discontinue use.

AVOID CAFFEINE.   Caffeine tends to aggravate the severity of symptoms. Try eliminating—or at least minimizing—any food and drinks containing caffeine in your diet. This includes not just coffee, but also tea, colas and many other sodas, and chocolate. But taper off slowly. If you are habituated to caffeine, stopping abruptly may cause headaches and irritability.

MANAGE STRESS.   Exhaustion, unresolved emotions, overwork, and any form of excessive stress, any time during the month, tend to affect your period. So do your best to reduce stress in your life. Take time every day for some meditation, a quiet walk, listening to music, dancing, or whatever you have found that works for you.

EXERCISE DAILY.   Half an hour of walking every day, and/or 15–30 minutes of Yoga postures or tai chi, is all most people need to keep the energy flowing smoothly in the body. The Sun Salutation, a cycle of 12 Yoga postures, is excellent for toning the entire body, inside and out. Other helpful Yoga postures include the Shoulder Stand, Plow, Cobra, and Forward Bend. But: exercise or Yoga during your period is NOT recommended. Rest and relax as much as your responsibilities permit.

AMENORRHEA (ABSENCE OF MENSTRUATION)

Amenorrhea means either that you have never had a period, or that your period has stopped for more than three months and you are neither pregnant, breastfeeding, nor in menopause. From a Western perspective, a cessation of menstruation is most often due to (1) intensive athletic training; (2) insufficient body fat (often related to 1, as well as to eating disorders such as anorexia); and (3) stress and anxiety. There is also a phenomenon known as "post-pill amenorrhea," which occasionally occurs when a woman stops taking birth control pills.

From the perspective of Chinese medicine, not having periods is seen primarily as a deficiency condition, especially of the energies of the Liver and Spleen meridians. The Acupressure points recommended are similar to the prescription for dysmenorrhea, but with a greater emphasis on tonification or strengthening.

Acupressure (for Amenorrhea)

The first two points (Sp 6 and St 36) are described in the section, "Ten Master Pressure Points" (beginning on page 49) where you will find illustrations of the precise point locations and suggestions on how to press for maximum benefit.

1. (Sp 6, Three Yin Meeting) This is an extremely important point for any "female" problems. It helps to stop pain and improves blood circulation in the uterus.

2. (St 36, Three Mile Foot) This is the most powerful point to nourish the *ch'i* and blood; it's excellent to rebuild any deficiency condition.

3. (St 29, Returning) Please see step 5 for Dysmenorrhea, on page 283.

4. (B 18, 20, 23, Back-associated points of the Liver, Spleen and Kidney) These points are located approximately 1-½ inches on either side of the spine. They start in the area just above the level of your belly button, and continue up to the middle of your back. Even if you have long and flexible arms, the best way you can press these points on your own is to lie on your back on the floor with a tennis ball behind you. Slowly roll up and down on the ball, first on one side then on the other. Or you can put two balls in a sock and do both sides at the same time. There are other valuable points right next to the spine on both sides that you will stimulate with this technique.

   Spend several minutes stimulating the points on each side. Be sure to let the tennis ball roll the whole distance from the lower back to the middle of the back several times.

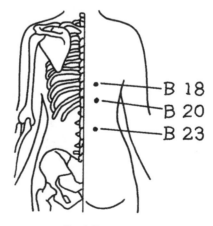

Fig. 143

Reflexology and Shiatsu techniques for Amenorrhea are the same as for Dysmenorrhea (see pages 284 and 287).

UTERINE BLEEDING (MENORRHAGIA/METRORRHAGIA)

This term covers several conditions characterized by excessive loss of menstrual blood, ranging from a prolonged menses (lasting as long as several weeks) to exceptionally heavy bleeding during menstruation, to heavy bleeding in between normal cycles. There are many different possible causes—including the use of an IUD (intrauterine device for birth control)—but we have selected points that will help curtail the excessive bleeding no matter what the cause.

Acupressure

Caution: Acupressure is helpful for uterine bleeding, but it is not strong enough, by itself, to correct the problem. Combined with the herbal remedies in the "Additional Suggestions" section, it becomes highly effective. But unusual bleeding should never be ignored. We urge you to get an evaluation from a Western M.D.

1. (Sp 1, Hidden White) Sp 1 is just off the outside corner of the cuticle of the big toe toenail. It is useful to stop bleeding in any part of the body, but it's especially helpful for uterine bleeding. Use your thumb to apply firm pressure. (See Fig. 139)

2. (Sp 4, Grandfather Grandson) Start at the joint where the big toe connects to your foot. Slide along the underside of this bone. From the center of the joint, go approximately two thumb widths. Sp 4 is not on the side of this bone, but just below it. This point has a very beneficial effect on any type of menstrual disorder. When paired with Pc 6 (below), the two points open what is called the Penetrating meridian, said to be the energetic source of all the other meridians in the body. Use your thumbs to apply moderate pressure for about 1 minute.

3. (Pc 6, Inner Gate) You will find this point on the palm side of your wrist, two thumb widths above the wrist crease in the center of the arm. It should be stimulated immediately after Sp 4 to open the Penetrating meridian. Use your thumb to apply moderate to firm pressure. Remember to always build up gradually, hold about a minute, and gradually release. Be sure to do both hands. (See Fig. 139.)

4. (Sp 8, Earth Pivot) See Step 4 under Dysmenorrhea, page 000 for point location and instructions for pressing.

Reflexology and Shiatsu techniques for Uterine Bleeding (Menorrhagia) are the same as for Dysmenorrhea (see pages 284 and 287).

Additional Suggestions: (Uterine bleeding)

The most effective treatment to stop uterine bleeding is a tea made from *Artemesia argyi,* also known as mugwort leaf. The chinese name is *ai ye.* This is the ingredient used to make moxa, which is used extensively in Chinese medicine. As moxa, it is formed into rolls or cones and lit near Acupressure points for its warming and energizing effects. Note: If it has already been formed into moxa sticks or cones, *do not use it* to make tea.

Loose moxa is available in the Chinatowns of many cities or from some Acupuncturists and herb suppliers. Many natural food stores carry mugwort, but be sure it is *Artemesia argyi,* as there are many species of artemesia; stores typically stock *Artemesia vulgaris,* which is not what you want.

Place 6–9 grams (about ⅓ ounce) of the herbs in a pan with 2 to 3 cups of water and bring to a boil. Turn down the heat and simmer for 10–15 minutes. Strain out the loose herbs with a wire mesh strainer and drink the remaining tea over the course of a day, a little at a time. Bleeding usually stops within 2–3 days. Again, any unusual bleeding should not be ignored. If it continues or recurs, please see a doctor.

Migraines

See "Headaches"

Morning Sickness

See "Nausea and Vomiting"

Motion Sickness

See "Nausea and Vomiting"

Nausea and Vomiting

Nausea is treated very effectively by pressure point therapy. Recent research has confirmed this, both for morning sickness in pregnancy, as well as chemotherapy-induced nausea. It can also be used to dispel motion sickness, and for nausea caused by chronic diseases. Mainstream medicine is beginning to acknowledge this, and Acupuncture is now used in increasing numbers of American hospitals for this purpose. You can use the same points at home.

ACUPRESSURE

1. (Pc 6, Inner Gate) This point is on the palm side of your wrist, two thumb widths above the wrist crease and in the center of the arm. This is the king of points to treat nausea. Use the thumb of the opposite hand to apply moderate to firm pressure. Breathe deeply while pressing.

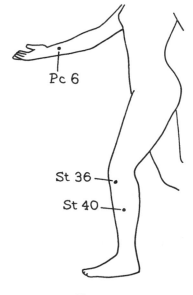

Fig. 144

The next two points (St 36 and St 40) are fully described beginning on page 49 ("Ten Master Pressure Points") where you will find illustrations of precise point locations and suggestions on how to press them for maximum benefit.

2. (St 36, Three Mile Foot) In addition to its powerful rejuvenative properties, St 36 also helps settle the stomach.

For morning sickness, add St 40:

3. (St 40, Abundant Splendor) This point is very helpful for reducing mucus, phlegm, and congestion, and it also has a beneficial effect on the stomach.

REFLEXOLOGY

To help settle nausea, we will focus on reflex areas for the throat, stomach, and digestive system, adding a few additional points for motion sickness.

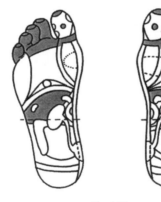

Fig. 145

1. As always, we recommend that you start your session with the Reflexology Warm-Up on page 69 for a sequence of steps to help you relax, tone the energy of the whole body, and prepare your feet to be worked on.

2. Since much of the feeling of nausea often originates in the throat, work the neck and throat reflexes located at the base of the toes and especially at the base of the big toe. Work the base of the big toe by rubbing and pressing. The finger or thumb walk technique is best here.

To stimulate the neck reflexes, "walk the ridge" at the top of the ball of the foot (at the base of the toes). Pull the flesh of the pad of the foot down and away from the ridge with your other hand. Walk in both directions.

3. Spend a minute or so on the pituitary gland reflex, located in the center of the pad of the big toe. Known as the "master gland," the pituitary

regulates the secretion of hormones and controls body temperature and metabolism, among its hundreds of functions. To press it most effectively, use the "hook and back up" technique described on page 68.

4. Next, work on your stomach reflex, in the center of the arch of your *left* foot. To help send energy to the liver, which is responsible for detoxifying the blood and manufacturing bile, work on your *right* foot, in the same general area as the stomach reflex on the left foot. We recommend that you simply work the entire area in the arch of each foot, from the pelvic line up to the diaphragm line. This will also stimulate the duodenum, pancreas, gallbladder, spleen, adrenals, and kidneys, sending healing energy to most of your digestive system. Use the thumb walk to thoroughly cover this area, moving up, down, and/or diagonally.

For motion sickness, add the following:

5. To work on the brain reflex, place the tip of your index finger on the tip of each toe, and roll the finger back and forth to press on the toe. You can also use your thumbnail to roll across the tops of the toes.

6. Motion sickness usually originates as a disturbance in the inner ear. To help settle this area, spend some extra time working on the inner ear reflex, which is located in the area you already worked in step 2, the ridge at the top of the ball of the foot. Spend some extra time there.

SHIATSU

As in the Acupressure exercise, the most important point to stimulate is Pc 6. But instead of the steady pressure suggested, try using a press and release technique. Press for 6–7 seconds and release. Repeat 5–6 times on each wrist. This might be more effective for you.

Because of the beneficial effect of the Spleen meridian on settling the stomach, we will stimulate this channel as well. (See Fig. 142 on page 288.) The Spleen meridian starts at the big toe. The first point is very close to the nail cuticle at the inside corner of the big toenail. From there, the meridian follows along the side of the big toe bone, at the inside of the foot, up the side of the ankle and the inside of the leg. Along the leg it follows just below the bone. Use the press and release technique from the big toe to just below the knee. When you're finished with one foot and leg, be sure to repeat the entire procedure on the other side.

ADDITIONAL SUGGESTIONS

THE GINGER CURE.   Ginger has long been known in Oriental medicine for its anti-nausea properties, and in recent years, Western research has verified its effectiveness. You can swallow powdered ginger as capsules (available at the health food store; follow recommendations on the bottle) or make a tea from fresh ginger. If you are traveling and have a problem with motion sickness, take some capsules with you.

To make ginger tea, use fresh ginger root from the grocery store. Cut a one-inch section into thin slices and bring it to a boil in a cup and a half of water. Turn the heat down and let it simmer 10–15 minutes. Sip the tea as needed to settle your nausea. If it tastes too strong, just add more water to dilute it.

Some natural food stores and Oriental grocery stores also sell freeze-dried ginger granules for making tea. Although this is convenient, fresh ginger tea will give better results. For future reference, ginger also has anti-inflammatory properties and has been used to help provide relief in rheumatoid arthritis. It's also helpful in colds.

TRY FASTING.   Vomiting is your system's way of clearing out toxins, whether from illness or some food you've eaten. Fasting—just drinking room temperature water or some juice, such as cranberry or *sweet* pineapple—will give your digestive system a chance to rest and heal.

LET YOURSELF VOMIT.   Though most of us hate throwing up, the fact is that once you do, you almost always feel better. So don't struggle to hold it down.

Neck and Shoulder Tension and Pain

Many of the body's meridians run up our arms and trunk and converge at the neck, making this area a kind of Grand Central Station for our *ch'i* or Life Energy. Because most of us hold a lot of stress and tension in and around our neck and shoulders, the flow of *ch'i* can easily be obstructed; the blocked or stagnant *ch'i* may cause stiffness or pain.

Tension causes us to involuntarily contract the muscles in this area; stress, tension, and tight muscles, continuing day after day, may lead to a state of chronic muscle rigidity. This, in turn, may pinch the nerves, leading not only to headaches, but, if the condition is severe, to pain and tingling in the arms and hands. Over time it can adversely affect the healthy curvature of the spine and the alignment of the cervical vertebrae. So, it's time to do something about that tension in your shoulders and neck!

The following pressure point prescriptions will help relieve those sore and stiff muscles. Even if you don't have neck pain, pressing these points will help you unwind after a busy day. Or you can use them at the office, especially if you spend extended periods of time in front of a computer screen. You can do a quick version (use just one or two points) at intervals throughout the day to prevent neck tension from building up.

ACUPRESSURE

This first sequence will help relieve pain and tension in both your neck and your shoulders.

1. (Li 4, Adjoining Valley) For an illustration of the exact location of this important point, and instructions on how to press it most effectively, please see page 49 for the beginning of "Ten Master Pressure Points." Li 4 not only relieves pain, it also helps release blocked *ch'i* along the Li meridian, which traverses the side of the neck.

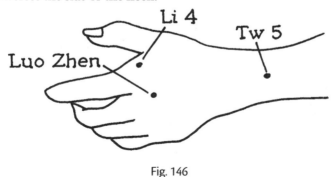

Fig. 146

2. (Tw 5, Outer Gate) Hold your left arm in front of you with the palm down, facing the floor. Measure two thumb widths above the wrist. The point is right in the center between the two forearm bones. Press firmly with your thumb or middle finger for about a minute. The Tw (triple warmer)

channel runs up the back of the arm to the shoulder and neck, and is therefore widely used in any type of arm, shoulder or neck complaints.

3. (SI 11, Heavenly Attribution) This point is on your back, over the scapula (shoulder blade). It's in the center of the scapula, ⅔ of the way from the bottom to the top. Wait—don't go away! We know this sounds too difficult to locate, but it's easy when you use the following tennis ball technique to stimulate it:

Lie on your back with a tennis ball underneath your left shoulder blade. Slowly slide your body up and down on the ball, so that the ball stimulates the whole scapula area. After working on the left side, do the right side.

The effectiveness of this point is related to the Small Intestine meridian pathway, which runs from this point up along the neck. Pressure on this point can do wonders for both neck and shoulder complaints. Stimulate this point for about a minute, longer if it feels good.

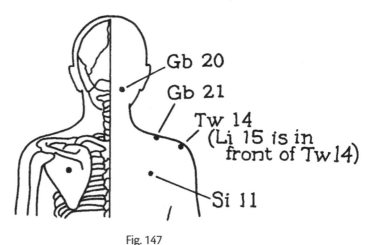

Fig. 147

4. Gb 21 (Shoulder Well) Place your right hand on your left shoulder. Midway between the neck and the outer edge of the shoulder on the highest point of the shoulder is Gb 21. This point is tender on most people. Use your middle finger to press firmly on the point with firm pressure. Or you can press both shoulders at the same time by curving your left hand over your left shoulder and right over the right. This point helps relieve muscle tension which can contribute to neck discomfort.

If you feel the pain and tension mostly in your neck, add "Luo Zhen" and Gb 20, as follows:

5. (Luo Zhen) This is one of the "extra points" that are not associated with specific meridians but have been found effective in clinical experience. This one is excellent for relieving neck pain and stiffness. It is located on the back of the hand in the channel between the index and middle finger. Start in the space between the knuckles of the two fingers. Move about one finger's breadth up toward the wrist. Feel for a natural depression. The point is close to the knuckles, but on the wrist side. It can be tender, especially when your neck is bothering you. Use your index finger or thumb to apply moderate to firm pressure for about a minute. Take some deep breaths while you press this and the other points in this section.

6. (Gb 20, Wind Pool) For an illustration of the precise location of Gb 20, and instructions on how to press it most effectively, please see page 49 for the beginning of "Ten Master Pressure Points."

If the pain and discomfort is mostly in your shoulders, add Li 15, Tw 14, and St 38, as follows:

7. & 8. (Li 15 and Tw 14) Both these points, which are located next to each other on the shoulder, have a major influence on the whole shoulder area. To locate them, first raise your arm to your side, parallel to the floor. Place your other hand on the top of the shoulder near the joint at the arm. You will feel two depressions, one on each side of a tendon that runs through the shoulder muscle. Li 15 and Tw 14 are in these depressions. Press both of them at the same time, using your thumb and index finger. You can use stronger than normal pressure on these points.

9. (St 38, Narrow Opening) St 38 is located halfway between the ankle bone on the outside of the foot and the center of the kneecap. At the halfway point, find the shin bone (tibia) and then go 1 thumb width off the bone to the outside. You can stimulate this point with either thumbs, knuckles, or the heel of the opposite foot. Use moderate to firm pressure for about a minute. Despite its distance from the shoulder, St 38 is one of the most effective points for relieving shoulder pain. You will derive maximum benefit if you slowly move your shoulder through its range of motion while stimulating this point.

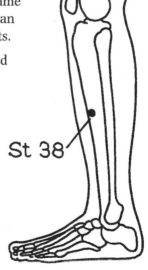

St 38

Fig. 148

REFLEXOLOGY

Most of the neck and shoulder pain we experience is not from injuries, but from accumulated tension from long hours sitting at desks, in front of computers, driving, and other basically sedentary jobs. Reflexology can significantly help relax these tense areas and relieve the discomfort.

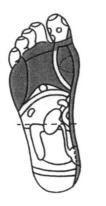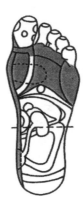

Fig. 149

    1. To begin the relaxation process, turn to the Reflexology Warm-Up on page 69. This important sequence helps you relax, tones the energy of the whole body, and prepares your feet to be worked on; please don't skip it!

    2. To help relax your chest and lungs and facilitate deep breathing, use the lung press (also called "metatarsal kneading"). (Please see Fig. 21 on page 64.) Wrap your left hand around your left foot, just below the base of the toes. Make your right hand into a fist, and press the flat backs of the fingers of the fist (not the knuckles) into the fleshy part of the foot. This is the area of the foot that corresponds to the chest and lungs.

Work both hands in a rotating, kneading motion. Relax some of the pressure of your fist, at the same time squeezing with your supporting hand on the top of the foot. Alternate between pressure and squeezing, but keep both hands in contact with your foot. Repeat several times with each foot.

While you are doing this, and for a minute or so afterwards, take some slow, deep breaths. You might want to close your eyes for deeper relaxation.

    3. The reflex zones for your shoulders are located on the bottom of your foot below your little toe, continuing out along the outside edge of your foot. To help relax your shoulders, work both horizontally and vertically along this zone. You'll probably find it most effective to use the thumb walk.

4. Next, work the neck reflexes on both feet by thumb walking along the ridge at the top of the ball of the foot (at the base of the toes). Pull the flesh of the pad of the foot down and away from the ridge with your other hand. Walk in both directions.

5. To further relax and loosen the neck, do some toe rotations. Stretch and rotate each toe, one at a time, using your thumb and index finger to grasp the toe near the base. Then use a slight lifting or pulling motion to gently stretch the toe and rotate it first in one direction several times, then in the opposite direction several times. Repeat with each toe. (See Fig. 23 on page 65.)

6. Thumb walk along the spine reflexes, located on the inside edge of both feet (zone 1), extending from the heel nearly to the top of the big toe. Work the entire spine, first moving slowly up the foot, then walking down; then take some time to walk across small areas horizontally. Pay particular attention to the cervical area of the spine (at the neck and shoulders) located along the big toe. If you don't have much time, concentrate on this area only.

7. Finish your session by comfortably rubbing your feet, wiggling them a little if you like. You can also use the thumb press on the solar plexus point for 15 to 30 seconds.

SHIATSU

1. Start with both hands on your neck, toward the back of the neck. With circular motions of the fingertips, massage around the base of the skull from the earlobes toward the spine. Take extra time at any tender areas. Then massage on either side of the spine down towards your shoulders. After a minute or two of warming and loosening up the muscles well, do the following series of stretches, which will open up the meridians along the back.

2. Stand straight, with arms hanging loosely at your sides, feet a comfortable distance apart. Bend your head forward a little and be aware of the weight of your head. Let the weight slowly bend your neck forward until your chin is close to your chest. The movement should be very slow and deliberate.

Now slowly bend the top of your body forward, and be aware of the weight of your shoulders as well as your head. Keep bending forward very slowly. Try to imagine one vertebra at a time moving, starting from the top of your spine as you bend forward and proceeding gradually to the lower back.

As you bend slowly forward, be aware of the weight of your head and arms, and let the weight slowly stretch the muscles as you go forward. Don't rush. Slower is better, even if it takes several minutes to be fully bent forward. Stand next to a soft chair or sofa that you could grab if you need the extra balance.

Return to a standing position in a slow and deliberate manner also.

3. Next, stretch your neck in the other direction. To do this lie on a bed on your back, with your head and neck hanging over the edge. Again, let the weight of your neck do the stretching. In this exercise it is best to let your neck stretch out for 30–45 seconds or so and then return it to a level position and hold it level for 10 seconds. Then let it stretch out again. Repeat this 3–5 times.

4. Finally, either standing or seated, let your neck gradually fall to one side and let gravity stretch the muscles for 10–15 seconds. Slowly return to an upright position, then stretch to the other side. Alternate side to side 3 times.

ADDITIONAL SUGGESTIONS

KEEP YOUR HEAD UP. Proper posture is one of the keys to keeping your neck and shoulders free of tension and pain. When the head is leaning forward, so that your ears are in front of your shoulders, tension builds up in the neck muscles. So try to keep your head back and level, with your chin tucked in. When working at a computer terminal, keep the screen at eye level rather than having to look up or down. Try to keep your head up, not lowered, while reading or working at your desk. And don't tuck the telephone between your neck and shoulder. These adjustments will help a lot to prevent stiffness and pain.

FOLLOW THESE SLEEP SUGGESTIONS. Sleep time should help to dissolve tensions and stress, not exacerbate them. Sleeping on a soft mattress, or using a pillow that is too thick, or sleeping on your stomach, can all cause or complicate stiff and sore necks and shoulders. So try curling up on your side to sleep, and use a thin pillow or none at all. Or try a special cervical pillow.

DO NECK EXERCISES.   (See the Shiatsu section.) You can also try doing some shoulder rolls. Start by pulling your shoulders up to your neck, hold, then drop them down. Make a shrugging motion while rolling your shoulders up and back, up and back. Then reverse, moving from back to front.

USE MUSCLE RELAXANTS.   Over the counter anti-inflammatories and muscle relaxants such as aspirin or ibuprofen may help. Or try an herbal remedy such as chamomile tea or licorice tea. These may not have as powerful an immediate effect as drugs, but they work gently and effectively.

TRY MASSAGE.   A gentle self-massage of the neck and shoulder with a few drops of warm oil (such as sesame, which has a warming effect) will definitely help to soothe aching neck and shoulder muscles. Of course, it's wonderful to have someone else perform the massage, if you have that option!

Pain

See also, "Angina," "Arthritis," "Back Pain,"
"Neck and Shoulder Tension," etcetera

Like it or not, pain is one of the facts of life. It may come from a bruise, a sprain, a pull or tear, or it may originate within, from an illness or troubled organ. It may be dull or sharp, generalized or very specific; it may burn, stab, ache, throb, or shoot. In this section we include pressure point self-treatments helpful for relieving pain in general, as well as some very specific treatments for alleviating pain in various parts of your body: elbow, wrist, fingers, along the spine, hip, thigh, knee, and lower leg. There's no reason for you to read through the entire section; just look ahead for the part you need to treat your pain.

You will find suggestions for relieving pain and stiffness in your neck and shoulders in the section, "Neck and Shoulder Pain," and other remedies in "Arthritis." For chest pain, see "Angina."

ACUPRESSURE

If the pain moves around:

If your pain has a quality of changing or moving around—sometimes it seems to be in one place, sometimes in another—use the following two points:

Gb 20 (Wind Pool)

Sp 10 (Sea of Blood)

Illustrations of the exact locations of these points, and instructions on how to press them most effectively, begin on page 49, "Ten Master Pressure Points."

Elbow Pain

The following points will help relieve "tennis elbow" or any similar pain in your elbow.

1. (Li 4, Adjoining Valley) See "Ten Master Pressure Points" beginning on page 49 for the precise location of this point and instructions for pressing most effectively. Li 4 is recommended here for its ability to relieve pain and to circulate the *ch'i* through the elbow area.

2. (Tw 5, Outer Gate) Hold your left arm in front of you with the palm facing down. Measure two thumb widths above the wrist. The point is right in the center between the two forearm bones. Press with your thumb or middle finger for about a minute. The Tw (triple warmer) channel runs up the back of the arm to the shoulder and neck, then moves around to the side of the neck; this point is widely used to treat any type of arm, shoulder, or neck pain.

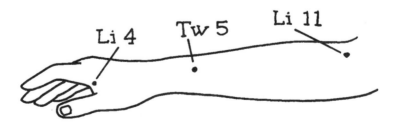

Fig. 150

3. (Li 11, Pool at the Crook) Like Li 4, this point is fully described in "Ten Master Pressure Points" (beginning on page 49) where you will find an illustration of the precise location and suggestions on how to press for maximum benefit. Li 11, because of its location, acts directly on the elbow.

4. (Tw 10, Heavenly Well) This point, located one thumb width directly above the tip of the elbow, toward the shoulder, helps relieve elbow pain and stiffness. Press firmly for about a minute with your thumb or middle finger, whichever is easier.

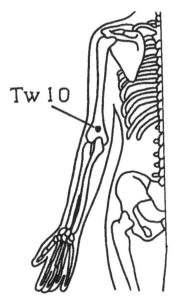

Fig. 151

Wrist Pain

1. Grab your wrist with the thumb and middle fingers of the opposite hand in this way: Put your thumb in the depression below the thumb at the wrist crease. Put your middle finger in the depression at the wrist crease on the little finger side. Use moderate to firm pressure, depending on how sensitive the points are, for about a minute.

2. Next, press the same three points recommended for elbow pain: Li 4, Tw 5, and Li 11. (See Fig. 150.) Li 4 is a potent pain reliever; Tw 5 is widely used to treat any type of arm, shoulder, or neck pain; Li 11 helps open the flow of *Ch'i* through the arm, thereby benefiting the wrist.

If your wrist pain is from carpal tunnel syndrome, add a point on the palm side of the wrist right in the center of the wrist crease, and a second point two thumb widths directly above the first (toward the elbow.) These points help reduce pain along the median nerve.

Finger Pain

1. A simple and helpful technique is simply to press in the webbing next to the painful finger or between painful fingers. Go up from the end of the webbing to the space between the joints. With the thumb or index finger, press directly into the joint area between the fingers. These points stimulate the *ch'i* flow to the fingers, and are helpful in both pain and numbness.

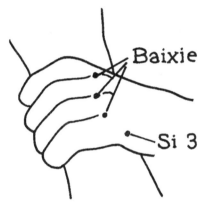

Fig. 152

2. (Li 4, Adjoining Valley) For an illustration of the exact location of Li 4 and instructions on how to press it most effectively, see page 49 for the beginning of "Ten Master Pressure Points."

Pain Along the Spine

1. (Gv 26, Man's Middle) Put your index or middle finger in the space between your upper lip and the bottom of the nose. The point is closer to the nose than the lip (about ⅓ of the distance from the bottom of the nose to the lip). You can press with your fingernail to more vigorously stimulate this point.

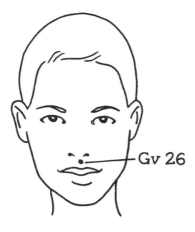

Fig. 153

2. (Si 3, Back Stream) Si 3 is on the back of your hand, at the joint of the little finger where the finger joins the hand. More specifically, it is on the side of the joint closest to the wrist, just below the bone. (See Fig. 152.) Use your thumb, or your index or middle finger. This point is intimately connected with the *yang* energy that flows up the spine in the Governing Vessel meridian. It is helpful for pain relief and disorders affecting the spine.

3. (B 62, Extending Vessel) This point is just below the ankle bone on the little toe side of the foot. (See Fig. 154.) Put your finger on the prominence of the ankle bone and slide off it into a depression right underneath it. If you find yourself on a tendon, slowly rock your finger until you go deeper into the depression. B 62 may be quite sensitive. Try working it while sitting on a chair, with your foot on a stool in front of you to help you reach it. This point reinforces the influence of Si 3 (above) on the spine. Si 3 followed by B 62 is used by professionals to open and stimulate the energy in the Governing Vessel meridian.

Hip Pain

1. (Li 4, Adjoining Valley) For an illustration of the exact location of Li 4 and instructions on how to press it most effectively, see page 49 for the beginning of "Ten Master Pressure Points."

2. (Gb 34, Yang Hill Spring) At the lower border of the kneecap, slide your finger off the shinbone toward the outside (little toe side). Two bones come together here. Press in the soft tissue area between them, using your index or index and middle fingers together. This is a major point in Acupuncture for nourishing the tendons and joints. It also promotes the flow of *ch'i* and blood in the legs and hip area.

3. (Gb 30, Jumping Circle) This point is the single most important point for relieving hip pain. It also stimulates circulation in the entire leg and low back. The point is located on the buttocks, about a third of the distance between the hip bone and the tail bone. Press this point quite strongly, using your thumbs or your fist. For even more pressure, lie down on the floor with your fists under your hips and slowly rock back and forth to stimulate these points on both sides.

4. (Gb 29, Squatting Crevice) Put your hands on either side of the waist at about belt level. Now slide down halfway toward the hip bone. Press firmly with the thumbs. In conjunction with Gb 30, this point is very effective for relieving hip pain.

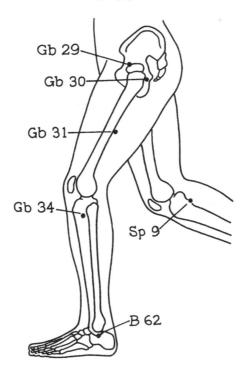

Fig. 154

Thigh Pain

1. (Li 4, Adjoining Valley) For an illustration of the exact location of Li 4 and instructions on how to press it most effectively, see page 49 for the beginning of "Ten Master Pressure Points."

2. (Gb 31, Wind Market) Locate this point standing up, but you can stimulate it either standing or sitting. It's on the outside of your thigh, at the point where your fingers touch the thigh when you let your arms hang loose at your sides. Press firmly for a minute with your thumb, or you can use your index and middle fingers together for firm pressure.

3. (Gb 34, Yang Hill Spring) See Step 2 under Hip Pain.

4. (B 36, Receiving Support) This helpful pain relieving point is on the back of the thigh, in the center of the crease that separates your buttocks from your thigh. Press with your middle finger, or lie on the floor with a fist under this point. (See Fig. 155.)

Lower Leg Pain (or numbness)

1. (Gb 34, Yang Hill Spring) See Step 2 under Hip Pain.

2. (B 57, Support the Mountain) You'll find this point in the center of the "V" formed by the lower border of your calf muscles. It's approximately halfway between the ankle bone and the point directly behind your knee. Use your thumb if you are sitting cross legged or holding one leg on the opposite knee. Otherwise, reach down and press with your middle finger. This point helps relieve leg pain and stiffness. It's also useful for hemorrhoids.

3. (B 58, Soaring Upwards) This point is about one thumb width below and to the outside of B 57. Treat it in just the same way.

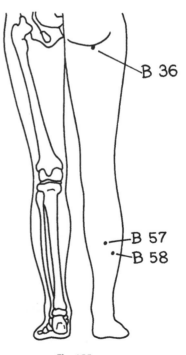

Fig. 155

Knee Pain

1. (Li 4, Adjoining Valley) For an illustration of the exact location of this important point, and instructions on how to press it most effectively, please see page 49 for the beginning of "Ten Master Pressure Points."

2 (Gb 34, Yang Hill Spring) See Step 2 under Hip Pain (on page 308). This is a major point in Acupuncture for nourishing the tendons and joints. It is used here to increase circulation in the tissue around the knee.

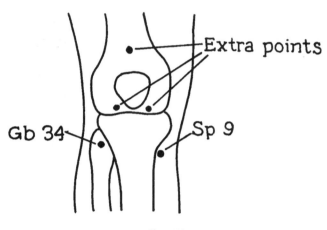

Fig. 156

3. There are three Acupressure points located around the knee. One is two thumb widths directly above the center of the kneecap. Two more points are in the "dimples" on either side of the lower border of the kneecap.

If there is swelling and water on the knee, add Sp 9:

4. (Sp 9, Yin Mound Spring) Bend your leg at the knee. On the inside side of the shin bone, slide your index finger up along the lower border of the shin bone until you are a few inches below the upper leg bone and your finger falls into a natural depression. Sp 9 is in this depression, right below a rounded prominence in the top of the leg bone (tibia). (See Fig. 154.) Pressing on this point will help reduce the swelling. The point helps regulate water metabolism, especially in the lower half of the body.

REFLEXOLOGY

Reflexology can be very helpful to control or relieve pain. That is because much of the pain we experience is not from injuries, but from accumulated stress that produces muscle tension and strain; Reflexology promotes deep relaxation, which helps relieve some of the discomfort. When pain *is* from illness or injury, Reflexology treatments can improve circulation to the injured area, by inducing relaxation that relieves cramped muscles and allows the blood and energy to flow. In addition, stimulation of the pituitary gland (by pressing the pituitary reflex) promotes production of endorphins, the body's natural painkiller that experts say may be anywhere from 10 to 200 times more powerful than morphine.

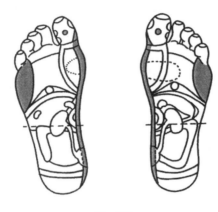

Fig. 157

1. Start by massaging your feet gently for a few minutes to help you settle down. Then use the relaxation techniques described in the Reflexology Warm-Up on page 69. Please don't skip this step: it helps you relax, tones the energy of the whole body, and prepares your feet to be worked on.

2. Many pain programs taught at pain clinics teach "breathing into the pain." To help relax your chest and lungs and facilitate deep breathing, use the lung press (also called "metatarsal kneading"). Wrap your left hand around the left foot, just below the base of the toes. Make your right hand into a fist, and press the flat backs of the fingers of the fist (not the knuckles) into the fleshy part of the foot. This is the area of the foot that corresponds to the chest and lungs. (See Fig. 21 on page 64.)

Work both hands in a rotating, kneading motion. Relax some of the pressure of your fist, at the same time squeezing with your supporting hand on the top of the foot. Alternate between pressure and squeezing, but keep both hands in contact with your foot. Repeat several times with each foot.

While you are doing this, and for a minute or so afterwards, take some slow, deep breaths, filling the diaphragm first and then the chest. Close your eyes for deeper relaxation.

3. Next, we recommend working on the area on your feet that corresponds to the area of pain on your body. Study the foot "maps" starting on page 45. Work most areas with the thumb walk; if the area is sensitive, such as the breast area on the top of the foot, use the finger walk (with your index finger), which places less pressure on the tender spot(s).

4. To help relax your shoulders, seat of much tension and stress, use the thumb walk on the bottom of your foot in zone 5, under your little toe and continuing out along the outside edge of your foot. Work both horizontally and vertically along this zone.

5. The nerve conduits of the spine fan out to reach all areas of the body. To nourish and relax this vital energy center, work on the spine reflexes located on the inside edge of both feet (zone 1), extending from the heel nearly to the top of the big toe. Work the entire spine, first moving slowly up the foot using the thumb walk technique, then walking down; take some time to walk across small areas horizontally. Pay particular attention to the part of the spine that corresponds to the area of the body where you feel pain. For neck or head pain, work the cervical spine points near the toes; for mid or low back pain, concentrate on the area in the arch of the foot and toward the heel.

6. Now work the pituitary gland reflex, located in the center of the pad of the big toe. This "master gland" regulates the secretion of hormones, controls metabolism, governs energy level, and appears to have a key role in the production of endorphins, the body's natural pain killer. To press on this point, massage with your thumb or use the "hook and back up" technique described on page 68.

7. Finish your session by comfortably rubbing your feet, wiggling them a little if you like. You can also use the thumb press on the solar plexus point for 15 to 30 seconds.

ADDITIONAL SUGGESTIONS

WARM IT.   Warmth is often very soothing to pain. Try putting a hot water bottle between your belly button and the pubic bone (for a general soothing effect, even if that's not the area that hurts) and see how it feels. If you notice that your pain is better with warmth, continue and repeat this treatment. You might also try it on the low back. Not only will you find this soothing, but pain-relieving points in these areas will be stimulated by the heat.

RELAX YOUR MUSCLES.   Most sudden pains and aches are muscular. Even headaches are frequently due to muscle tension in the neck and shoulders (see "Neck and Shoulder Pain"). To help muscles relax, try over-the-counter anti-inflammatories and muscle relaxants such as aspirin or ibuprofen. Or try an herbal remedy such as chamomile tea or licorice tea. These may not have as powerful and immediate an effect as drugs, but they work gently and effectively. Yoga stretching exercises, or tai chi, are also helpful.

RELAX YOUR MIND.   The stress of chronic pain, and the stresses of daily life, build up tension and increase feelings of suffering, even of being hopelessly trapped in suffering with no end in sight. (Chronic pain sufferers will know exactly what we mean.) To meet the challenge of pain with a more even mind, try meditation, deep breathing, Progressive Relaxation, even hypnosis.

ICE IT.   For immediate injuries, such as a twisted wrist or ankle, use an ice pack, or a home-made version such as a bag of frozen peas wrapped in a washcloth or small towel. (Don't apply ice directly to your skin.) Apply for about 20 minutes, remove for at least 20, then apply again, alternating for a couple of hours. You can then use ice for a few minutes every hour for the next couple of days to keep swelling down.

MOVE IT OR RUB IT.   Massaging tense or spasming muscles will help work out the pain; some movement should also help, such as walking or careful stretching. Of course, if pain gets significantly worse when you move, stop!—and consult a medical practitioner.

Pregnancy Problems

See also, "Nausea and Vomiting"

There is nothing more natural than pregnancy, and for many women, the time of carrying a child is joyful and problem-free. For other mothers-to-be, however, the joy is tarnished by problems like back pain, constipation, fluid retention, high blood pressure, leg cramps, varicose veins, nausea, sore breasts, and feelings of exhaustion.

The best way to avoid health problems during pregnancy is to begin living a healthy lifestyle long before conceiving. Regular exercise, a nourishing diet, meditation for stress management and spiritual upliftment, a tobacco-free environment, and moderate or no alcohol use will give you a big head start toward an easy pregnancy and a healthy baby.

The main source of problems is simply that pregnancy puts a lot of strain on the body. In the language of Oriental medicine, carrying and nourishing a baby in the womb makes greater demands on the body's *ch'i* or vital energy. Right from the start, the unborn child requires huge amounts of nutrients and energy that would otherwise be available to the mother. This drain on energy reserves can be especially stressful for women who are constitutionally weak or have a deficiency condition. Any such weakness or deficiency will cause fatigue, and may contribute to the problems mentioned previously as well as being a key factor for women who may be prone to miscarriage.

The root treatment for all these problems is to nourish the fundamental *ch'i* of the body. This is primarily accomplished by building the Spleen *ch'i*, as Spleen meridian energy underlies the energy of the entire system.

A common complaint during pregnancy is morning sickness. This can be very effectively treated with Acupressure. Please see the section, "Nausea and Vomiting."

ACUPRESSURE

1. (Sp 3, Supreme White) You will find it easiest to work this point if you sit cross-legged, or can comfortably put one foot on the opposite knee while sitting in a chair. You can also put your foot up on a stool. Place your right thumb on the outside edge of your left big toe, and slide it slowly up

until it goes over the big joint at the base of the big toe, where the toe is connected to the foot. On the heel side of the joint, find the bone that connects to the joint. Sp 3 is on the heel side of the joint, just off the lower border of the bone. This point is frequently tender, so you may not be able to use firm pressure. Most people find it easiest to use the thumb for this point.

Sp 3 is considered the "source point" of the Spleen meridian. It has a powerful revitalizing effect on the Spleen meridian, which in turn nourishes the entire body.

A related function of Spleen *ch'i* is to hold things in place or to hold things up. Any type of sinking or prolapse in the body is considered to be a condition known as "Spleen *ch'i* not holding." Miscarriage is included in this category, as are hemorrhoids and varicose veins. Sp 3 along with St 36 (see next point) strongly rebuilds the Spleen *ch'i*.

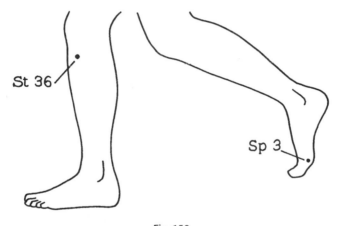

Fig. 158

2. (St 36, Three Mile Foot) This point is described in the section, "Ten Master Pressure Points" (beginning on page 49) where you will find an illustration showing its location and suggestions on how to press for maximum benefit. This is the most powerful point on the entire body for nourishing and rejuvenating the *ch'i* and blood. According to legend, soldiers in China relied on this point to sustain themselves when they were exhausted or weakened by lack of food. You may not be a foot soldier, but pregnancy can certainly be exhausting. This point can help keep you strong and healthy.

3. *For low back pain:* Fatigue and low energy can cause back pain by themselves, even without the added weight and pressure of pregnancy. The previous points will help ease low back pain indirectly, by rebuilding your

underlying energy. Also try the points recommended in the "Back Pain" section of the book. But, during your pregnancy, skip Li 4 and the "Extra Points" next to Li 4 described in that section. Li 4 is contraindicated during pregnancy, as it can start premature contractions.

REFLEXOLOGY

The following Reflexology routine will help you relax and dissolve stress, so you can maintain physical and emotional balance during your pregnancy. It will aid in the production and circulation of much-needed energy, and will tone your digestion, to provide more nourishment for both you and your child. It will stimulate the reflex areas for the reproductive system, to increase blood and energy flow. We suggest you spend about half an hour on this sequence, at least two or three times a week. This is a long procedure—the longest in the book, for a very important time of life! If you don't have time for all of it, do the opening relaxation and the steps that seem most suited to what you need.

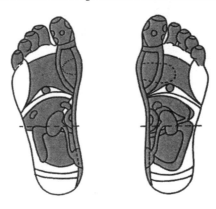

Fig. 159

1. Get started by sitting comfortably cross-legged on a bed or sofa. Massage your feet and relax them with the Reflexology Warm-Up on page 69. This will help you settle down and prepare your feet to be worked on.

2. To help relax, dissolve stress, and facilitate deep, regular breathing, work on the chest/lung/breast areas on both the bottom and top of your foot. First, thumb walk the chest and lung reflex zones on the ball of the foot (between the diaphragm line and the base of the toes). Then finger walk the related reflexes on the top of the foot. Use your index finger to work up from the webbing toward your ankle, pressing in the troughs between the toes.

This will also help reduce or prevent sore breasts. It may be quite tender, so don't press too hard. Remember to take some deep breaths!

3. Next, work all around the base of your big toe (at the webbing, where it joins the foot). This will stimulate more balanced and healthy activity of the thyroid and parathyroid glands, governors of metabolism, growth, energy level, and muscle tone. The thumb walk technique is best here, though some general rubbing and massaging will also be beneficial.

4. On the bottom of your foot, work the fleshy part of all the toes, especially the big toe. Use the thumb walk for maximum benefit. Work down the toe from the tip to the base, making three passes—both sides, and the center. Be especially thorough with the big toe. If you can, take five separate trips down that toe with your thumb, covering each of the five zones. (See Fig. 8 on page 27.) Reflex zones for the hypothalamus, pineal gland, pituitary gland, and brain are all located in the toes. Use the "hook and back up" technique (see page 68) on the pituitary reflex in the center of the pad of the big toe.

5. Continuing with your toes, work on the brain reflex (located at the very tip of each toe) by placing the tip of your index finger on the tip of the toe, and rolling your finger from side to side to press on the toe. You can also use your thumbnail to roll across the tops of the toes. It hardly needs saying that the brain is the ultimate control center for all mind/body activity and holds the key to physical and emotional balance.

6. Thoroughly work the large area on the bottom of your foot between the diaphragm and the heel. This area contains the liver, stomach, small intestines, kidneys, adrenals, and other internal organs. Work this entire area to help detoxify the blood, avoid nausea, regulate fluid retention, promote production of new blood, and stimulate digestion. Use the thumb walk, moving up, down, and diagonally.

7. Next, to enliven the nervous system and the flow of Life Energy throughout the body, work on the spine reflexes. These are located on the inside edge of both feet (zone 1), extending from the heel nearly to the top of the big toe, opposite the root of the toenail. Work slowly up the foot using the thumb walk technique. You will need to use a little extra strength on the thick skin of the heel area.

Then thumb walk all the way down, taking some time to walk across small areas horizontally. Remember that the upper spine is reflected near the toes, the lower spine from the middle of your foot down to the heel. To prevent or relieve lower back pain, work on the sacral area near the heel.

8. To promote more efficient digestion, absorption, and elimination, spend a little time pressing on the colon reflexes. Note on Fig. M, on page 45, that the reflexes for various aspects of the colon (ascending and descending colon, sigmoid colon, transverse colon) are divided between the two feet, and be sure to work all the appropriate areas thoroughly.

9. Now we will focus on improving energy circulation to the female organs, starting with the uterus. To locate the uterus reflex, make an imaginary line between the high point of your ankle bone (on the inside—big toe side) of your foot, and the very back and bottom of your heel. The uterus reflex is at the midpoint of that line. (See Fig. 37, on page 74.)

This point is likely to be very sensitive. Feel around for a tender spot with your index finger, and when you've found it (it may be in a slight indentation), work it gently with a circular motion. You can use your index finger, middle finger, or thumb.

10. The reflex for the ovaries is located in the same position, but on the *outside* (little toe side) of your foot. Again, when you find the spot (midway between the high point of the ankle bone and the back of the heel) work it with a slight circular motion. If these spots hurt a lot, ease off on the pressure; even stop for a few seconds, and then try again. Don't press too hard and hurt yourself.

11. The reflex for the fallopian tubes is located in a band around the top of your foot, where the foot joins the ankle. It doesn't run in a circle around the ankle, but at an angle. Just as the actual fallopian tubes connect the ovaries to the uterus, the fallopian tube reflex connects these two reflex points. This also tends to be tender, so work it gently. Try the finger walk using your index finger.

12. On both the inside and outside of each foot, along the Achilles tendon, is a long narrow zone that can help direct energy to the uterus. Hold your foot at the toes with the opposite hand (right foot with left hand and vice versa), tilt the foot away from you a little, and work the inside using the thumb walk. Start about six inches above the ankle bone and work down to the heel. Then walk up or down the outside of the foot in the same area, next to the tendon. Use the finger walk rather than thumb walk if the area is very tender (it exerts less pressure).

13. Frequent urination is almost unavoidable during pregnancy, as the internal space fills up with your new baby and pressure increases on the bladder. But it is helpful to work a bit on the kidney and bladder reflexes, to make sure these organs are functioning efficiently and are as toned as they

can be. You've already worked the kidneys at step 6. The reflex zone for the bladder is on the inside of your foot, in the arch, in zone 1 (beneath the big toe). It also continues up onto the side of your foot (pages 45 and 46).

14. As you can see, the vagina reflex extends from this part of the bladder reflex (on the side of the foot) all the way to the uterus reflex, which is midway between the ankle bone and the heel. Use the thumb walk technique, unless this area is too tender; then use your index finger with lighter pressure.

15. Congratulations on using this extensive procedure! A nice way to complete the process is to take a few minutes just to relax. Rub your feet and, if you like, repeat the relaxation techniques starting on page 64. Finish with the thumb press on the solar plexus point for 15 to 30 seconds.

NOTE: Ask your partner to do some Reflexology on your feet during labor. Particularly helpful: reflexes for your lungs, chest, and diaphragm (steps 1 and 2); spine (step 7), and gentle rotation on the uterus point (step 9).

SHIATSU

1. To build energy and strength and nourish the body's *ch'i*, we will stimulate the Spleen meridian.

This meridian starts at the big toe. The first point is very close to the nail cuticle at the inside corner of the big toenail. From there, it follows along the side of the big toe bone, at the inside of the foot. Use the press and release technique. Press firmly for 6–7 seconds, release, move about ½ inch along the meridian, and press again.

As you may know, the meridian then goes up the side of the ankle and

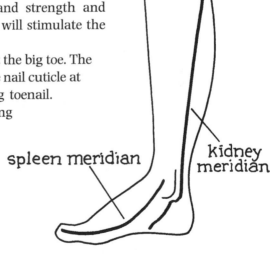

Fig. 160

the inside of the leg, but we are only going to stimulate the segment that lies on the foot. Stop at the ankle. We don't want to stimulate the meridian past the ankle because Sp 6, which is located above the ankle, is contra-indicated during pregnancy.

When you are finished with one foot and leg, be sure to repeat the entire procedure on the other side.

2. Next, stimulate along the Kidney meridian. Start on the sole of your foot, just below the ball of the foot, in the soft fleshy area. Use a circular rubbing motion with your thumb, using mild to moderate pressure.

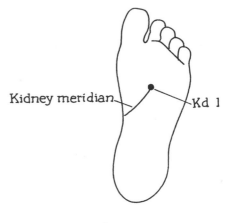

Then work in a line down the center of the sole of the foot to just in front of the heel. Continue using the same circular rubbing motion, rubbing at one spot and gradually moving up the foot.

Fig. 161

Now shift over to the area directly below your ankle bone on the big toe side of the foot. Switch to a press and release technique—press firmly for 6–7 seconds and release, then move a little further along the channel pathway and repeat the press and release. From here work out toward the Achilles tendon, paying special attention to any sore spots (work on them a little more). (See Fig. 160 on page 319.)

Finally, move slowly up the leg in the space between the ankle bone and the Achilles tendon. Move in a straight line. You can stop once you get near the vicinity of the knee. Do both legs.

ADDITIONAL SUGGESTIONS

NOURISH YOURSELF LIKE A PRINCESS.   Stock up on vitamins and top-quality food. If ever there was a time to be extra good to yourself nutritionally, this is it, as your nutritional needs are increased during pregnancy. Your own body needs more nourishment—and your baby needs it too.

Be sure to take a good quality supplement. Vitamin and mineral deficiencies (including Vitamin C, magnesium, calcium, and folic acid) have been linked to increased complications of pregnancy, as well as to birth defects. Seek out good medical advice. Your best, safest bet is to avoid unhealthy foods—refined white flour and sugar, fatty foods such as red meats and full-fat dairy products, fried food, etc.—and to include as many whole grains and fresh organic fruits and vegetables in your diet as possible.

BE CAUTIOUS ABOUT HERBS AND MEDICINES.   A number of herbs and herbal compounds are frequently recommended during pregnancy by Oriental medicine practitioners (and Western herbalists as well). However, we advise you to get personal advice from a qualified practitioner before using any herbs or medications. Many substances which are relatively safe for an adult body can have harmful effects on a growing fetus. Err on the side of caution during your pregnancy. This advice also holds for Western medications, which are much stronger and have more powerful side effects.

GET REGULAR EXERCISE.   Unless your doctor advises you to be more sedentary (which some women need), daily exercise is very important. For most women, a half hour walk every day will take care of it. More vigorous aerobic exercise is fine, but only if you are used to it. Certain Yoga postures are excellent for pregnancy, but others—any postures that put pressure on the abdomen, for example—are absolutely NOT helpful! This is something to discuss with your doctor. Exercise will make you feel more clear-minded and energetic, and is a definite mood-booster.

Premenstrual Syndrome (PMS)
See also, "Menstrual Difficulties"

The monthly onslaught of premenstrual symptoms endured by a large percentage of women (estimates vary from 30% to 80%) include irritability, depression, anxiety, insomnia, increased emotional volatility, fatigue, water retention and bloating, cramps, low backache, food cravings (especially for sugar), breast tenderness, headaches, and more. But the fact is, *suffering from PMS is not necessary.* The President's Council on Fitness estimated that 70 to 80 percent of women who suffer from various types of menstrual discomfort have unhealthy lifestyle habits such as poor diet or insufficient exercise. Reversing these habits can change your life!

Acupressure, Shiatsu, and Reflexology are very effective for PMS and other menstrual problems, but by themselves they will not remove all your symptoms. Regular exercise, a few simple dietary changes, and the use of herbs will also help. Even so, you may never eliminate every single discomfort. But if you follow the suggestions in this section, your monthly struggle with PMS can become a thing of the past.

From the point of view of Chinese medicine, the Liver (not the organ only, but the entire meridian and its energy) initiates the menstrual cycle. Thus the most common cause of PMS symptoms is disharmony in the Liver meridian and stagnation of the Liver *ch'i*, which is frequently accompanied by a deficiency of Liver *yin*.

The following pressure points and exercises will be helpful regardless of the origin of your specific symptoms. We suggest you use them for prevention, using as much of this program as you have time for as a regular routine several times a week. You can also use them for symptom relief.

ACUPRESSURE

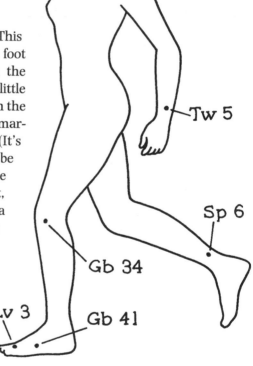

1. (Gb 41, Falling Tears) This point is on the top of the foot in the channel between the little toe and 4th toe, a little less than halfway between the ankle bone and the web margin between the toes. (It's closer to the toes.) Don't be surprised if it is quite tender. Once you locate it, press firmly for about a minute with your index or middle finger. This point is effective in restoring the smooth flow of *ch'i*, even more powerful when immediately followed by Tw 5.

Fig. 162

2. (Tw 5, Outer Gate) Hold your left arm in front of you with the palm down facing the floor. Measure two thumb widths above your wrist. Tw 5 is right in the center, between the two forearm bones. Press firmly with your thumb or middle finger for about a minute. When paired with Gb 41 this point is very helpful for smoothing out the effects of stress on the body. Repeat with the right arm.

The next two points (Lv 3 and Sp 6) are fully described in the section, "Ten Master Pressure Points" (beginning on page 49) where you will also find illustrations of the precise point locations and suggestions on how to press for maximum benefit.

3. (Lv 3, Bigger Rushing) This point can be sensitive in general, but can be even more so with PMS. Press on both feet simultaneously if that is comfortable, or one at a time. Press for about 1 minute.

4. (Sp 6, Three Yin Meeting) Located at the crossing of three *yin* meridians (Spleen, Liver, and Kidney), Sp 6 nourishes the *yin* of the entire body and is like a communication center connecting all the female organs.

5. (Gb 34, Yang Hill Spring) At the lower border of the kneecap, slide your finger off the shinbone toward the outside (little toe side). Two bones come together here. Press in the soft tissue area between them. Use firm pressure. The thumb works best, but if you can't get a good angle, use your index and middle fingers together. Remember to build up slowly, hold about a minute, and then gradually release. This point promotes the smooth flow of *ch'i* throughout the body. Obstruction to the flow of *ch'i* causes much of the pain and discomfort experienced with PMS.

For breast tenderness that is not responding with the above points, add Pc 6:

6. (Pc 6, Inner Gate) You will find this point on the palm side of your wrist, two thumb widths above the wrist crease and in the center of the arm. Pc 6 is very effective for any pain or discomfort of the chest, as it regulates both *ch'i* and blood in the chest. Tenderness in the breasts is caused primarily by blocked and stagnated *ch'i*, so it responds well to this point. Use moderate to firm pressure. Be sure to do both hands.

REFLEXOLOGY

Begin your Reflexology self-treatment for PMS at least a week before you expect your flow to begin. Spend 15 or 20 minutes, up to half an hour, every day if you can. These steps are also effective for relief of PMS symptoms. You don't need to do all of them if you don't have time.

1. Before you treat specific reflex areas, begin with the Reflexology Warm-Up on page 69. This is an important step that helps you relax, tones the energy of the whole body, and prepares your feet to be worked on.

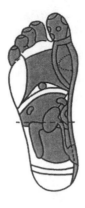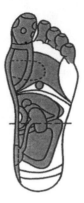

Fig. 163

2. To help you relax, dissolve stress, and relieve tenderness in your breasts, work the chest/lung/breast areas on both the bottom and top of your foot. First, thumb walk the chest and lung reflex zones on the ball of the foot (between the diaphragm line and the base of the toes). Then, on top of your foot, finger walk up from the webbing toward your ankle, pressing in the troughs between the toes. Start in zone 1 at the base of the big toe and go up about 2 inches. Continue working each zone, ending in zone 5 near the outside edge of your foot. Press with your index finger. This area may be quite tender, so don't press too hard. And take some deep breaths!

3. Press all around the base of your big toe (at the webbing, where it joins the foot). This will stimulate more balanced and healthy activity of the thyroid and parathyroid glands, governors of metabolism, energy level, and muscle tone. The thumb walk technique is best here, though some general rubbing and massaging will also be beneficial.

4. On the bottom of your foot, work the fleshy part of all the toes, especially the big toe. Use the thumb walk for maximum benefit. Work down each toe from the tip to the base, being especially thorough with the big toe. Try to do five separate trips down that toe with your thumb, covering each of the five zones. (See Fig. 8 on page 27.) Reflex zones for the hypothalamus, pineal gland, pituitary gland, and brain are all located in the toes. Use the "hook and back up" technique (see page 68) on the pituitary reflex in the center of the pad of the big toe.

5. Continuing with your toes, work on the brain reflex (located at the tip of each toe) by placing the tip of your index finger on the tip of the toe, and rolling your finger from side to side. You can also use your thumb-

nail to roll across the tops of the toes. The brain, as the ultimate control center for all mind/body activity, holds the key to physical and emotional balance.

6. Thoroughly work the large area on the bottom of your foot between the diaphragm and the heel. This area contains reflexes for the liver, stomach, small intestines, kidneys, adrenals, and other internal organs. Work this entire area to help detoxify the blood, regulate fluid retention, promote production of new blood, and stimulate digestion. Use the thumb walk, moving up, down, and diagonally.

7. Next, to enliven the nervous system and the flow of Life Energy throughout the body, work on the spine reflexes. These are located on the inside edge of both feet (zone 1), extending from the heel nearly to the top of the big toe. Work slowly up the foot using the thumb walk. You will need a little extra strength on the thick skin of the heel.

Then thumb walk all the way down, taking some time to walk across small areas horizontally. Remember that the upper spine is reflected near the toes, the lower spine from the middle of your foot down to the heel. To prevent or relieve lower back pain, work on the sacral area near the heel.

8. To promote more efficient digestion, absorption, and elimination, spend a little time pressing on the colon reflexes. Note in Fig. M (page 45) that the reflexes for various aspects of the colon (ascending and descending, sigmoid, transverse) are divided between the two feet, and be sure to work all the appropriate areas thoroughly.

9. Next let's focus on improving energy circulation to the female organs, starting with the uterus. To locate the uterus reflex, make an imaginary line between the high point of your ankle bone (on the inside—big toe side) of your foot, and the very back and bottom of your heel. The uterus reflex is at the midpoint of that line. (See Fig. 37 on page 74.)

This point is likely to be very sensitive. Feel around for a tender spot with your index finger, and when you've found it (it may be in a slight indentation), work it gently with a circular motion. You can use your index finger, middle finger, or thumb.

10. The reflex for the ovaries is located in the same position, but on the *outside* (little toe side) of your foot. Again, when you find the spot (midway between the high point of the ankle bone and the back of the heel) work it with a slight circular motion. If these spots hurt a lot, ease off for a few seconds, and then try again. Don't press too hard and hurt yourself.

11. The reflex for the fallopian tubes is located in a band around the top of your foot, where the foot joins the ankle. It doesn't run in a circle around the ankle, but at an angle. Just as the actual fallopian tubes connect the ovaries to the uterus, the fallopian tube reflex connects these two reflex points. This too tends to be tender, so work it gently. Try the finger walk using your index finger.

12. After this long workout, take a few minutes just to relax! Rub your feet gently and use the techniques starting on page 64. Finish with the thumb press on the solar plexus point for 15 to 30 seconds.

SHIATSU

1. Stand with your feet shoulder width apart, arms hanging loosely at your sides. With a deep, slow inhalation, slowly lift your arms over your head, then turn the palms to face the ceiling, with the fingertips pointing together. Look at the space between the tips of the fingers. On the exhalation, slowly lower the arms. Continue repeating this for 3 full minutes. If your balance is good, raise your heels off the ground as you lift your arms. Stretching the arms above you and standing on the toes helps open the channels and circulate the *ch'i.*

2. Next, stand in the horse posture for 2–3 minutes. See instructions on page 193. This is one of the best exercises to improve circulation and cultivate Kidney *ch'i.* In Chinese medicine, the Kidneys are considered the root of vitality.

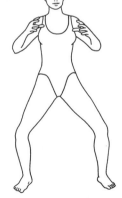

3. End by stimulating the Liver meridian. Sitting down now (after the previous two standing exercises), press on the top of your foot, beginning in the center of the top of the big toe. (See Figs. 141 and 142, pages 287 and 288.) Use the press and release technique—press for 6–7 seconds, release, move a little way along the channel, and press again.

Fig. 164—Horse Posture

Continuing with the press and release technique, move to the web margin between the big toe and second toe, and keep going up the channel between those toes. From the ankle the channel proceeds up the inside part of the leg along the bone. Use only mild to moderate pressure along the bone.

About halfway up the leg, the meridian comes off the bone and continues up the middle of the inside of the leg. Continue up the inside portion of your thigh, still pressing and releasing along the middle of the leg. Stop at the groin. On the thigh above the knee, you can use strong pressure. Don't forget to do both legs.

ADDITIONAL SUGGESTIONS

EXERCISE IS CRUCIAL. Be sure to get regular aerobic exercise (walking, jogging, swimming, whatever you enjoy) during the entire month, up until your period. Physical activity helps promote *ch'i* and blood circulation and can do a great deal to prevent physical symptoms and smooth out unwanted emotions. We recommend the Sun Salutation, a series of 12 Yoga postures that help to tone the entire body, inside and out. Other helpful Yoga poses include the Shoulder Stand, which also helps tone the entire body, and the Plow, Fish, and Forward Bend which massage and stretch the abdominal area. During your actual period, skip vigorous exercise and Yoga; rest and relax as much as your schedule and responsibilities permit.

BUST STRESS. Stress and anxiety definitely aggravate the situation. Stress may be unavoidable in life, but you need a program to help you deal with it. Exercise helps, but supplement it with Yoga, tai chi, ch'i gong, or meditation. Make the time even if you think you're too busy. Even 10-15 minutes a day of deep relaxation will make an enormous difference.

FINE TUNE YOUR DIET. What you eat is an important factor in whether you get PMS symptoms or not. Try to base your diet around whole grains and cooked vegetables. Avoid or at least minimize oily and fried foods, dairy products, wheat, and sweets. Watch out for chocolate cravings, and don't give in to them! Cut down on hot, spicy foods, alcohol, and stimulants such as caffeine.

These suggestions are not meant to torture you; there are good reasons behind them. For example, alcohol can exacerbate headaches and depression; caffeine contributes to breast tenderness, irritability, and anxiety. But if you are habituated to caffeine, stopping abruptly can cause headaches and irritability, so taper off slowly. Excess intake of refined sugar and salt can also aggravate symptoms.

Calcium is important to help muscles and nerves relax, so if cramps or backache are a problem for you, eat calcium-rich foods (but go for leafy green vegetables rather than dairy) or consider a supplement. Low levels of magnesium have been linked in some studies to more severe PMS symptoms. Magnesium also aids absorption of calcium. Many supplements contain the two minerals.

STOP SMOKING. Most medical practitioners, both Oriental and Western, would tell you that if you smoke, quitting is the best thing you can do for your health. Many helpful books and videos have been created with programs to help people kick the habit. Buy one, or borrow one from the library, follow the suggestions, and get free of this self-destructive habit! It is difficult, but it is possible, and well worth the effort.

TRY HERBS. If you can, have a consultation with an Acupuncturist who is also certified in Chinese herbology. Or purchase a pre-made herbal formula. One that is commonly prescribed for PMS is known as Xiao yao wan, a well-known formula which can also be used for stress. It eases Liver *ch'i* stagnation as well as nourishing the Liver function. For PMS it is typically taken during the last half of the menstrual cycle. Xiao yao wan—which, along with many other herbs, contains dang kuei, frequently prescribed for women's health—is available at some natural food stores. Chamomile tea is also soothing and helpful.

CONSIDER PROGESTERONE. Natural progesterone creams have become very popular to relieve the symptoms of both PMS and menopause. They are an alternative to the synthetic forms of progesterone (progestin) which are sometimes prescribed in Western medicine. Some of the symptoms of PMS are considered to result from a temporary estrogen/progesterone imbalance. Although many women have obtained good results with these products, be sure to get advice and evaluation from a qualified health practitioner before using them.

Prostate Problems

The prostate is a walnut-sized gland located below a man's bladder, midway between the scrotum and anus. It manufactures and secretes the milky fluid that accompanies the sperm, insulating and protecting it on its journey to the cervix. In ways yet to be understood, it also communicates to the cervix, coaxing it to relax and open to admit the sperm.

The prostate surrounds the urethra, the tube that carries urine from the bladder to the penis. Enlargement, the most common prostate problem (known technically as benign prostatic hyperplasia or BPH) affects approximately half of all men. The enlarged gland chokes the urethra, restricting the flow of urine, so that a man may wake several times during the night to urinate, or the flow of urine may be slow, difficult to start, or may "dribble" at the end. He may feel the need to urinate suddenly, or unusually often.

These, along with a burning sensation while urinating, are also symptoms common to prostatitis, an inflammation of the prostate.

A further problem, which we will not deal with here, is prostate cancer, which affects 1 out of every 8 men. Needless to say, with such a high percentage of men falling prey to this condition, it is wise for all men over 50 to have their prostate regularly checked, both by a digital/rectal exam, and the PSA (prostate-specific antigen) test.

ACUPRESSURE

The first two points (Sp 6 and St 36) are fully described in "Ten Master Pressure Points" (beginning on page 49) where you will also find illustrations of the exact point locations and suggestions on how to press them for maximum benefit.

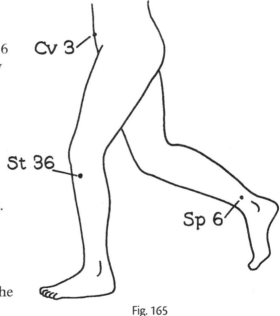

Fig. 165

1. (Sp 6, Three Yin Meeting) One of the most important Acupressure points, Sp 6 can nourish the *yin* energy of the body by simultaneously nourishing the *yin* of the Spleen, Liver, and Kidney meridians. In combination with St 36, it rejuvenates both *ch'i* and blood and brings vitality.

2. (St 36, Three Mile Foot) This is the most effective point to nourish the *ch'i* and blood of the body. In combination with Sp 6 it strongly revitalizes the entire body.

3. (Cv 3, Central Pole) First locate Cv 4, which is 4 finger widths directly below the navel (belly button). Cv 3 is one thumb width below Cv 4. Its influence is specific to bladder dysfunction. Use moderate pressure with your thumb or middle finger for about a minute. You can add a small circular motion along with steady pressure. Empty your bladder (if you need to) before pressing on abdominal points.

4. (B 28, Associated point of Urinary Bladder) B 28 is located approximately 1 and ½ inches on either side of the spine, in the mid-sacral area of the back. The best way to stimulate the B 28 points is to lie on your back on the floor, with a tennis ball beneath you. Slowly roll up and down on the ball, first on one side then on the other. Or, put two balls in a sock and line them up so they are on both sides of the spine, and slide up and down. You'll stimulate a number of valuable points adjacent to the spine with this technique. Spend several minutes working these points.

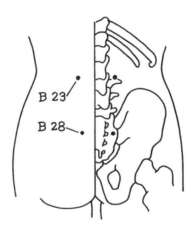

Fig. 166

For prostatitis, add Lv 3:

5. (Lv 3, Bigger Rushing) For an illustration of the exact location of this important point, and instructions on how to press it most effectively, please see page 49 for the beginning of "Ten Master Pressure Points."

The Liver meridian circles the reproductive organs and will stimulate the flow of *ch'i* or Life Energy in and around the prostate to help restore healthy functioning.

REFLEXOLOGY

Laura Norman, author of *Feet First* and one of the nation's leading Reflexologists, says that "Prostate problems in men seem to have been ready made for Reflexology! Most reflexologists will attest to a high success rate with this ailment." So give the following sequence a try several times a week for a week or two, and see if you don't start experiencing results.

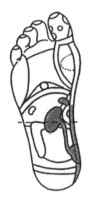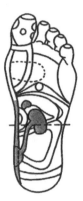

Fig. 167

1. Before you treat specific reflex areas for your prostate problems, begin with the Reflexology Warm-Up on page 69. This is an important step that relaxes you and prepares your feet to be worked on; please don't skip it!

2. To energize the lower back, bladder, and reproductive system, start by stimulating the lower spine reflexes, on the inside edge of both feet (zone 1). We are concerned primarily with the lumbar and sacral areas, between the heel and the midline of the foot. When you work the spinal reflexes, work slowly up the foot to around the midline, using the thumb walk technique, then start in the middle and walk down toward the heel. If you have time, you can also walk across small areas horizontally.

Oriental medicine (and Reflexology) tend to see problems not as isolated symptoms, but as part of an interconnected, larger whole. The prostate is clearly connected to both the urinary and reproductive systems. So the next several steps will involve working these two systems to bring improved circulation and healing.

3. First, press on the reflex areas for the kidneys and adrenals. These areas are in the center of the foot, above and below the waistline and on the inside of the large tendon running up the foot. Use the thumb walk.

4. Next, massage the bladder and ureters. Their reflex zone is on the bottom of the foot, mostly in zone 1 (beneath the big toe). Arch your foot slightly backwards to extend the tendon while working on the ureters. Use the thumb walk to work up from the bladder, then cross the big tendon and work up or across the kidney reflex.

5. The specific reflex for the prostate is often very tender, especially if symptoms are present. To locate it, make an imaginary line between the high point of your ankle bone on the inside (big toe side) of your foot, and the very back and bottom of your heel. The prostate reflex is at the mid-point of that line. (See Fig. 37 on page 74.)

Feel around for a tender spot with your index finger, and when you've found it (it may be in a slight indentation), work it gently with a circular motion. You can use your index finger, middle finger, or thumb. Again, these spots may be very tender. Back off if it starts to hurt a lot; wait a bit, and try again. Or come back to it tomorrow.

6. On both the inside and outside of each foot, along the Achilles tendon, is a long narrow zone that can help with chronic problems related to the prostate. Hold your foot at the toes with the opposite hand (right foot with left hand), tilt the foot away from you a little, and work the area using the thumb walk or, if it is very tender, use the finger walk, which exerts less pressure. Start about six inches above the ankle bone on the inside (big toe side) and work down to the heel. Then work either up or down the corresponding area on the outside of your foot.

7. End by taking a few minutes to relax. Stress has been correlated with prostate problems, so this is not a meaningless step! Rub your feet and use the relaxation techniques described on page 64.

SHIATSU

Prostate problems are usually associated with the Kidney and Liver meridians. The following Shiatsu routine will give some stimulation and enlivenment to both.

1. Begin with the Liver meridian, which starts in the center of the top of your big toe. Use the press and release technique: Press for 6–7 seconds, release, move a little way along the meridian, and press again.

Starting at the top of the big toe, move along the toe to the web margin between the big and second toe, then continue up the groove between those toes. From the ankle, the meridian proceeds up the inside part of the leg, along the bone. Use only mild to moderate pressure along the bone. About halfway up the leg the meridian comes off the bone and continues up the middle of the inside of the leg. Above the knee, the pathway travels slightly higher than the middle of the inside portion of your thigh. Stop at the groin. On the thigh above the knee, use strong pressure.

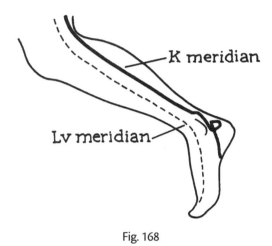

Fig. 168

2. To stimulate the Kidney energy, use the press and release technique in exactly the same way, along the Kidney meridian. Start in the center of the sole of your foot (see Fig. 161) and slowly work up to the knee.

3. We also recommend the exercise known as the horse posture, one of the best exercises to cultivate Kidney *ch'i*. This posture is widely used in almost all martial art forms. When done properly it builds stamina, cultures *ch'i*, and promotes circulation. Please see Fig. 100 and the instructions on page 193.

ADDITIONAL SUGGESTIONS

HERBAL HELPERS. The herb saw palmetto (*serenoa repens*) has been used effectively for helping to shrink an enlarged prostate. Get a standardized extract from your health food store. Sometimes it comes combined with the herb *Pygeum africanum*; the combination has been found helpful. You can also drink a tea made of ginseng, hibiscus, or horsetail several times a day.

GET MOVING.   As in virtually any health condition, exercise is helpful. Research verifies that men who are physically fit have less prostate trouble than those who are not. We recommend a baseline of half an hour of vigorous walking a day, for everyone; if you are fit for it, some more energetic aerobic exercise (swimming, jogging, bicycling, etc.) is fine, though you should consult your doctor before beginning any exercise program, especially if you are over 40 —which you are likely to be if you have prostate symptoms!

GO WHEN YOU HAVE TO.   Don't retain urine unnecessarily. Holding back can strain the prostate.

GET OFF YOUR BOTTOM.   Sitting puts pressure on the prostate. If you sit a lot—and that means driving as well as sitting at a desk—get up and walk around regularly.

CUT THE FAT.   A diet high in fat has been correlated with increased risk of prostate cancer (as well as heart disease and other types of cancer). So restrict your fat intake. As we've noted, leading-edge researchers such as Dean Ornish say that if you keep your daily calories from fat to about 10% of your daily intake, you would virtually eliminate all danger of heart disease and cancer! A vegetarian or almost-vegetarian diet, with plenty of fresh fruit and vegetables and lots of whole grains such as rice, oats, and whole wheat and only a little bit of chicken, fish, or turkey, is an ideal low-fat, high-fiber diet.

VITAMINS A, C, AND E ARE HELPFUL.   Try a supplement if your diet isn't rich in fresh fruit and vegetables.

Sexual Problems

See also, "Stress," "Anxiety"

It seems amazing, in a culture that expends so much time, attention, and financial resources on sex, that so many people continue to have so many sex-related problems. Despite vastly increased openness about sex, and the availability of far more information than ever before, including books, videos, and classes on improving intimacy and communication, Tantric sex, sexual positions, Mars and Venus, achieving orgasm, etc., sexual dissatisfaction still remains one of the primary causes of discord and disharmony in intimate relationships.

Some sexual problems are organic and biological, including many instances of low sex drive, certain cases of impotence, and most instances of infertility—an increasingly common problem, and perhaps the most distressing of all sexual difficulties. Stress is another major culprit in sexual dysfunction. Tension and anxiety about one's personal appearance or performance, fear of sexually transmitted diseases, and stored up, relationship-related resentments block free and open expression and response.

This short section is far from a complete guide to solving your sexual difficulties! But with the help of pressure point therapies and some lifestyle recommendations, you can definitely overcome many sex-related issues and begin to enjoy a richer and more fulfilling sex life.

This section is really four sections in one. We will look at four troublesome sexual problems:

- Low libido
- Infertility
- Impotence
- Vaginal dryness

First, we offer specific Acupressure points for each of the four. Then we add Reflexology and Shiatsu techniques that will be helpful for all sexual concerns, and some additional suggestions. This information can be extended to help you understand and deal with other sexual difficulties.

LOW LIBIDO

Sexual energy relies on the underlying *ch'i* of the body to be healthy and active. Low libido is frequently a sign of fatigue or debility, of simply being exhausted and run down. The following points, while not magical aphrodisiacs, can help restore your vital energy, which in turn can help recharge your sexual batteries and renew your sex drive.

The first three points (Sp 6, St 36, and Kd 3) are described in the section, "Ten Master Pressure Points." Please turn to page 49 for illustrations of the precise point locations, and suggestions on how to press for maximum benefit.

1. (Sp 6, Three Yin Meeting) This is an excellent point to nourish the *yin* energy of the body. We recommend it here for its revitalizing properties.

2. (St 36, Three Mile Foot) In combination with Sp 6, this point, excellent for energizing the *ch'i* and blood, strongly rejuvenates the entire body.

3. (Kd 3, Supreme Stream) In Chinese medicine, the kidneys are intimately involved with reproduction and sexual function. Kd 3, considered the "source point" for the Kidney meridian, exerts a powerful, nourishing effect on the meridian and all that it influences.

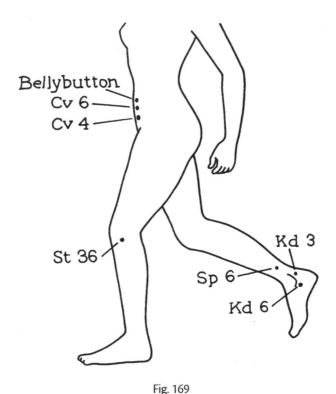

Fig. 169

4. (Cv 6, Sea of *Ch'i*) This point is about one and a half finger widths directly below the navel. Place the middle finger of both hands there, and press inward with the fingertips of both hands to a depth of about an inch. Use moderate pressure, and hold for a minute or two, breathing deeply.

As the name implies, this point has a powerful tonic effect on the body's *ch'i* and helps circulate it throughout the system. **Caution:** Pregnant women should not use pressure on this or any other abdominal points.

5. Ear Point. Please see the Ear illustration (Fig. I) on page 41. This point helps enliven libido.

INFERTILITY

Many factors, far too complex for this book, may be involved in infertility. It is due to the man about 35 percent of the time (low sperm count; poor motility); to the woman another 35 percent (failure to ovulate; endometriosis; infections); the remaining 30 percent is due to a combination of the two or to unknown causes.

Among the many other factors identified as possible causes of infertility are hormonal imbalances, smoking, habitual alcohol or marijuana use, anti-hypertensive drugs such as beta blockers, antibiotics, steroids, antidepressants, and tranquilizers such as diazepam (Valium). A previous history of venereal diseases such as gonorrhea and syphilis, and repeated genital herpes infections, may also lead to infertility.

To diagnose the cause of infertility and decide on a course of action to treat it, expert medical advice is needed. However, relieving stress is an important component of any strategy, as high levels of stress may not only cause or contribute to the problem, but may also result from repeated failure to conceive. So please see the "Stress" section for suggestions.

From the perspective of Chinese medicine, reproduction is governed by the Kidney energy. Therefore points to boost Kidney *ch'i* will be helpful.

For illustrations of the exact location of the first three points offered here (Sp 6, Kd 3, and B 23), as well as instructions on how to press them most effectively, please see page 49 for the beginning of "Ten Master Pressure Points."

1. (Sp 6, Three Yin Meeting) One of the 12 most important Acupuncture points on the body, Sp 6 is the meeting point of the three *yin* meridians of the leg (Spleen, Liver, and Kidney). It nourishes both *ch'i* and blood and brings vitality to the *yin* of the entire body. Sp 6 is used for all types of gynecological disorders. **Caution:** Pregnant women should not press this point.

2. (Kd 3, Supreme Stream) As mentioned before, in Chinese medicine the Kidneys are considered crucial to reproduction and the health of the reproductive system. As the "source point" for the Kidney meridian, this point exerts a powerful rejuvenating influence on the entire Kidney channel.

3. (B 23, Back-associated Kidney point) A number of points valuable for treating infertility and other sexual problems are located on the lower back (along the spine) and along the sacrum. The best way you can stimulate these points is to put a couple of tennis balls in a sock, and slowly roll up and down on them. (A couple of tightly rolled socks will also do the job.) This point, in combination with Kd 3 strongly invigorates the Kidney *ch'i*.

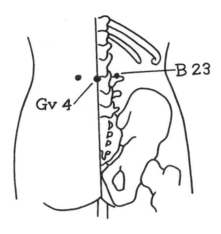

Fig. 170

4. (Gv 4, Vitality Gate) This point is located on the spine, below the second lumbar vertebra, at the same level on the back as B 23.   Be sure to press it as you roll on your tennis balls! This point is a strong tonic for the kidneys and energizes the source *ch'i.*

5. (Cv 4, Gate of Original *Ch'i*) Located 4 finger widths directly below the navel (See Fig. 169), Cv 4 is looked upon as one of the major points on the body. As its name implies, Cv 4 stimulates your original or constitutional *ch'i.* (The combination of Sp 6 and St 36 mentioned in "Low Libido," stimulates the *ch'i* your body produces from the food you eat and the air you breath.)

Cv 4 is often used to help promote strength in individuals with weak constitutions or who are run down from chronic illness. It is helpful for chronic, deep-seated fatigue, rather than ordinary day-to-day tiredness.

This point is the *dan tien* that various forms of martial arts, such as *tai chi* and *ch'i gong*, cultivate for power, centeredness and well-being. **Reminder:** Pregnant women should not use pressure on this or any other abdominal points

IMPOTENCE

For many years, the common understanding about impotence —failure to achieve or sustain an erection—was that it was primarily a psychological problem, caused by anxiety, fear of failure, hidden resentments, or other mental or emotional states. While these issues are certainly involved in many instances, in recent years both research and clinical experience have clearly shown that many, if not most cases of impotence are due to medical, biological reasons.

Foremost among these causes is vascular disease: clogged arteries, caused by a high-fat diet, which restrict blood flow. Erections are caused by the filling-up of the penis with blood. When the blood vessels are narrowed by accumulated fat, erections become difficult or impossible. Also, alcohol and various "recreational" drugs such as marijuana, cocaine, or heroin may cause impotence, as well as literally *hundreds* of prescription medications which warn that impotence or reduced sex drive may be a side effect.

However, when there is not a specific, known biological condition, Chinese medicine would likely classify it as a Kidney deficiency. The best Acupressure points to boost the Kidney energy are precisely the ones recommended in the section on Infertility: Sp 6, Cv 4, Gv 4, B 23, and Kd 3. Please refer to that section and use the information.

VAGINAL DRYNESS

This problem, which typically appears in the menopausal years when estrogen levels decrease, may cause a woman discomfort or pain during intercourse. It is usually classified as a *yin* deficiency condition by Oriental medicine. The following points to help remedy this condition are famous for nourishing *yin*.

1. (Lu 7, Broken Sequence) Hold one hand out in front of you with the palm facing down. Start from the 'V' shape formed by your thumb and index finger, and use the index finger of the other hand to trace along the top of the thumb to the wrist. Your finger will fall into a natural depression where the base of your thumb joins the wrist. Keep going another inch and a half and you will be on Lu 7. Maintain firm pressure (you can use your thumb or index finger) for about a minute, then switch hands. Lu 7, in combination with Kd 6 rejuvenates the body's *yin* energy and opens the Conception Vessel meridian. By nourishing *yin*, the bodily fluids are also nourished.

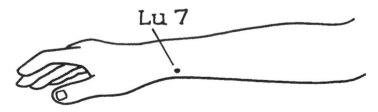

Fig. 171

2. (Kd 6, Shining Sea) Find the ankle bone on the inside of the foot (the big toe side). Kd6 is straight down (toward the sole of the foot) one thumb width. This is the primary point on the Kidney channel to energize Kidney *yin*. It has a moistening, nourishing, and cooling influence. (See Fig. 169.)

3. (Sp 6, Three Yin Meeting) As mentioned before, this is one of the most powerful Acupressure points for nourishing *yin* and revitalizing the system. The meeting point of three *yin* meridians, it nourishes *ch'i* and blood and brings vitality to the *yin* of the entire body. See page 49 ("Ten Master Pressure Points") for an illustration of the exact location of Sp 6, and instructions on how to press it most effectively. **Caution:** Pregnant women should not press on this point.

REFLEXOLOGY

The following Reflexology sequence will help to dissolve some of the stress that invariably accompanies—and often precipitates—sexual problems. Even infertility may be stress-related, as the biochemistry of the body can be severely disrupted by a continuously stressful life. These techniques promote deep relaxation. In addition, they release blocks in the flow of energy to the reproductive regions of the body.

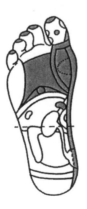 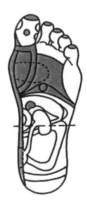

Fig. 172

1. Before you treat any specific reflex areas, please begin with the Reflexology Warm-Up on page 69. This is an important step that helps you relax, tones the energy of the whole body, and prepares your feet to be worked on.

2. Use your thumb to walk across the narrow diaphragm line on the sole of your foot. To go deeper into this reflex, try holding your toes with one hand and rotating or flexing your foot into your thumb.

3. To open up the chest area for deeper breathing and increased relaxation, thumb walk the chest and lung reflex zones on the ball of the foot (between the diaphragm line and the base of the toes). You can also finger walk the chest and lymph gland reflexes on the top of the foot between the toes. And take some deep breaths!

4. Next we will focus on the endocrine glands, to help balance and energize hormone activity in the body. First, stimulate the reflex zone for the thyroid (around the base of the big toe) by rubbing and pressing. The finger or thumb walk technique is best here.

5. The pituitary gland in the center of the pad of the big toe, known as the "master gland," regulates the secretion of hormones. Massage with your thumb or use the "hook and back up" technique (see page 68) for greater accuracy.

6. You'll find the reflex area for the adrenal glands (which produce sex hormones) above the kidneys, on the inside of the large tendon running up the foot. Use the thumb walk and, for best results, the "rotation on a point" technique. (See page 68.)

7. To enliven the reflex for the brain, place the tip of your index finger on the tip of the toe, and roll your finger back and forth to press on the toe. You can also use your thumbnail to roll across the tops of the toes.

8. Working the spine reflex, especially in the lumbar and sacral regions will send life energy (*ch'i* or *prana*) to the sexual organs and reproductive system. The spine reflex is located on the inside edge of both feet (zone 1), extending from the heel nearly to the top of the big toe.

Spend a little time on the entire spine, working slowly up and then down the foot using the thumb walk technique. Then focus on the lower spine area from about the middle of your foot down to the heel. Many experts in sexual problems say that a relaxed lower back and pelvic area is essential to healthy sexual functioning; working this area will help.

9. Next we will focus on increasing circulation and the flow of energy to the sexual/reproductive area. To locate the reflex for the uterus (the same spot in men is the prostate reflex) make an imaginary line between the high point of your ankle bone on the inside (big toe side) of your foot, and the very back and bottom of your heel. (See Fig. 37, on page 74.) The uterus reflex is at the midpoint of that line.

This point is likely to be very sensitive. Feel around for a tender spot with your index finger, and when you've found it (it may be in a slight indentation), work it gently with a circular motion. You can use your index finger, middle finger, or thumb.

10. The ovary and testes reflexes are located in the same position as the uterus reflex, but on the *outside* (little toe side) of your foot. Again, when you find the spot (midway between the high point of the ankle bone and the back of the heel) work it with a slight circular motion. (See page 46.)

11. The reflex for the fallopian tubes (on women) and seminal vesicles (on men) is located in a band around the top of your foot, where the foot joins the ankle. It doesn't run in a circle around the ankle, but at an angle. This too tends to be sensitive, so work it gently.

12. To find the reflex for the penis and vagina, first locate the uterus/prostate point on the inside (big toe side) of your ankle. This zone runs at about a 45 degree angle between that point and the bladder reflex.

13. Conclude your session with a few minutes of relaxation techniques (see Step 1) and just give your feet a gentle rubbing.

SHIATSU

1. In Chinese medicine, as we've been discussing, potency and sexual activity are governed by the Kidneys, which are also considered the root of vitality. One of the best exercises to cultivate Kidney *ch'i* is the horse posture. When done properly it builds stamina, cultures *ch'i*, promotes circulation, and increases sexual vitality. Please see the description and illustration of the horse pose on page 193.

2. To further enliven the Kidney energy, press along the Kidney meridian, starting on the sole of your foot, just below the ball of the foot, in the soft fleshy area. Use a circular rubbing motion with your thumb, using mild to moderate pressure. (See Fig. 161, page 320.)

Then work in a line down the center of the sole of the foot to just in front of the heel. Continue using the same circular rubbing motion, rubbing at one spot and gradually moving up the foot. Shift over to the area directly below your ankle bone on the big toe side of the foot, and switch to a press and release technique—press firmly for 6-7 seconds and release, then move a little further along the channel pathway and repeat the press and release. From here work out toward the Achilles tendon, paying special attention to any sore spots (work on them a little more).

Finally, move slowly up the leg in the space between the ankle bone and the Achilles tendon. Move in a straight line. You can stop once you get near the vicinity of the knee. Do both legs. (See Fig. 168, page 333.)

ADDITIONAL SUGGESTIONS

For all conditions:

- A nourishing diet, strong digestion, a lifestyle free from excessive stress, and sufficient exercise to energize the body but not tire yourself out, are all central to sexual and reproductive health. Please see the 11 Simple, Universal Guidelines for Good Health on page 77.
- Helpful Yoga postures include the Shoulder Stand, Plow, Bow, and Fish.
- Consider counseling. Fertility problems definitely require professional medical guidance, to diagnose the problem and choose a course of action. In addition, since satisfying sex is so bound up with harmony in relationship, if you have ongoing sexual problems such as impotence, premature ejaculation, or failure to enjoy sex or experience orgasm, we urge you to seek some professional help, not just about sex alone, but about your relationship. Counseling can often uncover an underlying problem and help you resolve it.

For impotence:

- The herb ginkgo biloba improves blood circulation. If the impotence is related to circulation insufficiency, ginkgo may be helpful.
- A low-fat, low-cholesterol diet will help keep arteries from becoming lined with the fatty plaque that blocks blood flow. Follow the same diet you would follow to prevent heart disease: plenty of fresh fruits and vegetables and whole grains, and a minimum of meat, dairy (other than non-fat or low-fat milk products), and fatty fried foods.

For low libido:

- Various foods are considered strengthening to sexual vitality. These include beans (especially kidney, black, and azuki); almonds (try blending 10 blanched almonds in a cup of warm milk with a teaspoon of sugar); dates; apples (better cooked); and figs. Avoid an excess of white sugar. Garlic and onions added to the diet will also be helpful.

For infertility:

- Astralagus (huang ch'i) has been shown to increase sperm motility.
- Vitamin C and other anti-oxidants such as Vitamin E and beta-carotene may be helpful, especially for male infertility. These are said to increase sperm count and motility.
- A low-fat diet may be important, as fat deposits in arterial linings may prevent sufficient oxygen and nutrients from reaching the testicles (resulting in low sperm count) and the ovaries (preventing full maturation of the ova).

For vaginal dryness:

- The most famous *yin* tonic in Chinese medicine is *Liu wei di huang wan.* It is available at some natural food stores and in Chinatown pharmacies in major cities.
- Estrogen replacement therapy will almost certainly help, but it also has potentially serious drawbacks. This is a decision to make with medical advice. You might consider natural estrogen precursors, such as the herbs shatavari (a widely used Ayurvedic herb available in natural food stores) and wild yam (diascorea).

Shoulder Pain

See "Pain"

Shoulder Tension

See "Neck and Shoulder Tension"

Sinus Problems

See also "Colds" and "Allergies"

Our sinuses are small air-filled spaces in the bone structure of our face, on either side of the nose. They are lined with a fine layer of mucus, to keep the nasal cavity moist and to filter the air we breathe to remove dust, smoke, pollen, and other pollutants before they reach the lungs.

Due to such factors as allergens, environmental irritants, bacterial infections, and colds, the sinuses may become clogged, swollen, or infected, resulting in pain, pressure, headaches, and/or a runny nose. Another type of sinus problem occurs when the cavity becomes dry and crusty, whether from hot, dry air, or from an infection.

From the standpoint of Oriental medicine, the smooth flow of *ch'i* through the nasal area becomes impeded by these various causes; finger pressure can be used to restore the flow, which helps heal the painful, inflamed sinuses.

ACUPRESSURE

1. (Li 4, Adjoining Valley) For an illustration of the exact location of this important point and instructions on how to press it most effectively, see page 49 for the beginning of "Ten Master Pressure Points." In addition to its great ability to relieve pain, Li 4 is known as the command point for the face.

2. (Lu 7, Broken Sequence) This point on the Lung meridian helps relieve nasal obstructions. Hold one hand in front of you with the palm facing down. Start from the V shape formed by your thumb and index finger. Use the index finger of the other hand to trace along the top of the thumb to the wrist. Your finger will fall into a natural depression where the base of your thumb joins the wrist. Keep going another inch and a half and you will be on Lu 7. (See Fig. 171, page 339.) Maintain firm pressure (you can use your thumb or index finger) for about a minute, then switch hands.

3. (Li 20, Welcome Fragrance) This is a very beneficial point for any nasal symptoms, including sinusitis, stuffy nose, and sinus headaches. Place your index or middle fingers in the grooves right next to each nostril and press, directing the pressure upward. Use moderate pressure. Build up gradually, hold about a minute, and release.

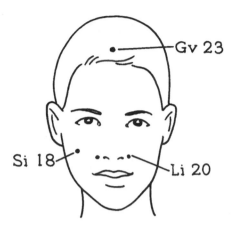

Fig. 173

4. (Si 18, Cheek Bone Crevice) This is another good point for sinus and allergy-type symptoms. Drop straight down from the outside edge of the eye socket, until you are on the lower border of the cheek bone. There is a natural depression there. Use medium pressure and hold for about a minute before releasing. Use your middle finger or thumb.

5. (Gv 23, Upper Star) Located one thumb width inside the hairline of the forehead directly above the nose, this point is specific for nose disorders.

   If you have a lot of congestion, add St 36.

6. (St 36, Three Mile Foot) Please see page 49 for the beginning of "Ten Master Pressure Points," for a description and illustration of this point and how to press it most effectively. St 36 helps relieve congestion by nourishing the Spleen energy, a key factor in digestion. When Spleen energy is weak, the digestive system suffers, producing an excessive "damp" condition in the body, which aggravates the sinus congestion.

REFLEXOLOGY

Reflexology can be very helpful in clearing clogged and even infected sinuses. However, it may take several sessions before you have significant relief, so be patient.

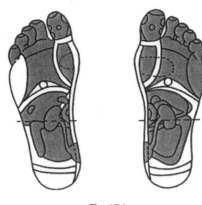

Fig. 174

1. Before you start to press specific reflex areas for your sinus condition, be sure to begin with the Reflexology Warm-Up on page 69. This will not only relax your feet, but will also enliven all the reflex zones.

2. To facilitate deep and unobstructed breathing, start by working on the two main chest/breast/lung reflex areas. First, thumb walk the chest and lung reflex zones on the ball of the foot, between the diaphragm line and the base of the toes. Then, press the *top* of your foot; work up from the webbing toward your ankle, pressing in the troughs between the toes. Work this area with your index finger, using the finger walk. And take some deep breaths!

3. Next, work on improving the circulation of blood and energy to your head by relaxing the neck area. To do this, thumb walk the ridge at the top of the ball of the foot (at the base of the toes). Pull the pad of the foot down and away from the ridge with your supporting hand. Walk in both directions. This area also influences the eyes and ears, which may be affected by your sinus problems.

4. Your toes present a gold mine of opportunities to influence the sinuses. Specific sinus reflexes are located on the 4 smaller toes; reflexes for the sides of the neck, for key glands (pineal, pituitary), and for the upper spine, are on your big toes.

On the bottom of your foot, work the fleshy part of all the toes, especially the middle third of each of the smaller toes, to help open the sinus cavities and nasal passages. Use the thumb walk for maximum benefit. Work down the toe from the tip to the base, and be especially thorough with the big toe. If you can, make five separate trips down that toe with your thumb, covering each of the five zones. (See Fig. 8 on page 27.) Use the "hook and back up" technique on the center of the pad of each big toe to stimulate the pituitary gland.

5. Healing also involves elimination of toxins. To strengthen and balance the immune system, purify the blood, and reduce inflammation, work on the reflexes for the liver, small intestines, kidneys, adrenals, and other internal organs. These are in the arch of your foot, from the mid or waistline up to the diaphragm line. Use the thumb walk to thoroughly cover this area, moving up, down, and diagonally.

6. Finally, to promote efficient elimination so any infection can be quickly thrown out of the body, work on the various colon reflexes, which are divided between the two feet in the soft area between the heel and the midline of the foot. Study Fig. M on page 45 and be sure you work these areas thoroughly, using the thumb walk.

SHIATSU

The following sequence of Shiatsu points around the nose, eyes, and forehead can help relieve sinus headaches, pressure, and congestion.

1. First, use your index fingers to firmly press the 3 points along both sides of your nose. Press simultaneously on both sides, 3–5 seconds at each point. Then repeat twice.

2. Press the 3 forehead points in the same way.

3. Press each point around the eyesockets, using your thumbs for the upper points and your middle finger for the lower points. Do NOT press hard around the eyes. You will find several natural depressions that help locate the points for you! Press both sides simultaneously for 3–5 seconds, release, and repeat twice.

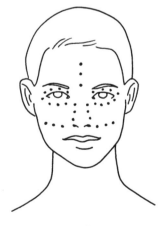

Fig. 175

4. Press the points along the bottom edge of the cheekbones. Press with 3-finger pressure on both sides. Again, press for 3–5 seconds, release, and repeat twice.

5. Use 3 fingers to press on the temples, in a straight line from the corner of the eye toward the ear. Use medium pressure at most, pressing and releasing.

ADDITIONAL SUGGESTIONS

HERBAL FORMULAS. *Bi Yan Pian* and *Pe Min Kan Wan* are effective Chinese herbal formulas for sinus conditions. Some natural food stores and many Chinatown pharmacies carry them.

NASAL WASH. One of the best ways to help clear up sinus congestion is to make a mild saline solution (about ¼ teaspoon salt added to ¼ cup pure, warm water) and snuff it. Pour a little in a small cup (an eye cup or shot glass works well) or in the palm of your hand, and sniff it up into your nostrils, one nostril at a time. You may tilt your head back and let the salt water slip down into your throat; then spit it out. If this is uncomfortable, just sniff it in, then gently blow your nose. Or, you can use an eye dropper and instill 5 or 6 drops into each nostril. You can repeat this several times a day.

STEAM IT. Another amazingly simple, effective way to help clear up painful, congested sinuses is to humidify them several times a day. Boil up a small pan of water with a few drops of eucalyptus oil or a little powdered ginger in it. Turn off the heat, cover your head with a towel, lean over the pot, and inhale the steam. Just standing a while in a hot shower is also effective.

YOGA. Helpful postures include the Fish, Plow, and Bow.

PREVENTION. To avoid future sinus problems, follow these four simple guidelines:

- Minimize dairy products in your diet, especially yogurt, ice cream, and cheese.
- Avoid iced drinks.
- Minimize exposure to cold and/or very dry weather.
- Stop smoking.

Skin Problems

See also, "Acne," "Beauty Secrets"

The skin is your body's largest organ. It serves as the immune system's first line of defense against external "invaders" such as bacteria, and, through its thousands of tiny sweat glands (about 600 per square inch), helps the body purify itself. If the kidneys are not adequately eliminating toxins through the urinary system, or if we are constipated, the excess toxins may find their way to the skin.

Problem skin—whether acne, dermatitis (including eczema and psoriasis), oily skin, dry skin, skin rashes—has a multitude of causes. Poor diet, weak digestion, poor functioning of internal organs, insufficient exercise, hormonal imbalance, all can contribute. Even something as simple as not drinking enough water can lead to skin problems. Stress is also a major factor. For example, the emotional pressures of adolescence, combined with major hormonal changes, frequently break out on the skin as acne.

To prevent or fully heal skin disorders, a multi-faceted approach works best, involving diet, exercise, and stress management as well as herbs or other medications. But a great deal can be accomplished using finger pressure therapy, especially for disorders caused or aggravated by stress.

In the following sections, we will consider treatment strategies for several conditions. For treatment of acne, please see "Acne."

CONTACT DERMATITIS

This condition is considered a delayed hypersensitivity to irritants such as soaps, detergents, or pollen, but it may be due to any number of causes. For instance, many common prescription drugs cause itching as a side effect. The symptoms—itching, redness, swelling—are caused by the immune system's inflammatory response. The standard Western treatment, corticosteroids, are effective in relieving symptoms, but also have well-documented negative side effects.

Chinese medicine considers inflammatory responses as excess "wind" and "heat." Balancing these excesses helps eliminate the underlying cause of the hypersensitivity itself, and thus treats the root of the problem. Although it helps with symptom relief, Oriental medicine is usually not as fast as Western medications, but produces fewer side effects and more long-lasting results.

Acupressure

1. (Tw 5, Outer Gate) Hold your left arm in front of you with the palm down. Measure two thumb widths above the wrist. The point is right in the center, between the two forearm bones. It aids in expelling wind and heat. Use your thumb to apply moderate to firm pressure for about a minute.

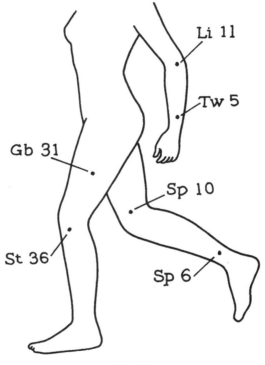

Fig. 176

2. (Li 11, Pool at the Crook) This point also clears wind and heat and is widely used for many skin conditions. Please see page 49 for the beginning of "Ten Master Pressure Points," for a description and illustration of Li 11 and how to press it most effectively.

3. (Gb 31, Wind Market) Locate this point standing up, but you can stimulate it either standing or sitting. It's on the outside side of your

thigh, at the point where your fingers touch the thigh when you let your arms hang loose at your sides. This is a point where the knuckles work well. Use firm pressure. Pressing this point helps expel excess wind and relieves itching.

4. (Sp 10, Sea of Blood) About 2 thumb widths above the top edge of the knee you will feel a bulge in your thigh muscles. It's on the top of your leg, toward the inside. Press firmly for a minute with your thumb or the knuckle of your middle finger. Sp 10 helps dispel excess heat from the blood which can contribute to skin disorders. It also helps promote better circulation.

ECZEMA

Eczema is a form of dermatitis that produces crusted, dry lesions along with the itching and redness of ordinary rashes and contact dermatitis. Individuals with this condition often have dry skin, which can aggravate the itching. In Chinese medicine, the person with eczema is usually treated as having an excess of wind and damp heat, along with Blood deficiency.

Acupressure

1. (Li 11, Pool at the Crook) See step 2 on page 351.
2. (Sp 10, Sea of Blood) See step 4 above.
3. (B 40, Supporting Middle) This point is located at the back of the knee, in the crease that forms when you bend the knee and right in the center between the two tendons. B 40 is better known for relieving back pain, but we recommend it here for its healing effect on skin conditions caused by heat in the blood. (See Fig. E, page 38.)

For illustrations of the precise location of the next two points, and instructions on how to press them most effectively, see page 49 for the beginning of "Ten Master Pressure Points."

4. (St 36, Three Mile Foot) This is the most powerful point to revitalize the *ch'i* and blood. In combination with Sp 6, it helps rejuvenate the entire body.
5. (Sp 6, Three Yin Meeting) **Caution:** Pregnant women should not press on this point.

Reflexology

1. Since stress is at the root of many skin disorders (as well as being an aggravating factor) we suggest that you begin by giving your feet a good massage and relaxing them—and yourself—with the Reflexology Warm-Up on page 69.

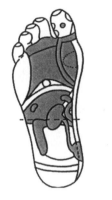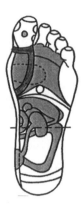

Fig. 177

2. Then work the reflex for the thyroid gland (around the base of the big toe) by rubbing and pressing. The finger or thumb walk technique is best here.

3. Work the neck reflexes on both feet by walking the ridge at the top of the ball of the foot (at the base of the toes). Pull the flesh of the pad of the foot away from the ridge with your other hand, and walk in both directions.

4. Thumb walk the chest and lung reflex zones on the ball of the foot (between the diaphragm line and the base of the toes).

5. Use the finger walk on the neck, lymphatics, and chest area on *top* of your foot, in the solid part of the foot above the toes. Work up from the webbing toward your ankle, and in the troughs between the toes. Start in zone 1—at the base of the big toe—and go up about 2 inches. Continue working each zone. Work this area with your index finger, using the finger walk. And remember to take some deep breaths!

6. To help regulate hormonal action, work the pituitary gland in the center of the big toe, using the "hook and back up" technique (page 68) for pinpoint accuracy.

7. To stimulate the liver, spleen, bladder, colon, and other internal organs in order to facilitate elimination, work the entire area in the arch of your foot, from the pelvic line up to the diaphragm line. Use the thumb walk to thoroughly cover this area. At the sensitive kidney and adrenal reflexes, use the "rotation on a point" technique. (See page 68.)

ADDITIONAL SUGGESTIONS

EAT FRESH, HEALTHY FOOD.   To keep the skin healthy you need a diet rich in fiber, which keeps the colon clean and elimination regular. Fresh fruits and vegetables are important; everyone should eat several servings each day.

DRINK PLENTY OF WATER.   Water helps your kidneys eliminate toxins, which your body might otherwise try to eliminate through the skin. And it moisturizes your skin.

QUIT SMOKING.   Smoking decreases blood flow to the skin and causes premature wrinkling and aging of the skin.

EXERCISE REGULARLY.   Aerobic exercise keeps the organs healthy and promotes healthy digestion and elimination.

USE A HUMIDIFIER   in a dry climate or when the heat is on during the winter. Dry air actually draws moisture out of the skin.

WATCH YOUR DIET.   Some foods that typically aggravate skin conditions are fried foods; chocolate; salty and greasy foods such as potato chips; dairy products; and spicy food. Especially avoid saturated fats, found in meat and dairy. Experiment with cutting some of these out of your diet and see if it helps. Alcohol, coffee, and tobacco can also aggravate symptoms. (From a Chinese medicine perspective, all three create heat.) Aspirin may also aggravate symptoms.

MASTER STRESS.   Stress can aggravate the symptoms of many skin disorders. Be sure to have a stress management program that works for you: a way to deal with frustration, anger, and pressure; a regular program of relaxation, meditation, nature walks, etc.

HERBS AND VITAMINS. To help minimize the inflammatory response, try Vitamin C—1000 mg/day; quercetin—600 mg/day, and bromelain—600 mg/day. Chinese herbs are also helpful for these conditions but a formula needs to be tailored individually by a qualified practitioner. Note: If you have any moles, freckles, or other skin blemishes that are growing or changing in shape or color, see your physician.

Sore Throat

One of our most common ailments, sore throats are the reason for 40 million doctor visits a year by adults, not to speak of the millions of childhood sore throats. The soreness, redness, and swelling may have several causes, including bacterial infections, viruses (like common cold and flu bugs), and allergens, such as animal hair and numerous pollens. Smokers may suffer from an ongoing dry, scratchy throat along with their smoker's cough.

Unless caused by a bacterial infection such as strep, which requires a doctor's care and generally calls for antibiotics, sore throats are usually easy to remedy. The following finger pressure methods and additional suggestions should help you.

ACUPRESSURE

The first two points (Li 4 and Li 11) are beneficial for all sorts of sore throats, whether acute (the type that comes with the common cold or flu) or chronic (persistent and ongoing, such as smoker's throat). Additional points for various conditions follow. For location illustrations of these two points, as well as instructions on how to press them most effectively, please see page 49 for the beginning of "Ten Master Pressure Points."

1. (Li 4, Adjoining Valley) In addition to being a "command point" for any disorders of the face, Li 4 is extremely helpful to relieve pain. It helps clear excess heat and regulates the smooth flow of *ch'i* throughout the body. We also suggest it here because the pathway of the meridian goes directly through the neck.

2. (Li 11, Pool at the Crook) Combining this point with Li 4 helps clear heat from the throat.

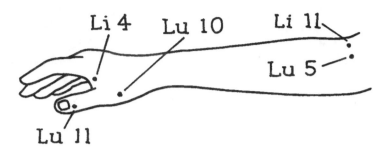

Fig. 178

For an acute sore throat, add:

3. (Lu 11, Lesser Metal) The last point on the Lung meridian, Lu 11 is used to clear excess heat and is thus very helpful to relieve a sore throat. It is located on the thumb, at the bottom corner of the nail (the corner farthest away from your little finger).

Stimulate the point by holding your right thumb between the thumb and first two fingers of your left hand; press with the thumb. You want the pressure to be right where the cuticle meets the nail corner. To properly stimulate this point, you need to press hard. Slowly rock the thumb that you're pressing back and forth as you press. Remember to build up pressure, hold about a minute, then gradually release. Repeat with the other hand.

4. (Lu 10, Fish Border) This point is on the meaty part of your hand below your thumb. It's right in the center between the wrist and the first thumb joint, in a depression along the bone. Like Lu 11 (above) it clears heat from the Lung and is used for sore throat. You'll have to go fairly deep into the flesh to find it, and you'll need strong pressure, holding for about a minute.

If the sore throat is very severe or accompanied by high fever, add St 44:

5. (St 44, Inner Courtyard) This point is located on the top of the foot, in the web margin between the 2nd and 3rd toes. It is right in the center of the web. Use your thumb, and with firm pressure angle into the 'V.' Or, put your thumb underneath your foot, with the middle finger on the point. Apply pressure by squeezing the thumb and finger together. This is the most powerful point on the Stomach meridian to clear heat. And the pathway of the meridian passes directly through the neck.

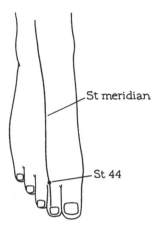

Fig. 179

For Chronic Sore Throat

A chronic sore throat is a persistent one, lasting more than 2–3 weeks. It may take the form of chronic hoarseness, or be mild and accompanied by dryness. An ongoing smoker's sore throat is in this category. Chinese medicine treats this condition primarily by nourishing the underlying *yin* and fluids of the body, with a secondary emphasis on clearing heat. Use Steps 1–3 for heat clearing, and then add:

6. (Lu 5, Cubit Marsh) Let your right arm hang in front of you with the palm up. Put the fingertips of your left hand on the elbow crease (of the right arm). Keep your palm facing up and slowly raise your forearm. Feel for the tendon in the elbow crease that pops out as you raise the forearm. Lu 5 is in the elbow crease on the thumb side (with the palm up) of the tendon. Either the thumb or middle finger works well here. Use moderate to strong pressure. This point helps clear heat and moisten the throat.

7. (Kd 6, Shining Sea) From the ankle bone on the inside of your foot (the big toe side), slide one thumb width straight down toward the sole of the foot. Kd 6 is located here. This is the primary point on the Kidney channel to strengthen Kidney *yin*. Pressing this point has a moistening, nourishing, and cooling influence. This point helps carry the Kidney *yin* energy upward. Since the Kidney channel also runs through the neck, this point brings a cooling, moistening effect to the throat. (See next page.)

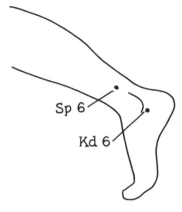

Fig. 180

8.   (Sp 6, Three Yin Meeting) For an illustration of the exact location of Sp 6, and instructions on how to press it most effectively, see page 49 for the beginning of "Ten Master Pressure Points." This is one of the 12 most important pressure points on the body. **Caution:** Pregnant women should not press Sp 6.

REFLEXOLOGY

1.   Before you treat specific reflex areas for your sore throat, please be sure to begin with the Reflexology Warm-Up on page 69.

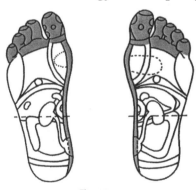

Fig. 181

2.   Start specific treatment by working the neck reflexes on both feet. Thumb walk along the ridge at the top end of the ball of the foot—at the base of the toes. Pull the flesh of the pad of the foot down and away from the ridge with your supporting hand, and walk in both directions.

3. Next, work all your toes, especially the big toe. Reflex zones for the hypothalamus (which regulates body temperature), pineal gland, pituitary gland, and brain are all located here. On the bottom of your foot, work the fleshy part of all the toes. Use the thumb walk for maximum benefit. Work down the toe from the tip to the base, making three passes—both sides, and the center. Be especially thorough with the big toe. If you can, make five separate trips down that toe with your thumb, covering each of the five zones. (See Fig. 8, on page 27.)

4. To help heal swollen lymph glands in your neck, use Reflexology on the lymph drainage area on *top* of your foot. Work up from the webbing toward your ankle, pressing in the troughs between the toes. Start in zone 1, at the base of the big toe, and go up about 2 inches. Work each zone, ending in zone 5 near the outside edge of your foot. Press with your index finger, using the finger walk. This area may be quite tender so don't press too hard.

5. To stimulate more balanced and healthy thyroid activity (located at the base of the throat), work the reflex zone for the thyroid gland (around the base of the big toe) by rubbing and pressing. The finger or thumb walk technique is best here.

6. Next, press the spine reflexes, especially for the cervical area. The spine reflexes are located on the inside edge of both feet (zone 1), extending from the heel nearly to the top of the big toe. To send healing energy to the neck and throat, use the thumb walk to move slowly up the spine reflex from about the ball of the foot to the middle of the toes. Thumb walk down, and finally criss-cross the area by walking across small areas horizontally.

ADDITIONAL SUGGESTIONS

GARGLE.   Probably the easiest home remedy, and one that is quite effective, is gargling. Use 1 cup of warm water (as hot as you can comfortably handle) with ½ teaspoon of salt added.

AVOID DAIRY PRODUCTS.   Stay away from yogurt, ice cream, cheese, and other dairy foods.

TRY HERB TEA.   A soothing and healing herbal tea recommended by Ayurvedic expert Vasant Lad is a mixture of ginger, cinnamon, and licorice root. Mix the herbs and use ½ teaspoon per cup of hot water.

STEAM IT. Dry air, whether from forced heat in the winter or a desert climate, can irritate your throat. Use a humidifier for prevention or, if you already have a sore throat, boil up a pint of water, shut off the heat, put a towel over your head, and breathe normally through your nose as you lean over the pot and inhale the steam.

WARM IT. Wear a scarf, or wrap a towel around your throat. The warmth may not heal, but it's definitely soothing.

YOGA POSTURES. Good postures for your sore throat include the Shoulder Stand, which puts pressure on points around the throat; the Locust and Fish, which stretch the meridians connected with the throat, and the Lion, justly famous for its healing action on sore throats.

Stiff Neck

See "Neck and Shoulder Tension"

Stress

We all experience stress every day. Although we do our best to cope with it, it's one of the most significant health hazards in modern life. Experts estimate that between 70 and 80 percent of all health disorders—and doctor visits—are stress-related. Stress may be due to physical causes such as fatigue, polluted air, excessive noise, chronic pain, or prolonged exposure to extreme heat or cold. It may also come from mental/emotional sources like divorce, time pressure at work, school exams, family and relationship problems, a sense of being overloaded and overwhelmed, uncertainty, disappointment, the death of loved ones, and so on.

The body's biochemical responses to stress cause and aggravate any number of conditions, including allergies, arthritis, asthma, back pain, colitis, diabetes, emphysema, headaches, high blood pressure, hypoglycemia, menstrual disorders, and many more, including the two great killers, cancer and heart disease. Stress affects the digestive tract, causing inadequate digestion and absorption. Chronic stress suppresses the immune system, which leads to increased susceptibility to many illness. Psychologically, stress produces anxiety and may lead to depression.

It is true that some people seem to thrive on high pressure, high speed, deadlines, and other aspects of life that leave other people exhausted. We all respond differently to life's challenges, based on our physical stamina and psychological temperament. "One man's meat is another's poison." One person's great joy, such as loud heavy metal music or caring for a baby, may be another person's stressful nightmare. But even someone who feels exhilarated by high-pressure situations may discover that they were taking a damaging toll on their physiology.

Few of us can manage to avoid stressful situations. The key is what is commonly known as "stress management"—taking action to counteract the harmful effects of stress through exercise, meditation, relaxation techniques, Yoga, tai chi, qi gong, dietary changes, etc. Pressure point therapies can be very effective and beneficial.

From the perspective of Chinese medicine, the main effect of stress on the body is the disruption of the smooth flow of *ch'i* or Life Energy, which is the forerunner of many illnesses. Finger pressure therapy eliminates blockages and restores the harmonious flow of Life Energy.

ACUPRESSURE

The first two pressure points for stress management (Li 4 and Lv 3) are fully described in the section, "Ten Master Pressure Points" (beginning on page 49) where you will also find illustrations of the precise point locations and suggestions on how to press them for maximum benefit.

1. (Li 4, Adjoining Valley) One of the most important Acupressure points, Li 4 helps to reduce muscular tension and harmonize the flow of *ch'i* in the body. (See also Fig. 178, page 356.)

2. (Lv 3, Bigger Rushing) The Liver meridian is adversely affected by stress. Lv 3 is the best point to help rebalance Liver *ch'i* that becomes stuck or stagnant as a result of stress. (Fig. 184, page 365.)

3. (PC 6, Inner Gate) You will find this point on the palm side of your wrist, two thumb widths above the wrist crease in the center of the arm. This point, especially in combination with Lv 3, has a powerful effect on counteracting the harmful physical and emotional effects of stress. You can press with your thumb, or wrap your middle finger around your arm to apply moderate pressure.

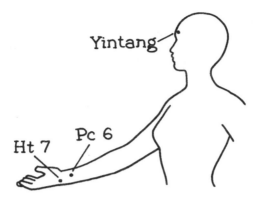

Fig. 182

4. (Yin Tang, "Extra Point") This point, which is above the bridge of your nose and between the eyebrows, is famous for its calming effect. Use your thumb or middle finger to press with moderate pressure.

5. (Ht 7, Mind Door) You will find this point on the palm side of your hand, on the wrist crease, directly below the little finger. Find the bony knob on the outside of your left wrist (the little finger side). The point is next to that, in a small indentation. Press for 30 seconds with your thumb using moderate to firm pressure; release gradually; switch hands. This point has a calming effect on the mind and emotions and is an effective antidote to stress.

6. Ear Point. See Fig. I on page 41 for an effective anti-stress point on the ear.

REFLEXOLOGY

Perhaps the greatest contribution of Reflexology is its ability to dissolve tension and stress simply by working with the feet. Some of the most important reflex areas to press and massage for stress relief include the spine, neck and shoulders, chest and lungs, and the endocrine glands.

But before you treat specific reflex areas for stress management, please begin with the Reflexology Warm-Up on page 69. This important step helps you start to relax and prepares your feet to be worked on.

1. Work the entire chest area (including the lung and heart reflexes) to help regulate breathing and heart rate, which both get out of balance when we

are stressed. Thumb walk the chest and lung reflex zones on the ball of the foot (between the diaphragm line and the base of the toes). Spend some more time walking across the diaphragm line. Then rotate or flex your foot (with your holding hand) to help work this key area. And take some deep breaths!

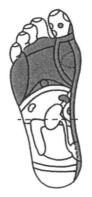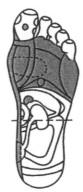

Fig. 183

2. Now work on the chest and lymph gland reflexes on the top of your foot. Work up from the webbing toward your ankle, pressing in the troughs between the toes. Start at the base of the big toe (zone 1) and go up about 2 inches. Continue working each zone, ending in zone 5 near the outside edge of your foot. Press with your index finger, using the finger walk.

3. Almost all of us hold a great deal of tension in our necks and shoulders. To promote relaxation of this vital area, start by walking the ridge at the top of the ball of the foot (at the base of the toes). Pull the pad of the foot down and away with your other hand. Walk in both directions.

4. The reflex zone for your shoulders is on the bottom of your foot in zone 5, under your little toe, continuing out along the outside edge of your foot. It extends from the base of your little toe down to the diaphragm line. To relax your shoulders (and improve circulation to your head), work both horizontally and vertically along this zone.

5. Next, press the all-important spine reflexes, to relieve tension and promote energy flow through the nervous system into all parts of the body. These reflexes are on the inside edge of both feet (zone 1), extending from the heel nearly to the top of the big toe.

When you work the spinal reflexes, work slowly up the foot using the thumb walk technique. You will need a little extra strength on the thick skin of your heel. Then walk all the way down, from heel to toes. Take some time to walk across small areas horizontally as you move up the foot.

6. To help balance your energy level and the hormonal secretions of the endocrine glands, work the reflexes for the key endocrine glands, including the pituitary (in the center of the bottom of the big toe), the thyroid (at the base of the big toe), and the adrenals (between the waistline and the diaphragm line, toward the inside of the foot). Working these areas will create balance in the body and nervous system and help relieve stress and anxiety.

7. Finish by giving your entire foot some wiggles and gentle twists, and rubbing them gently all over. You will find this soothing and relaxing. Return to the solar plexus point and press for a full minute, keeping your eyes closed and breathing deeply for extra relaxation.

SHIATSU

1. Deep breathing helps tremendously to re-establish the healthy flow of *ch'i* in the body. Stand with your feet shoulder width apart. Start with your arms hanging loosely at your sides. With a deep, slow inhalation, slowly lift your arms over your head, then turn your palms to face the ceiling with the fingertips pointing together. Look at the space between the tips of the fingers.

On the exhalation, lower your arms. Repeat 5–6 times. If your balance is good, raise your heels off the ground as you lift your arms. Stretching your arms above you and standing on your toes helps open the meridians and circulate the *ch'i.*

Next we will work on the two meridians most affected by stress, the Liver and Gallbladder. (See Fig. J on page 42, and Fig. 184 on page 365 for location of meridians.) Use the press and release technique. Press for 6–7 seconds, release, move about half an inch along the channel, and press again.

2. To stimulate the Liver meridian, start in the center of the top of your big toe. Using the press and release technique, progress along the toe to the web margin between the big toe and second toe, then move up the channel between the two toes. From the ankle, the channel proceeds up the inside part of the leg, along the bone. Use only mild to moderate pressure along the bone. About halfway up the leg the meridian comes off the bone and continues up the middle of the inside of the leg. Above the knee, the pathway travels slightly higher than the middle of the inside portion of your thigh. Stop at the groin. On the thigh above the knee, you can use strong pressure.

3. Find the space in your foot between the 4th and 5th toes. This is Gallbladder meridian territory. Start at the web margin and stimulate the channel with the press and release technique. Continue about halfway up the foot to where you no longer feel a space between the toe bones.

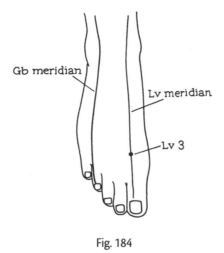

Fig. 184

4. End by taking five or six slow, deep breaths. Sit up straight and breathe from the diaphragm, first filling the belly, then the chest.

ADDITIONAL SUGGESTIONS

A HOLISTIC APPROACH.   Stress isn't something you can take a pill to combat. Effective stress management requires a comprehensive program, including a healthy diet, adequate exercise, meditation or relaxation, Yoga stretching, etc. For a simple approach to a healthy lifestyle, please see the 11 Simple, Universal Guidelines for Good Health on page 77.

HERBS.   The Chinese herbal formula Xiao Yao Wan counteracts the effects of stress (especially stuck *ch'i* in the Liver meridian). It also has some blood rejuvenating effects, and is well-suited to women or anyone under stress who tends towards deficiency type conditions. However, if you're a Type A personality, another formula, Xiao Chai Hu Tang, is better suited for you.

FOOD SMARTS.   In addition to the general dietary suggestions in the "11, Simple Guidelines," we recommend that you avoid foods that tend to create *ch'i* stagnation, such as heavy, greasy foods and excess alcohol and sweets. Some spices that help move *ch'i* are ginger, black pepper, and garlic. Use your common sense. Avoid overeating and eating right before bed. Make sure to have an adequate intake of vitamins and minerals, especially B-complex.

Swelling and Water Retention (Edema)

See also, "PMS"

Edema (swelling due to water retention) is caused by water build-up in the space between the cells. It may affect almost any part of us. Feet and ankles may swell. Cheeks and eyes may suddenly appear puffy; rings may become tight on swollen fingers. Premenstrual women may find their bellies and thighs bloated and their breasts swollen and tender. Swelling during pregnancy is equally common. The following point sequences will help with all of these. For premenstrual swelling, please see our section on "PMS."

In Chinese medicine, water metabolism is said to be governed by many factors but the most important here are the Spleen and Kidney meridian systems. By stimulating various points along these meridians and those that interact intimately with them, pressure point therapy can help regulate water metabolism and restore the body's fluid balance.

ACUPRESSURE

1. (Cv 6, Sea of *Ch'i*) This point is about one and a half finger widths directly below the navel. (See Fig. 193, page 378.) Place the middle finger of both hands there, and press inward with the fingertips of both hands to a depth of about an inch. Use moderate pressure and hold for a minute or two, breathing deeply. This point has a powerful effect on strengthening *ch'i* and circulating it throughout the body. You might try lying on your back to work it. Start by taking a few deep breaths to relax. **Caution:** Pregnant women should not use pressure on any abdominal points.

The next two points (St 36 and Sp 6) are fully described in the section, "Ten Master Pressure Points" (beginning on page 49) where you will find point location illustrations and suggestions on how to press for maximum benefit.

2. (St 36, Three Mile Foot) The key point for rejuvenating the *ch'i* and blood of the entire body, it is even more powerful in combination with Sp 6. We are also recommending it for its effect on the digestive system.

3. (Sp 6, Three Yin Meeting) This one point nourishes the overall *yin* of the body by simultaneously nourishing the *yin* of the Spleen, Liver, and

Kidney meridians. Use it here for its ability to regulate dampness, and for its strengthening effect on the Spleen meridian. **Caution:** This point should be avoided by pregnant women.

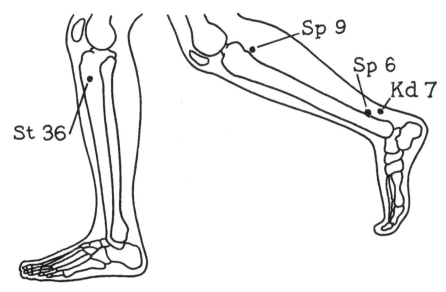

Fig. 185

4. (Sp 9, Yin Mound Spring) Bend your leg at the knee. On the inside of the shin bone, slide your index finger up along the lower border of the shin bone until you are a few inches below the upper leg bone and your finger falls into a natural depression. Sp 9 is in this depression, right below a rounded prominence in the top of the leg bone (tibia). Pressing on this point will help reduce the swelling. The point is also very involved with the regulation of water metabolism, especially in the lower half of the body.

5. (Kd 7, Returning Current) The easiest way to locate Kd 7 is to first find Kd 3. On the inside of the ankle (big toe side), Kd 3 is halfway between the ankle bone and the Achilles tendon. Place your thumb on the prominence of the ankle bone, and let it slide down toward the Achilles tendon. Kd 3 is in the depression, approximately halfway between the bone and the back of the ankle.

From Kd 3, go up two thumb widths toward the knee. This is Kd 7. Press with your thumb using medium to firm pressure, for about a minute.

Kd 7 is specific to the *yang* aspect of Kidney *ch'i* which is what we want to strengthen.

REFLEXOLOGY

1. Before you start to treat specific reflex areas for water retention, begin with the Reflexology Warm-Up on page 69. This is an important step that relaxes you and prepares your feet to be worked on; please don't skip it!

Please note that when the feet are swollen, they may be quite tender, so this is a time you might choose to use hand Reflexology rather than work on the feet. Since working with the feet is generally more effective, we're giving our recommendations in terms of zones on the foot. Check Fig. Q and Fig. R (pages 47 and 48) for locations on the hand.

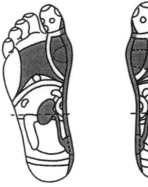

Fig. 186

2. Because poor circulation (especially to the extremities) can be at the root of edema, start by stimulating the heart and cardiovascular system. The reflex zones for the heart are on your left foot, reaching across from the ball of the foot (under the big toe) to the middle of your foot (under the middle toe); some Reflexologists hold that there is an additional area on your right foot, primarily on the ball of the foot; there's no harm working here also. Use the thumb walk to go up, down, and across. Take plenty of time to work this area thoroughly.

3. Massage the chest and lung reflex zones, also on the ball of the foot, between the diaphragm line and the base of the toes. You can also finger walk the chest and lymph gland reflexes on the top of the foot (in the grooves between the toes) to help release any fluid congestion in the chest and lungs.

4. Work along the entire spine reflex to enliven the nervous system. These reflexes are located on the inside edge of both feet (zone 1), extending from the heel nearly to the top of the big toe, opposite the root of the toenail.

Work slowly up the foot using the thumb walk technique. You'll need a little extra strength on the thick skin of the heel. You will also have to switch your hand position a few times to get the right angle. Also walk down the spinal reflex area, and across small areas horizontally.

5. Now focus your attention on the urinary system—bladder, kidneys, and ureters—to stimulate elimination of water from the body. The kidney reflex zones are in the center of the foot, above and below the waistline and on the inside of the large tendon running up the foot. Use the thumb walk. Don't press on the tendon. While working here, press the adrenal reflex; for best results, use the "rotation on a point" technique. (See page 68.)

6. Finally, massage the bladder and ureter reflexes, located mostly in zone 1 (beneath the big toe). The ureters stretch down from the kidneys to the bladder, located where the heel begins. Work up from the bladder, then cross the big tendon and work up or across the kidney reflex. Use the thumb walk technique.

SHIATSU

1. Rub the palms of your hands together rapidly for 10–20 seconds, until they get nice and warm. Place your right hand on your abdomen right below your belly button. With a clockwise circular motion, massage with moderate pressure the area from your belly button to just above the groin area. This will stimulate the Conception Vessel points from Cv 6 down to Cv 3. This area is the *dan tien* that various forms of martial arts, tai chi and *ch'i gong* cultivate for power, centeredness, and well-being. It's like strengthening the root of a plant to bring nourishment to all parts of it. Massage for 1–2 minutes.

2. The next exercise can be done seated or standing. Place your palms on either side of your low back. (This will be over the kidneys.) Vigorously rub up and down. You should feel the heat generated from the friction of your hands. This will also help enliven the Kidney energy.

3. Now stimulate the Spleen meridian (see illustrations on pages 287 and 288) starting at the big toe. The first point is close to the cuticle at the inside corner of the big toenail. From there the meridian follows along the side of the big toe bone, at the inside of the foot, up the side of the ankle and the inside of the leg. Along the leg it follows just below the bone. Use the press and release technique (press 6–7 seconds, release, move a fraction of an inch along the channel, press again) from the big toe to just below the knee. Be sure to do both feet and legs.

4. The Horse posture will strengthen the Kidneys and help alleviate edema. Even two minutes a day will be helpful. Please see page 193 (Fig. 100) for complete instructions and an illustration of the Horse posture.

ADDITIONAL SUGGESTIONS

CUT DOWN ON SALT.   Sodium causes the body to retain water. Don't add salt to food as you cook it, or once it's on your plate. And try to avoid those salty snacks: chips, pretzels, salted nuts, etc.

EXERCISE.   Walking every day for 20 to 30 minutes will help improve circulation and reduce the swelling.

GIVE YOUR FEET A RAISE.   If the swelling is in your feet and ankles, lie down and put your feet up on a pillow. If lying down is not convenient, at least put your feet up on a footstool or a small table. Or put your feet up on your desk at the office; tell 'em, "Doctor's orders!"

Tinnitus (Ringing in the Ears)

See "Hearing Problems"

Toothache

Toothaches are most often due to untreated tooth decay that has allowed bacteria to penetrate to the pulp of the tooth. A cracked tooth or infection of the gums may also be the cause, or there may be pain due to an injury, an extraction, impacted wisdom teeth, or even physical exhaustion which allows a minor or latent inflammation to become acute.

The pressure point recommendations following CANNOT cure a toothache caused by infection or inflammation. You need to go to the dentist for proper treatment. But the pain can be greatly or even entirely relieved for a little while, until the tooth is worked on by a dentist.

From the perspective of Chinese medicine, most toothaches are due to excess heat in the Stomach channel; sometimes they may be due to "wind heat."

ACUPRESSURE

1. (Li 4, Adjoining Valley) One of the most important Acupressure points, Li 4 relieves headaches and other pain, relaxes muscular tension, and is known as the "command point" for the face. Please see "Ten Master Pressure Points" beginning on page 49 for precise location and an illustration.

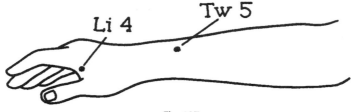

Fig. 187

2. (Tw 5, Outer Gate) Hold your left arm in front of you with the palm down. Measure two thumb widths above the wrist. The point is right in the center, between the two forearm bones. Press firmly with your thumb or middle finger for about a minute. The Tw (Triple Warmer) channel runs up the back of the arm to the shoulder and neck, then moves around to the side of the neck and along the jaw.

3. (St 6, Jaw Bone) To find this point, clench your teeth to find the center of the muscle that bulges at the jaw. Then relax, and press where the center of the bulge was. Press with the index and middle fingers of each hand. Use mild to moderate pressure.

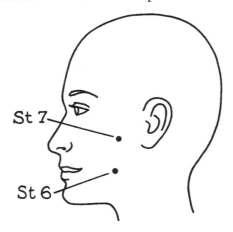

Fig. 188

4. (St 7, Lower Gate) Place your fingertips about an inch in front of your ears and let them move up and down across the hard bony ridge that goes across your face. (That ridge is your cheekbone.) St 7 is below this ridge about an inch in front of the ear and a little higher than the top of the earlobe on most people, in a large natural depression. Use your middle or index finger with mild to moderate pressure. Both St 6 and St 7 can help with local pain relief.

REFLEXOLOGY

As we said, the organic disorders that cause teeth to hurt—cavities, gum inflammation, etc.—cannot be healed by finger pressure techniques. You need to see a dentist. But, in addition to relieving pain, these techniques can help improve circulation around the affected area, which can improve gum health and may help reduce future problems.

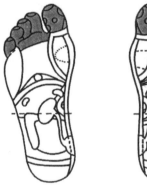

Fig. 189

1. Before you start to treat specific reflex areas around the mouth and gums, please take a few minutes for the Reflexology Warm-Up on page 69.

2. To improve general circulation to the head, work the neck reflexes on both feet by "walking the ridge" at the base of your toes. Pull the flesh of the pad of the foot down and away with your supporting hand. Walk in both directions.

3. All the reflex points and zones directly affecting teeth, gums, and jaws are on your toes. First, on the bottom of your foot, work the fleshy part of all the toes. Use the thumb walk for maximum benefit. Walk down the toe from the tip to the base, making three passes—both sides, and

the center. Be especially thorough with the big toe. If you can, make five separate trips down that toe with your thumb, covering each of the five zones. In the center of the pad of the big toe, use the "hook and back up" technique (page 68) on the pituitary reflex.

4. On top of your foot, work the specific reflexes for the teeth and gums. These run across the top of the big toe, between the base of the toe (at the webbing, where there's a groove) and the toe nail. Thumb walk in all directions to cover this area thoroughly. (See Fig. O, page 46.)

SHIATSU

In the following Shiatsu sequence, you will be stimulating the Large Intestine and Stomach meridians, to help clear heat from them.

1. The Large Intestine (LI) meridian begins at the tip of the index finger and runs along the thumb side of the finger bone to the wrist, up the forearm to the elbow, and then continues on. Start at the tip of your left index finger (on the thumb side) and use the press and release technique: Press for 6 or 7 seconds; release; move a fraction of an inch along the channel; press again. Use firm pressure with your thumb.

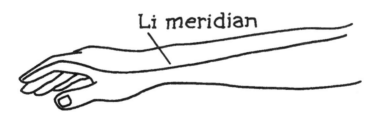

Fig. 190

When you come to the knuckles, press just under the bone on one side of the knuckle, then on the other; don't press on the knuckle itself. Follow the channel as it moves upward, close to the side of the finger bone in the hand up to Li 4 in the center of the webbing between thumb and index finger.

From here the meridian follows a virtually straight line to the outer edge of the elbow crease. To be sure you are on the right line, hold your arm in front of you with the palm facing your stomach about 4–5 inches away from your body. Imagine the line drawn on your arm in this position. Press and release along the entire length of your forearm to the elbow. Stop at the elbow crease. Be sure to do both arms.

2. Next, stimulate the Stomach Meridian, which runs between the 2nd and 3rd toes, across the top of the foot and up the front of the ankle. From the ankle it continues up the front of the leg, about 1 finger breadth to the outside (little toe side) of the shin bone. (See Figs. J and K, pages 42 and 43.) Start on the top of the foot, in line with the space between the 2nd and 3rd toe. Use the press and release technique and start working gradually toward the toes. Be sure you stay in the channel between the 2nd and 3rd toe, and work down to the webbing between them. From here go along the little toe side of the 2nd toe to the nail. Do both feet.

Now go the other way. Start at the second toe on the little toe side, and go back up the meridian using the press and release technique, moving between the 2nd and 3rd toes, across the top of the foot and the front of the ankle, up the front of the leg about ½ inch (1 finger breadth) to the little toe side of the shin bone. Stop just below the knee.

ADDITIONAL SUGGESTIONS

SPICE IT.   Placing a clove next to the aching tooth (between cheek and tooth) will help alleviate the pain. Chew the clove for a few minutes at first to release the juice, then just let it stay there. You can use clove oil also, or tea tree oil; use a cotton swab to place a little on the surrounding gums.

BRUSH AND FLOSS!   To prevent future problems, take good care of your teeth!

Weight Control

See also, "Eating Disorders," "Stress"

If you're worried about your weight, you're not alone. At any given time, about 40 percent of American women and 25 percent of American men are trying to lose weight. For some, the urge to slim down is largely psychological, conditioned by images in the media and the fashion industry. But the fact is that tens of millions of people—about one third of us—tip the scales beyond our optimal level for good health.

Our high-fat diet and sedentary lifestyle make it easy to put on the pounds, difficult to take them off. But getting to a healthy weight is one of the most important things you can do to avoid serious illness now and in the future.

We don't want to scare you, but the health risks of carrying around excess poundage are real. If you're only a few pounds overweight your increased risks are minor, but if you're more than 20 percent above your optimum weight or wearing more than 25 percent body fat, you're looking at an increased risk of heart disease, high blood pressure, adult onset diabetes, respiratory problems, as well as certain types of cancer, including breast cancer in women and colon, rectal, and prostate cancer in men.

The bottom line: obesity shortens the life span of both men and women. This is a scientific fact. So the quest to control our weight is significant.

You probably know a lot about typical Western methods of weight control: dieting, pills, hypnosis, exercise, etc. From the perspective of Chinese medicine, weight control is associated with the proper functioning of the digestive system and the metabolism of water in the body.

The following pressure point techniques are not going to magically melt away the pounds. But in combination with a program of sensible eating and regular exercise, they can be a potent ally in the battle of the bulge.

ACUPRESSURE

Three of the following five points (Sp 6, St 36, and St 40) are described in the section, "Ten Master Pressure Points" (beginning on page 49) where you will also find illustrations of the precise point locations and suggestions on how to press them for maximum benefit.

1. ("Appetite Control" ear point) See Fig. I, on page 41. Overeating is only one of many factors involved in weight gain, but it is important, and this appetite control point can help. It is located on the ear, and is easiest to find while looking in a mirror. Place your fingers on your jaw, in front of your ears. Open and close your mouth a few times until you feel your jaw bone moving underneath your fingers. Now try putting one finger where you feel the most movement of the jaw. Your finger should be right next to a little fleshy protrusion of the ear (not the ear lobe). Grab this part of the ear with your thumb and index finger and press with steady pressure.

2. (Sp 6, Three Yin Meeting) In combination with St 36 this point has a strengthening effect on the digestive system. **Caution:** Pregnant women should not press this point.

3. (St 36, Three Mile Foot) This is the best point to nourish the *ch'i* and blood; we recommend it here for its beneficial effect on the digestive system.

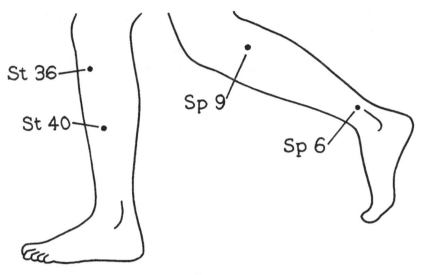

Fig. 191

4. (Sp 9, Yin Mound Spring) This point is a close neighbor of St 36. After pressing St 36, slide your finger across the shinbone until you are just off the shinbone on the inside side of the leg. Now slide your finger upwards along the shinbone towards the knee about an inch, until you fall into a natural depression. Sp 9 is in this depression, right below a rounded prominence in the top of the leg bone (tibia). This point is involved with the regulation of water metabolism in the body.

5. (St 40, Abundant Splendor) This is the best point in traditional Chinese medicine for clearing excess damp and phlegm; it is very helpful for eliminating excess weight.

6. End your Acupressure session by again stimulating the appetite control point on both ears.

REFLEXOLOGY

Our Reflexology session for weight control will center around two strategies: (1) energizing the endocrine glands to promote balanced hormone secretion and appropriate appetite; and (2) toning the entire digestive system, so you will gain maximum benefit from the food you eat. Since part of the problem with being overweight is psychological, such as emotional eating—for some people, it's the major part—we suggest you also look at our Reflexology "workouts" for Stress and Anxiety, for additional tips.

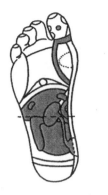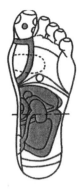

Fig. 192

1. Start with the Reflexology Warm-Up on page 69. This is an important step that helps you relax, tones the energy of the whole body, and prepares your feet to be worked on.

2. Next work on key endocrine glands, including the pituitary (in the center of the bottom of the big toe), the thyroid (at the base of the big toe), and the adrenals (between the waistline and the diaphragm line, toward the inside of the foot). Working these reflexes will help create balance in the body and nervous system and help you get a grip on your appetite and eating. Use the special "hook and back up" technique on the pituitary reflex. (See page 68.)

3. Rather than try to pinpoint specific aspects of the digestive system to work on, we suggest you use the thumb walk to work across the entire area in the arch of your foot, from the midline (waistline) up to the diaphragm line. The stomach reflex is on the left foot, the liver primarily on the right. Work both feet and thoroughly cover this area, moving up, down, and/or diagonally. In this way you'll also stimulate the pancreas, gallbladder, kidneys, and adrenals.

4. Moving lower, below the waistline, you'll encounter the reflex areas for the colon. Points for various aspects of the colon are divided between the two feet; don't worry about tracing the path of each and every part, such as the ascending colon or descending colon; simply work up, down, across, and diagonally in this area with the thumb walk.

SHIATSU

With the tips of the fingers of both hands, press on the point midway between your belly button and the bottom of your breast bone. On most people this will usually be just over four finger widths above the belly button. Do the press and release technique for 1–2 minutes. (Press for 6–7 seconds; release; press again.)

Then let your fingers slide downward and to the left, while giving moderate stimulation as you go. When you get to a point level with and about 2 inches to the left of the belly button, again take 1–2 minutes to stimulate this area.

Slowly circle down to a point about one and a half inches below your navel. Stimulate 1–2 minutes.

Finally, let your fingers come up to a point about 2 inches to the right of the navel. Stimulate 1–2 minutes.

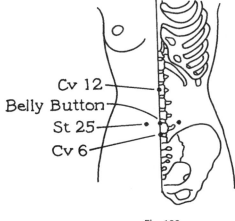

Fig. 193

ADDITIONAL SUGGESTIONS

Real, lasting weight loss is possible, though it will take some work and a long-term commitment.

USE REVERSE ECONOMICS.   Here's the bottom line: In order to lose weight and keep it off, you need to use up more calories than you take in—spend more than you earn—not just today or this week, but for the rest of your life. The following guidelines will help.

TAKE IT SLOW.   Diets—especially crash diets—don't work. Research shows that 90 percent of people who diet regain the weight they lost. Plan to lose weight gradually.

MAKE LIFESTYLE CHANGES.   You can lose weight and keep it off if you make a commitment to two things: a healthier, lighter, low-fat diet, and regular exercise.

MOVE IT. Aerobic exercise—sustained, rhythmic exercise using the large muscles of the body—helps you lose weight by increasing the rate at which your body burns fuel. Jogging, swimming, cycling, skiing, aerobic dancing, as well as action sports like basketball or tennis, are excellent ways to get your blood going and your fat burning.

DON'T FALL FOR THE HYPE. Getting more exercise doesn't require expensive equipment, special clothing, or health club memberships. It just means increasing your physical activity. Take a half hour walk every day, in the early morning, at your lunch break, or when you get home. Park a mile from work and walk the rest of the way. Household jobs like raking, sweeping, scrubbing floors, carrying bags of groceries, shoveling snow, moving furniture, which increase metabolism as well as toning your muscles, can accomplish all you need.

TRIM THE FAT. Along with regular exercise, cutting dietary fat is the key to your weight loss program. Some doctors say it's okay to get 30 percent of your daily calories from fat, but to lose weight, you'll probably have to cut down to 20 percent or even less.

When you shop, head straight for the fresh food in the produce section. Instead of packaged food, sweets, and meats, fill up with vegetables, fruit, legumes, whole grain breads and cereals. And forget about eating fast foods, which are notoriously off the chart in fat content.

Diet plans that work center around complex carbohydrate foods. Not only are they low in calories and packed with vitamins and minerals, but your body also has to work harder to digest them, burning more calories. And they're high in fiber. Follow these guidelines:

- Eat more salads and cooked vegetables.
- Increase your consumption of legumes such as lentils, kidney beans, pinto beans, and navy beans.
- Use whole grain bread rather than white breads.
- Eat more potatoes, baked or boiled.
- Choose whole grain cereals such as oatmeal.

DEAL WITH STRESS. If you feel your eating habits are stress-related—such as "emotional" eating when you feel pressured or unhappy—please look at our chapter, "Stress," for stress management strategies, and seek professional help if you need it.

Recommended Books on Pressure Point Therapy

General Books on Oriental Medicine and Acupressure:

Between Heaven and Earth: A Guide to Chinese Medicine, Harriet Beinfield and Efrem Korngold.

The Chinese Way to Healing: Many Paths to Wholeness, Misha Ruth Cohen.

The Handbook of Chinese Massage: Tui Na Techniques to Awaken Body and Mind, Maria Mercati.

The Web That Has No Weaver: Understanding Chinese Medicine, Ted J. Kaptchuk.

Reference Texts on Chinese Medicine:

A Manual of Acupuncture, Peter Deadman, Mazin Al-Khafaji, Kevin Baker.

> This is the definitive text for Acupuncture point locations. Beautiful illustrations, extensive historical references.

Acupuncture: A Comprehensive Text, Shanghai College of Traditional Medicine, translated and edited by John O'Connor and Dan Bensky.

The Foundations of Chinese Medicine: A Comprehensive Text for Acupuncturists and Herbalists, Giovanni Maciocia.

Acupuncture Point Combinations, Jeremy Ross.

Reflexology:

Better Health with Foot Reflexology, Dwight C. Byers.

> The author, director of the International Institute of Reflexology in St. Petersburg, Florida has trained most of the leading reflexologists in this country and abroad.

Feet First: A Guide to Foot Reflexology, Laura Norman.

> One of Dwight Byers's star pupils; extensively illustrated.

Indian Natural Medicine:

Ayurvedic Secrets to Longevity and Total Health, Peter Anselmo with James S. Brooks, M.D.

The Complete Book of Ayurvedic Home Remedies, Vasant D. Lad.

Beauty:

Asian Health Secrets, Letha Hadady, D. Ac.

> Several chapters on beauty.

Ayurvedic Beauty Care, Melanie Sachs.

Index